REVIEW OF
Hemodialysis

FOR NURSES AND DIALYSIS PERSONNEL

TENTH EDITION

REVIEW OF
Hemodialysis
FOR NURSES AND DIALYSIS PERSONNEL

JUDITH Z. KALLENBACH, MSN, RN, CNN
Clinical Educator and Writer
DaVita Kidney Care
Akron, Ohio

ELSEVIER

Elsevier
3251 Riverport Lane
St. Louis, Missouri 63043

REVIEW OF HEMODIALYSIS FOR NURSES AND DIALYSIS PERSONNEL,
TENTH EDITION

ISBN: 978-0-323-64192-0

Notice

Practitioners and researchers must always rely on their own experience and knowledge in evaluating and using any information, methods, compounds or experiments described herein. Because of rapid advances in the medical sciences, in particular, independent verification of diagnoses and drug dosages should be made. To the fullest extent of the law, no responsibility is assumed by Elsevier, authors, editors or contributors for any injury and/or damage to persons or property as a matter of products liability, negligence or otherwise, or from any use or operation of any methods, products, instructions, or ideas contained in the material herein.

Previous editions copyrighted 2016, 2012, and 2005.
Library of Congress Control Number: 2019955458

Content Strategist: Sandra E. Clark
Content Development Specialist: Brooke Kannady/Kathleen Nahm
Publishing Services Manager: Shereen Jameel
Project Manager: Manikandan Chandrasekaran
Design Direction: Brian Salisbury

Printed in India

Last digit is the print number: 9   8   7   6   5   4

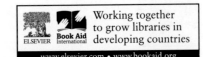

It is with gratitude and thanks that I dedicate this edition to Joanna Freeman, a trusted and respected leader, colleague, and friend. The experience gained by working with you is the gift of a lifetime.

REVIEWER

Dr. Felicia D. Lambert, DNP, CNN
Doctor of Nurse Practice, Master's in Nursing Education
Fresenius Kidney Care
Regional Quality Manager
National Kidney Foundation Medical Advisory
    Board Member of Central Ohio
American Nephrology Nurse Association Buckeye

PREFACE

The *Review of Hemodialysis for Nurses and Dialysis Personnel* provides an overview of dialysis therapies and care of patients with chronic kidney disease (CKD). This book is intended to be a practical resource for nurses and technicians and other dialysis personnel who have recently begun their nephrology careers, those preparing to take a nephrology certification exam, or any professional interested in learning more about the principles of dialysis and the complexities encountered when caring for this population. This edition is again written in a question-and-answer format to provide quick answers to questions you may have regarding the disease process and treatment.

With the shift to value-based integrated kidney care models, a new chapter is included which identifies the nurse's role in the case management of CKD patients. The essentials of providing patient-centric care are introduced along with a discussion on how to manage the risk factors and comorbid conditions common to this population.

I am very encouraged by the continued improvements we have seen in renal technology over the years that help to improve our patients' quality of life. After this edition went into production, an executive order was passed on July 10, 2019, dedicated to advancing kidney health for Americans with CKD. The executive order, *Advancing American Kidney Health,* is three-pronged and focuses on (1) preventing kidney failure through better diagnosis, treatment, and incentives for preventive care; (2) increasing patient choice through affordable alternative treatments for end-stage renal disease, moving more patients into home dialysis, and encouraging the development of artificial kidneys; and (3) increasing access to kidney transplants by modernizing the organ recovery and transplantation systems. This is surely an exciting time to be involved in the care of patients with CKD on any level!

You will find updated information on treating and monitoring kidney patients through all stages of CKD with strategies to improve their quality of life and activate them in their care. I am very excited to have included tools on motivational interviewing that can assist in engaging our patients and help them to modify their behaviors for improved health outcomes. Updates to Centers for Medicare & Medicaid Services quality measures and Centers for Disease Control and Prevention infection control initiatives are also included.

I would like to thank the authors and contributors from previous editions who helped to build the framework for this current edition and who shared their clinical experience and knowledge.

I would like to thank a few colleagues who shared their clinical expertise with me for content and organization, including Joan Fieldhouse, RN, for her expert consultation and sound advice on pediatric dialysis. Many thanks, Joan. A special thank you goes to a very dear friend and colleague, Gloria Wallace, RN, who provided consultation and a critical eye to the renal case management chapter of this book. Gloria, you have been an amazing teammate over the years, and your joyful presence, optimism, and wisdom are missed more than you can ever know.

Thank you to Sandra Clark and Brooke Kannady for editorial and publication support. I thank you all for your patience and understanding throughout this publication process.

Thank you to Felicia D. Lambert, DNP, CNN, an old friend found again, for reviewing the manuscript before publication and offering excellent and helpful suggestions. And finally, thank you to my family, Keith, Michael, and Maeve, for being there!

I hope that this edition will continue to provide quick answers sometimes needed to understand as well as to provide dialysis care to our patients.

ACKNOWLEDGMENTS

The publisher and authors wish to thank the contributors to past editions: Kathy Bender, RN, BSN, CNN; Lowanna S. Binkley, RN, MA, CNN; Christopher R. Blagg, MD, FRCP; Eileen D. Brewer, MD; Linda S. Christensen, RN, CNN; Kenneth E. Cotton, MA, MBA, MPA; Helen Currier, RN, CNN; Jim Curtis, CHT, CNCT; Lesley C. Dinwiddie, RN, MSN, FNP, CNN; Ronald Emerson, AD, CHT; Nancy Gallagher, RN, BS, CNN; Peter W. Gardner; Susan K. Hansen, RN, MBA, CNN; Mara Hersh-Rifkin, MSW, LCSW; Margaret S. Holloway, RN, MN; Martin V. Hudson, CNBT; Kathy Laws, RN, BS, CNN; Mary M. Macaluso, RN, BSN, CPDN, CNN; Gwen Elise McNatt, RN, MS, CNN, CFNP; Susan Montgomery, RN, MA, CNN, Allen R. Nissenson, MD, FACP; Patt Peterson, RN; Eileen Peacock, RN, MSN, CNN, CIC, CPHQ; Ginnette Pepper, RN, PhD; Christy A. Price, RN, MSN; Georgina Randolph, RN, MSN, MBA, CNN; Karen Robbins, RN, MS, CNN; Mark Rolston, CHT; Karen Schardin, RN, BSN, CNN; Jennifer Skero, FNP-BC, CDE, Sandra Smolka-Hill, RN, MSN, CNN; Julia Walsh Starr, RN, MSN; Beverly Wells Storck, RN, BSN; Jo Anne E. Strutz, RN; Cedric Tuck-Sherman, MBA; Philip M. Varughese, BS, CHT; Susan C. Vogel, RN, MHA, CNN; Ron Wathen, MD, PhD; Susan E. Weil, RD, CS; Gail S. Wick, BNS, RN, CNN; and Mary Ann Wierszbiczki, RN, MN. We are grateful for your commitment and desire to share your expertise with the nephrology community.

CONTENTS

CHAPTER 1

THE HEMODIALYSIS TEAM

Dialysis, the process by which accumulated waste products are removed from the blood, is a complex treatment requiring a team of highly trained individuals with a variety of skills. To ensure the success of this chronic treatment, the interdisciplinary team must work with the patients and their families to provide support in clinical and psychosocial needs. The team members include, but are not limited to, the physician, nurse, technician, dietitian, social worker, and administrator. Other team members might include a biomedical technician, psychologist, dentist, child development specialist, pharmacist, physician's assistant, vocational rehabilitation counselor, renal case manager, clergy member, nurse practitioner, and clinical nurse specialist or others with the special skills needed to help patients reach their maximum potential. The patients and their family members are integral components of the dialysis team; without their participation, all efforts of the other team members would be fruitless.

STRUCTURE OF THE DIALYSIS FACILITY

Every dialysis facility has a medical director who is ultimately responsible for the medical care provided by the facility. The medical director must have completed a board-approved training program in nephrology, must have at least 12 months of experience in nephrology, and must be certified in internal medicine or pediatrics. As long as a qualified nephrology training program has been completed, maintenance of a current board certification in internal medicine, pediatrics, nephrology, or pediatric nephrology should meet the qualification to become a facility medical director. The medical director is required to be knowledgeable of and responsible for the integrity of the water treatment system in the facility. The director must ensure that the system can produce water that meets the standards of the Association for the Advancement of Medical Instrumentation (AAMI). The medical director is also responsible for conducting the Quality Assessment and Performance Improvement (QAPI) program. Each dialysis facility has written policies and procedures to guide staff members in clinical practice and patient care. These policies and procedures address the established standards of care, quality assurance, equipment and maintenance standards, reuse, and any pertinent medication or treatment protocols. The policies and procedures of such facilities must be approved by the facility's governing body, which includes the medical director, director of nursing, and administrator, and must be in accordance with the laws of that state and the rules of the Centers for Medicare & Medicaid Services (CMS).

ROLE OF THE NEPHROLOGIST

The nephrologist assesses the patient and determines when chronic kidney disease (CKD) has advanced and requires the initiation of dialysis therapy. A nephrologist is an internist with an additional 2 to 3 years of specialty training in the field of nephrology. Increasing evidence has indicated the importance of having patients seen and followed by a nephrologist early in the course of CKD, long before progression to the point at which maintenance dialysis is required. With early nephrologic intervention, appropriate medical therapy can be instituted that may improve or at least maintain kidney function and delay the need for dialysis.

When the need for dialysis has been determined, the nephrologist is responsible for writing the orders for the dialysis prescription, which comprise the therapeutic components of the procedure. These include the specific dialyzer, blood and dialysate flow rates, anticoagulation requirements, duration or length of time of dialysis, frequency of dialysis, and other tailored instructions that may be required for specific vascular access.

ROLE OF THE NURSE

WHAT ARE THE FUNCTIONS OF THE DIALYSIS NURSE?

The dialysis nurse is required to receive additional training to provide the complex care required for a patient with either acute or CKD. Although nurses are responsible for the direct care of patients undergoing dialysis, technical staff members often perform much of this care under the nurse's supervision. The CMS requires that a registered nurse (RN) responsible for nursing care must always be present in the unit when in-center dialysis patients are being treated. The RN must meet all requirements of the state where she or he practices to be able to provide care in the dialysis facility. Patient and family education and ongoing reinforcement and support for self-care are additional critical services provided by the nurse. In addition, the nurse is responsible for ongoing assessment of the patient and generally initiates multidisciplinary care conferences when necessitated by the patient's physical, emotional, or social condition.

Nursing administration or nursing service organizations may differ among dialysis units. In facilities that use a primary nursing model, each patient has a specifically designated primary nurse who is responsible for overall patient care.

However, case management is also an appropriate approach for the care of dialysis patients. This model expands nursing care and responsibility beyond the dialysis unit to the hospital, ambulatory care or outpatient facility, and home. Case management ensures continuity of care from both the quality of care and economic perspectives. Whichever model is used, the goal of nursing is to serve as an advocate for patients who require assistance and to empower them to become their own advocates.

As continuous quality improvement (CQI) becomes increasingly important as a means of ensuring delivery of quality care to patients, nurses are taking the lead in this activity. In some settings, nurses also participate in the roles of a business manager or fiscal administrator and manage overall facility operations including financial outcomes and budget.

WHAT IS THE ROLE OF THE ADVANCED PRACTICE NURSE IN DIALYSIS?

Use of advanced practice nurses (APNs) in acute and chronic dialysis settings has become more common as the patient population continues to increase. Nurse practitioners and clinical nurse specialists focused on kidney care currently work in a diverse range of health care settings that cover all nephrology specialties. APNs can manage the care of patients with CKD at all stages. Some APNs function as clinician, educator, consultant, administrator, or researcher. Current trends indicate an increase in the number of patients with kidney disease and a decrease in the number of nephrologists available to provide care. Nurse practitioners can be used to help bridge this gap. APNs can work collaboratively with the health care team to ensure that all patients with kidney disease receive quality care and thus experience improved outcomes.

ARE THERE ESTABLISHED STANDARDS OF PRACTICE FOR DIALYSIS NURSES?

Regulations governing the administration of the end-stage renal disease (ESRD) program under the CMS describe a number of standards and criteria related to the qualifications of professional staff, acceptable patient care policies and procedures, and unit administration. However, the CMS does not issue standards of practice for dialysis nurses.

Professional nursing organizations promote high standards of nephrology nursing practice. In 1987, the Nephrology Nursing Certification Commission (NNCC) was established to develop, implement, and coordinate all aspects of certification for nephrology nurses in the United States; in 1988, the American Nephrology Nurses' Association (ANNA) published its first standards of care. A nephrology nurse who meets the qualifications and passes the NNCC's written examination is entitled to use the Certified Nephrology Nurse (CNN) as a professional credential. The Certified Dialysis Nurse (CDN) credential is available to RNs without a baccalaureate degree from the NNCC. Other options include the Certified Hemodialysis Nurse (CHN) and Certified Peritoneal Dialysis Nurse (CPDN) certifications, which are available to both RNs and licensed practical/vocational nurses (LPN/LVNs) from the Board of Nephrology Examiners Nursing and Technology (BONENT). The NNCC also offers the Certified Nephrology Nurse–Nurse Practitioner (CNN-NP) exam to those who have been nationally certified as nurse practitioners and possess a minimum of a master's degree in nursing. The Nephrology Nursing Scope and Standards of Practice published by ANNA (2017) describe competent nursing and APN care in nephrology and present competent behaviors associated with the role.

Certification, although required for some, is strongly encouraged for all nephrology care providers. Certification in a specialty practice such as nephrology indicates a higher degree of professional competence, which ultimately improves patient safety and care.

Since 1977, the Kidney Disease Outcomes Quality Initiative (KDOQI), put forth by the National Kidney Foundation (NKF), has offered clinical practice guidelines for all stages of CKD in the areas of anemia management, hemodialysis adequacy, peritoneal dialysis adequacy, and vascular access for dialysis care. KDOQI also offers an additional eight guidelines for CKD in the areas of diabetes, anemia, bone metabolism and nutrition in adults and children, hypertension, dyslipidemia, and classification of CKD. The intended goal of these guidelines is to improve the quality of care and outcomes for all people with kidney disease and to help reduce the risk of developing kidney disease. The clinical practice guidelines are evidence based and are not mandated nor intended to comprise the requirements of or to be specific to nursing practice; rather, these guidelines are intended for the general care of patients with CKD at any stage of the disease process and to guide health care professionals while making treatment decisions (see Appendix A for additional information on NKF KDOQI).

ROLE OF THE DIALYSIS NURSE MANAGER

The nursing leader or nurse manager responsible for patient care coordination may assume several titles depending on the facility's structure. Whether as the nursing administrator, director of nurses, clinical manager, charge nurse, or nursing coordinator, this nurse is primarily responsible for direct patient care. Supporting a professional practice model ensures that patients receive optimal care. The dialysis nurse manager is usually accountable for hiring, staffing, disciplinary action, labor and supply utilization, and quality and regulatory activities. The nurse manager must be a full-time employee of the facility, meet the particular state practice requirements, and have at least 12 months of experience in clinical nursing and an additional 6 months of experience in providing care to dialysis patients.

Modeling knowledgeable, skillful care of patients is a vital aspect of the role of the nurse manager, along with the recruitment and retention of an adequate number of well-prepared patient caregivers, both nurses and technicians. It is also the responsibility of the nurse manager to equip personnel with knowledge through learning opportunities and to provide resources in the form of supplies and time, thus enabling staff to provide the desired quality of patient care. The nurse manager ensures a high quality of care within a cost-effective environment while promoting patient and staff safety.

ROLE OF THE DIALYSIS UNIT ADMINISTRATOR

The dialysis unit administrator is responsible for ensuring the fiscal soundness of the dialysis facility. The administrator may make purchasing decisions, and it is desirable that these decisions be made with an understanding of their clinical implications. A unit administrator usually has either a clinical or a fiscal background. Occasionally, an administrator with a clinical background will also acquire a Master of Business Administration (MBA) degree or obtain other fiscal or business education. This individual is thus prepared with both the clinical expertise to make decisions in the best interest of patients and the business expertise to make decisions in the best interest of the facility.

ROLE OF THE DIALYSIS TECHNICIAN

The role of the dialysis technician varies from state to state because of differences in the practice regulations and mandates of different regulatory agencies. Some duties that may be permitted in some states but not in others include intravenous administration of heparin, cannulation of the vascular access, and provision of treatment to a patient with a central venous catheter. Because of these variations, it is always necessary to check the laws and rules of the state where the technician is practicing. Dialysis technicians have been integral members of the dialysis health care team since dialysis programs were initiated. Two major roles exist for dialysis technicians: one role focuses on assembly and maintenance of the equipment, and the other focuses on patient care. In some settings, technicians have both patient and equipment care responsibilities. Timely and accurate assembly of dialysis equipment is vital to any dialysis program. Ongoing maintenance of costly equipment is a highly valued element of a dialysis program. Dialysis technicians work with all members of the dialysis team; however, in most settings, they are most closely aligned with nurses. The technicians' patient care activities are delegated and supervised by professional nurses.

WHAT ABILITIES ARE REQUIRED OF DIALYSIS TECHNICIANS?

Knowledge of mechanics and technological skills are essential for technicians who assume responsibility for equipment setup and maintenance. Understanding of the principles of physics and computer technology is also desirable for technicians. Interpersonal skills are necessary for maintaining good relations with patients and their families. Dialysis technicians must have some understanding of human anatomy and physiology and the pathophysiology of CKD. They must have full understanding of the theories and principles of dialysis, treatment complications, and care of the vascular access. Math skills are essential for calculating weight gain and loss, fluid removal requirements, and medication administration. For patient safety, a technician also must have patient monitoring skills and clinical judgment.

ARE THERE ESTABLISHED STANDARDS OF PRACTICE FOR DIALYSIS TECHNICIANS?

Dialysis technicians are bound by the standards of practice issued by the state where they practice. The CMS also has requirements for dialysis technicians, and these requirements apply to technicians with any responsibility for direct patient care. Direct patient care is defined as any aspect of health care for a patient that is provided personally by a staff member, including but not limited to collecting data (e.g., vital signs, weights, symptoms since last treatment), setting up the dialysis machine, initiating and terminating treatment, care of the dialysis access, delivering any aspect of the hemodialysis or peritoneal dialysis process, responding to machine alarms, and administering medications as allowed (ESRD Conditions for Coverage: Frequently Asked Questions About Patient Care Technicians, April 2010).

The ESRD rules and regulations approved by the CMS Conditions for Coverage (CfCs) in 2008 imposed education requirements on dialysis technicians providing patient care. According to the final rule, dialysis technicians must be certified under a recognized state or national certification program within 18 months of hire and must meet all state requirements. They must also possess a high school diploma or equivalent, complete a training program, and have a validated competency checklist for clinical skills approved by the medical director and governing body of the dialysis facility. Different levels of regulation continue to exist at the state level; these include licensure, registration, and certification. The CMS has approved three national and commercially available dialysis technician certification exams: BONENT, NNCC, and the National Nephrology Certification Organization (NNCO). The CMS has approved all three of these national programs as meeting the CMS requirements for patient care technician (PCT) certification (Table 1.1). Some states require a certain exam; therefore, it is best to become familiar with the certification requirements mandated by the specific state. An advanced certification is offered for clinical dialysis technicians by the NNCC. The Certified Clinical Hemodialysis Technician–Advanced (CCHT-A) exam is for PCTs who hold national certifications such as CCHT, CHT, or CCNT and have 5 years of continuous employment and a minimum of 5000 hours as a clinical hemodialysis technician.

WHAT EDUCATIONAL OPPORTUNITIES ARE AVAILABLE TO DIALYSIS TECHNICIANS?

Dialysis programs offer on-the-job training for newly hired and inexperienced technicians. Some states mandate a minimum number of hours that the dialysis technician must complete in both the clinic and the classroom in order to practice. Certificate programs for dialysis technicians are available through some community colleges, and continuing education programs are offered by health care agencies, specialty organizations, and technical colleges.

The National Association of Nephrology Technicians/Technologists (NANT) and BONENT offer many educational programs, both locally and nationally. In addition, large nephrology meetings may provide advanced learning opportunities for technicians seeking expanded responsibilities or those functioning in expanded roles. These include but are not limited to the annual dialysis conference, NKF clinical meetings, the American Society of Nephrology meeting, the ANNA symposium, and meetings sponsored by the AAMI.

Table 1.1 Credentialing Programs for Dialysis Technicians

CREDENTIALING AGENCY	CERTIFICATION	ELIGIBILITY REQUIREMENTS	COGNITIVE OR PRACTICE DOMAINS	MEASURES
Nephrology Nursing Certification Commission (NNCC)	Certified Clinical Hemodialysis Technician (CCHT)	The applicant must possess a minimum of a high school diploma or its equivalent, the General Educational Development (GED). The applicant must have successfully completed a training program for clinical hemodialysis technicians that includes both classroom instruction and supervised clinical experience. Recommended 6 mo (or 1000 hr) of clinical experience	Clinical, 50% Technical, 23% Environmental, 15% Role, 12%	Basic competency for hemodialysis patient care technicians
Board of Nephrology Examiners Nursing and Technology (BONENT)	Certified Hemodialysis Technician/ Technologist (CHT)	The applicant must possess a state-accredited high school diploma or official transcripts. Minimum of 6 months of experience in nephrology patient care and current active participation in an ESRD facility	Patient care, 45% Machine technology, 12% Water treatment, 15% Infection control, 18% Education and personal development, 10%	Measures technical proficiency in certain skills and general areas of knowledge
National Nephrology Certification Organization (NNCO)	Certified Clinical Nephrology Technologist (CCNT)	The applicant must possess a minimum of a high school diploma or its equivalent OR 4 yr of full-time experience in the field of nephrology technology. Completion of a 1-yr nephrology technology training program[a] with clinical experience or completion of a combination nephrology technology training program[a] of <1 yr and work experience equivalent to 1 yr	Principles of dialysis, 10% Care of the patient with kidney failure, 18% Dialysis procedures and documentation, 17% Complications of dialysis, 15% Water treatment and dialysate preparation, 15% Infection control and safety, 20% Dialyzer reprocessing, 5%	Competency in the specialized area of practice of patient care for hemodialysis technicians

Table 1.1 Credentialing Programs for Dialysis Technicians (*Continued*)				
CREDENTIALING AGENCY	**CERTIFICATION**	**ELIGIBILITY REQUIREMENTS**	**COGNITIVE OR PRACTICE DOMAINS**	**MEASURES**
	Certified Biomedical Nephrology Technologist (CBNT)	The applicant must possess a minimum of a high school diploma or its equivalent OR 4 yr of full-time experience in the field of nephrology technology. Completion of a 1-yr nephrology technology training program with clinical experience or completion of a combination nephrology technology training program of <1 yr and work experience equivalent to 1 yr	Principles of dialysis, 10% Care of the patient with kidney failure, 18% Dialysis procedures and documentation, 17% Complications during dialysis, 15% Water treatment and dialysate preparation, 15% Infection control and safety, 20% Dialyzer reprocessing, 5%	Competency in the specialized area of practice of biomedical hemodialysis

[a]Clinical Nephrology Technician candidates in Ohio are required to have a minimum of 12 months of experience in dialysis care to take the examination.

ESRD, End-stage renal disease.

From Nephrology Nursing Certification Commission: *CCHT certification examination application booklet,* August 2015, NNCC; Board of Nephrology Examiners Nursing and Technology: *Candidate examination handbook,* January 1, 2018, BONENT; and National Nephrology Certification Organization: *Clinical nephrology technology and biomedical nephrology technology handbook for candidates,* December 6, 2017, NNCO.

ROLE OF THE RENAL DIETITIAN

A renal dietitian serves as a consultant to patients and their families as well as to other members of the dialysis team. The renal dietitian must be registered in the state and have 1 year of professional experience in clinical nutrition as a registered dietitian. Dietitians provide indispensable support to the patient through all phases of CKD, including in-center, home, and peritoneal dialysis. Dietary management is instrumental in delaying the need for dialysis. Furthermore, even after dialysis is initiated, the renal dietitian contributes through ongoing assessment of the nutritional status of the patient and education of the patient and his or her family. (See Chapter 14 for a more detailed description of the roles of nutrition and the renal dietitian in the care of patients with CKD.)

ROLE OF THE SOCIAL WORKER

WHAT ARE THE MAIN GOALS OF THE NEPHROLOGY SOCIAL WORKER?

Patients with CKD experience multiple losses and require significant psychosocial intervention at various stages throughout the course of their illness. The Council of Nephrology Social Workers describes their purpose as twofold:

* To assist patients and families in dealing with the psychosocial aspects of CKD
* To develop and implement methods for dealing with these problems and needs as a key to the role of the nephrology social worker

HOW DOES THE SOCIAL WORKER ACHIEVE THESE TWO GOALS IN A TREATMENT CENTER?

The social worker assists the patient and his or her family in adjusting to the illness both before and after initiation of maintenance dialysis. This involves psychosocial assessment, provision of emotional support, and educational reinforcement to help the patient cope with the challenges of CKD. Therefore, a thorough working knowledge of all available resources is essential. The social worker participates with other treatment team members in short- and long-term planning with the patient and his or her family. Evaluation of the patient's social background is important for successful development of the treatment plan. The social worker apprises other team members of special facets of the patient's or family's behavior, history, and functioning that may influence the individual patient's care and treatment course.

What Are the Necessary Qualifications of the Nephrology Social Worker?

A qualified social worker is defined by ESRD regulations as a person who is licensed, if applicable, by the state where he or she practices and who meets at least one of the following conditions:
1. Has completed a course of study with specialization in clinical practice and holds a master's degree from a graduate school of social work accredited by the Council on Social Work Education
2. Has served as a social worker for at least 2 years, of which 1 year was in a dialysis unit or transplant program before September 1, 1976, and has established a consultative relationship with a social worker qualified under condition 1
   Continuing education programs for social workers are available through the Council of Nephrology Social Workers.

What Other Difficulties Would Cause a Patient with Chronic Kidney Disease to Seek Psychosocial Intervention?

Awareness of one's own mortality and a life restricted by dependence on a machine are only two of the issues that confront patients on dialysis. The social worker assists patients and their families in adapting to illness-imposed lifestyle changes, such as alterations in family and societal roles. End-of-life care discussions including advance directives, identifying a health care agent, palliative care, and hospice may be initiated by the social worker.

Behavioral health consultations or team conferences with behavioral health staff are an important resource for the social worker and dialysis team for several reasons.

First, most dialysis patients are subjected to situational stress. Despite this fact, behavioral health intervention may be perceived by the patient as an unnecessary and unwelcome intrusion. The social worker assists patients in resolving their problems and dealing with crises, but behavioral health resources should be available for consultation or referral when needed.

Second, some patients become increasingly dependent or noncompliant during periods of their illness. During such times, the social worker should work with the patient, family, and other team members to help understand this behavior. Ultimately, the patient is responsible for much of his or her own management, and this should be emphasized by the social worker.

Finally, because sexual dysfunction can be a problem for patients undergoing maintenance dialysis, the social worker may be the team member whom the patient or his or her family members approach for counseling or referral.

ETHICS, RIGHTS, AND RESPONSIBILITIES

For a patient with CKD and his or her family, life with maintenance dialysis requires major activity and lifestyle changes. These disruptions are sometimes unpleasant as well as unanticipated. Frequently, the dialysis unit and involved personnel are perceived by the patient as causes of this unsatisfactory situation. Frustration and conflict are likely to develop and must be resolved.

Is Written Consent Necessary Before Starting Dialysis?

Informed written consent is always required for any invasive procedure, including dialysis. For emergency dialysis, if the patient is too ill to provide written consent, the next of kin or another person who has durable power of attorney may sign the consent for treatment.

It is important that staff members as well as patients and their families understand the importance of informed consent because patients and their families often have misconceptions or unrealistic ideas about dialysis and the procedures involved. The exact format of the consent form is determined by the provider's or institution's legal adviser. This form should clearly document that an adequate discussion and explanation of the benefits, complications, risks, and alternatives have been provided and understood by the patient. Separate consent is necessary for access procedures or modifications. Update of the dialysis consent form is necessary if there is a significant change in the procedure that might affect the patient, such as dialyzer reuse.

What Are Some of the Rights of the Patient?

- To be fully informed about his or her illness
- To be informed about the nature of the treatment and the usual risks
- To be fully informed about the alternative methods of treatment
- To expect that treatment will be tailored to individual health needs
- To know that personal privacy will be respected and professional confidentiality will be maintained
- To have input into the treatment regimen

Can a Patient Voluntarily Decide to Discontinue Dialysis?

Many, but not all, professionals believe that a rational adult with full understanding of the consequences should have the right to elect treatment cessation for reasons that are valid to the individual patient. If a patient believes that the dialysis treatment is no longer maintaining or contributing to his or her quality of life, the patient is encouraged to discuss this with the health care team, including the physician, as well as immediate family members. It is well within a patient's rights to choose to terminate dialysis. The patient would then be eligible for hospice care. The associated ethical and legal issues are complex; not all nephrology workers agree, and in some instances, courts have ordered dialysis to be continued.

WHAT ARE SOME RESPONSIBILITIES OF THE PERSONNEL TOWARD PATIENTS?

- To ensure that the patient is as fully informed as possible by his or her personal physician regarding his or her medical condition
- To ensure that all safeguards are met fully and to provide high-quality dialysis service
- To be supportive of the patient and his or her family in their adjustment to the illness, its treatment, and the accompanying changes in their lives. This involves teaching them about the disease and its treatment so that they can make informed decisions and set realistic goals.

WHAT ARE SOME RESPONSIBILITIES OF THE PATIENT?

- To understand and follow the instructions of the physicians, nurses, and other personnel providing care unless the patient is mentally incompetent. A medical care power of attorney would then be required to make decisions regarding the patient's treatment and health care
- To strive for a high degree of independence through learning and to assume responsibility for self-care as far as possible
- To respect the rights and privacy of other patients.

WHAT ARE SOME EXTERNAL AGENCIES INVOLVED IN DIALYSIS CARE?

Other agencies exist who make recommendations and provide guidance and resources for the safe delivery of care for the CKD patient in any stage of the disease or modality. The CMS, AAMI, and Centers for Disease Control and Prevention (CDC) provide additional guidelines and standards in the areas of infectious disease testing and monitoring, immunizations, dialysis treatment safety, quality standards, personnel requirements, infection control, water and dialysate standards, and interdisciplinary clinical care. More information can be found on these agencies in Appendix A.

CHAPTER 2

HISTORY OF DIALYSIS

Until the 1960s, maintenance dialysis was not an option for those who required treatment for chronic kidney disease (CKD), and treatment was limited to the relief of symptoms imposed by uremic syndrome. The development of adequate and dependable treatment for CKD spanned decades. Major barriers included the need to create a reliable dialyzer membrane, discover an effective anticoagulant, identify a suitable method for accessing the patient's bloodstream, and provide financial resources for treatment. Maintenance dialysis, a life-sustaining therapy, emerged from the results of many pioneering scientists who, through tenacity and risk taking, discovered a way to safely remove toxins and excess fluid from the bloodstream of a patient with CKD. Worldwide, many advances in dialysis delivery systems, dialyzer technology, vascular access, renal pharmacotherapy, and treatment options were made because of the work of these individuals.

An early pioneer in the development of the technologies and treatment used for maintenance dialysis was Thomas Graham, a professor of chemistry in Glasgow, Scotland. Graham formulated the law of diffusion of gases, known as Graham's law, and described the idea of selective diffusion. This selective *diffusion*, or separation of substances across a semipermeable membrane, gave rise to the term dialysis, which was first used by Graham in 1854 (Cameron, 2002). The science of clinical dialysis was not recognized for at least 50 years after Graham's death.

Some of the significant milestones in the history and development of dialysis are reviewed in this chapter.

WHO WAS CREDITED WITH CONSTRUCTING THE FIRST ARTIFICIAL KIDNEY?

Several well-known groups and individuals have contributed to the scientific development of the artificial kidney. The earliest written account describing the process of filtering a substance using an artificial device was published in 1913. John Abel and his colleagues Leonard Rowntree and Bernard Turner built a device known as the vividiffusion apparatus to remove toxicities from the blood. This device was made of hollow collodion tubes housed in a glass cylinder in which the dialysate was circulated. The collodion tubes contained microscopic pores that allowed substances to seep out of the tubes and into the circulating fluid. Hirudin, a substance extracted from leeches, was used as an anticoagulant. This was the first artificial kidney, and it debuted in 1913 at a medical conference in London. Abel and his colleagues demonstrated this device during a procedure in which salicylic acid was removed from the blood of an animal. The system did not use a pump to circulate the blood but rather used the force of the heart to pump the blood through the extracorporeal circuit (Cameron, 2002). The process of constructing this dialyzer was arduous, and the collodion tubes were very fragile. This device was never used on a human, although it served as a model for future dialyzer development.

WHEN WAS THE FIRST HUMAN DIALYSIS PERFORMED?

In 1924, Dr. Georg Haas, a German physician, first attempted to dialyze a human with uremic symptoms. The goal of this treatment was to remove toxic nitrogenous substances from the blood. Collodion membranes were constructed to perform the treatment and were used in a manner similar to that used by Abel and his associates. Haas used a venovenous approach whereby blood was removed from the body, passed through the collodion membrane, exposed to a dialyzing solution, and then reinfused into the bloodstream. The trial treatment was not highly successful and lasted only 15 minutes. Hirudin remained the only available anticoagulant to prevent the blood from clotting. Haas dialyzed four more patients in the following year, but the treatments never lasted long because of the toxic reactions provoked by hirudin. Haas later dialyzed a patient after the discovery of heparin in 1928.

WHEN WAS HEPARIN INTRODUCED?

A major obstacle encountered in the research and development of hemodialysis was the lack of a suitable anticoagulant. Hirudin was the principal anticoagulant used, but it caused many side effects and allergic reactions because it was insufficiently purified. Heparin was introduced in 1928 by Dr. William Henry Howell of Johns Hopkins Hospital, although it was discovered by a young medical student, Jay McLean. The discovery of heparin was a major milestone in the history of dialysis because it allowed systemic heparinization in humans without the severe allergic reactions frequently encountered with the use of hirudin.

WHEN WAS THE FIRST SUCCESSFUL TREATMENT PERFORMED WITH AN ARTIFICIAL KIDNEY?

Dr. Willem J. Kolff is often referred to as the "father of dialysis." Kolff was a Dutch physician who in 1943 created the first dialyzer suitable for human use, called the rotating drum dialyzer. Kolff used cellophane, a material not used by previous scientists, to construct the hollow tubes in his device. In his procedure, the patient's blood circulated in a spiral of cellophane tubing wrapped around a wooden drum. The drum rotated through a dialyzing solution housed in a porcelain tank (Friedman, 2009). Kolff dialyzed only patients with acute kidney injury (AKI), and dialysis with this device required a treatment time of nearly 6 hours. This artificial kidney was very awkward and had no safety features, but it marked the beginning of successful patient treatment as a result of advances in technology. In 1948, Kolff redesigned his device at the Peter Bent Brigham Hospital in Boston along with Dr. Carl Walters and Dr. John Merrill. The Kolff-Brigham artificial kidney was constructed of stainless steel with a Plexiglas hood. The dialyzer clearance volume could be modified by adjusting the number of cellulose tubing wraps. These dialyzers were used to treat AKI in injured soldiers during the Korean War. Kolff later developed a disposable coil dialyzer known as the twin-coil dialyzer.

When Was Continuous Renal Replacement Therapy Introduced?

Continuous renal replacement therapy (CRRT) is a technique commonly used to provide treatment to critically ill patients with AKI. This renal replacement therapy provides slow and constant fluid removal over a longer period of time, as opposed to the intermittent nature of conventional hemodialysis. Dr. Peter Kramer first described CRRT in 1977. The earliest form of CRRT was designated continuous arteriovenous hemofiltration (CAVH). The patient's blood was moved from an artery to a vein through a device called a hemofilter. This slower and less aggressive therapy is particularly useful for patients who are critically ill and unable to tolerate rapid fluid and electrolyte shifts and the concomitant hemodynamic compromise. See Chapter 18 for more information on AKI and related therapies.

Who Created the Arteriovenous Shunt?

Gaining access to the patient's bloodstream was a major dilemma when performing necessary treatments in the early years of dialysis. In 1960, Dr. George Quinton and Dr. Belding Scribner introduced the external arteriovenous (AV) shunt, making chronic dialysis a reality. Previously, a patient's blood vessel could be accessed only by way of surgical incision. Repeated vessel cutdowns precluded treatment for patients with CKD who required maintenance dialysis because their blood vessels quickly became exhausted. The AV shunt consisted of a small plate placed outside the body, usually on the forearm. A Teflon tube was placed in both the patient's artery and vein. The tubes were connected to the bloodlines of the dialysis machine during treatment. When not used during dialysis treatment, the loops were connected externally with a U-shaped device, allowing continuous blood flow through the loops to maintain patency. Hemodialysis treatment before this time was performed exclusively in patients with AKI. This breakthrough in vascular access development now permitted long-term treatment of patients requiring maintenance dialysis.

When Did Home Hemodialysis Become a Modality for Patients with Chronic Kidney Disease?

Home hemodialysis as a treatment modality in the United States was initiated in 1964 by Dr. Belding Scribner in Seattle and Dr. John Merrill in Boston. Maintenance home dialysis was a sensible answer to help keep the cost of treatment affordable while increasing the number of patients able to receive treatment. Patients were dialyzed using twin-coil and flat-plate dialyzers during this time. A single-patient dialysis machine with a proportioning system was developed for use at home. These early machines were large and cumbersome but became the prototype for the machines used today. Treatments were initially performed twice a week or, in some cases, whenever uremic symptoms developed.

When Was the Internal Arteriovenous Fistula Developed?

In 1966, Dr. Michael Brescia and Dr. James Cimino created the AV fistula, which was the first permanent internal vascular access. The AV fistula was constructed by joining the radial artery to the cephalic vein. Although the AV shunt opened the door for the treatment of end-stage renal disease (ESRD), the AV fistula became the premier vascular access. It continues to remain the access of choice for hemodialysis patients today. The Brescia-Cimino fistula had fewer complications, and the problem of accidental dislodgment and bleeding was not a concern as it was with the AV shunt.

When Did Medicare Begin to Pay for the Treatment of All Patients with Chronic Kidney Disease?

President Richard Nixon signed the Social Security Amendments of 1972, which extended Medicare coverage to those requiring kidney replacement therapies. Before the introduction of this landmark legislation, funding for chronic dialysis treatment was limited. Treatment was available only to those who met certain criteria or could afford to pay for their own treatment. The number of patients needing treatment far exceeded the available resources. Dialysis machines were scarce, and hospitals with the necessary equipment often set up patient selection committees to determine who would be eligible to receive dialysis treatment. The committees nominated patients who were considered worthy or eligible to receive treatment on the basis of criteria such as age, rehabilitation potential, position in the community, emotional status, and comorbid conditions.

The amendment was originally intended for those younger than 65 years of age but was later revised to include those 65 years of age and older. Federal funding allowed dialysis to be made available to patients without regard to age or comorbidities. Patient selection committees were no longer necessary because the majority of patients were eligible to receive federally funded treatments. As a result of this landmark legislation, outpatient dialysis centers proliferated across the country.

When Was the First Successful Kidney Transplant Performed?

Early endeavors in kidney transplantation were performed on humans using xenografts (transplants from one species to another). These early attempts were performed using organs from sheep, goats, and pigs. These grafts did not survive very long, and the recipients died soon after the procedure. The lack of immunosuppressive therapy and inadequate understanding of tissue typing constituted barriers to successful transplantation. It was not until 1954 that the first successful transplant was performed on identical twins at Peter Bent Brigham Hospital in Boston by Dr. Joseph Murray. Murray became interested in organ transplantation while attending to burn patients during his employment as a physician in the Army. He observed the rejection of foreign skin grafts as well as successful cross skin graft in a pair of identical twins. This compelling observation became the catalyst for Murray's study of organ transplantation. Much work was still needed to understand the nature of organ rejection to achieve long-term success in nontwin organ transplantation. Successful cadaveric transplants began in the 1960s. Long-term graft survival had to wait until the 1970s and 1980s when the immunosuppressants cyclosporine (Sandimmune) and tacrolimus (Prograf) were introduced.

WHEN WAS RECOMBINANT ERYTHROPOIETIN INTRODUCED?

The US Food and Drug Administration approved the use of epoetin alfa (Epogen) in 1989. Anemia was generally treated with frequent and multiple blood transfusions. Anabolic steroids such as nandrolone decanoate (Deca-Durabolin) were also used to ameliorate the anemia associated with CKD. These steroids were usually administered weekly by intramuscular injection. The introduction of recombinant human erythropoietin diminished, or in most cases precluded, the need to administer blood transfusions and anabolic steroids.

WHEN WERE THE NATIONAL KIDNEY FOUNDATION'S KIDNEY DISEASE OUTCOMES QUALITY INITIATIVE GUIDELINES PUBLISHED?

The National Kidney Foundation (NKF) first published the Kidney Disease Outcomes Quality Initiative (KDOQI) guidelines in 1997. These guidelines became the evidence based clinical practice guidelines that are in use today. The guidelines were revised in 2002 to establish the five stages of CKD, which classify kidney disease on the basis of the glomerular filtration rate (GFR). The new classification system eliminated the use of the terms *end-stage kidney disease, chronic kidney failure,* and *chronic renal insufficiency*. The new classification system is based on the markers of kidney disease, such as albuminuria, GFR, and duration of structural or functional alterations (Eckardt, Berns, Rocco, & Kasiske, 2009). Throughout this book, *CKD stage 5* and *ESRD* are used interchangeably. The NKF has published 18 sets of KDOQI guidelines since the ones first published in 1997, which address early identification of CKD, staging of CKD, prevention and management of CKD, and recommendations for the optimization of kidney replacement therapy. KDOQI continually updates its guidelines as new scientific evidence supports change in interventions. New guidelines in Vascular Access and Nutrition in CKD published in 2018 (NKF, 2017).

WHAT IS KIDNEY DISEASE IMPROVING GLOBAL OUTCOMES?

Kidney Disease Improving Global Outcomes (KDIGO) was originally established in 2003 by the NKF but became an independent nonprofit foundation organization in 2013. The goal of KDIGO is much like that of KDOQI in that the organization desires to promote awareness of kidney disease and to disseminate clinical practice guidelines but on a global level. KDIGO has volunteer members from around the world helping to promote and adopt guidelines and recommendations related to the prevention and or management of kidney disease. KDIGO has written evidence based guidelines in the following areas: AKI, anemia in CKD, blood pressure in CKD, CKD management, CKD mineral and bone disorder, diabetes and CKD, glomerulonephritis, hepatitis in CKD, lipids in CKD, and transplant.

WHAT ARE THE CENTERS FOR MEDICARE & MEDICAID SERVICES CONDITIONS FOR COVERAGE FOR END-STAGE RENAL DISEASE FACILITIES?

The Centers for Medicare & Medicaid Services (CMS), formerly known as the Health Care Financing Administration (HCFA), is a federal agency that administers Medicare, Medicaid, and the Children's Health Insurance Program. The role of the CMS is to ensure that the recipients of these programs are aware of the benefits to which they are entitled. The CMS also ensures that the program and services are made available and accessible to those in need and that the services are provided effectively. The CMS has developed the Conditions for Coverage (CfCs), which outline the minimum requirements or standards that providers must meet to participate in Medicare and Medicaid programs. The CfCs were first published in 1976 and have recently been updated to reflect advances in technology and standards of care. The new conditions, which were published on April 15, 2008, are patient centered, with emphasis on the quality of care. Medicare surveys are conducted about every 36 months to ensure that facilities comply with the federal standards. State agencies may also survey facilities in response to a complaint made by a patient or staff member.

In January 2019, CMS approved the National Dialysis Accreditation Commission (NDAC) LLC which is the first independent organization approved by CMS to conduct surveys for Medicare certification. The survey process conducted by NDAC mirrors the CMS ESRD CfCs. The NDAC survey process has deemed approval to be used as a certifying agency that permits the dialysis provider to be awarded as a certified Medicare provider in all 50 states. Potential benefits of accreditation through NDAC are faster approval of de novo dialysis clinics, predictable survey cadence, and timely surveys when adding expanded services such as increased stations or an additional modality.

WHAT IS THE BUNDLED PAYMENT SYSTEM?

When Medicare coverage was extended to patients with CKD in 1972, dialysis services were provided and paid for on a fee-for-service basis. In 1983, the first "bundled" composite rate payment system was set up to reimburse the costs of dialysis treatments. This bundled system provided a flat rate for the dialysis procedure, including both labor and supplies.

Both hemodialysis and peritoneal dialysis treatments were paid at the same rate. Monthly routine laboratory tests were included in this composite rate. Items excluded from this bundled or composite rate were erythropoietin-stimulating agents (ESAs), parenteral iron and vitamin D, antibiotics, and carnitine, as well as all other laboratory tests. These services were billed separately by the dialysis provider. In response to the increased number of patients requiring dialysis and the associated costs, Medicare reengineered the payment system. As the incidence of diabetes, hypertension, and obesity continues to increase, it is obvious that the number of patients with CKD requiring maintenance dialysis will also increase. This trend was the catalyst for designing a payment system to help control the treatment costs while ensuring the delivery of high quality care.

The new Medicare Bundled Dialysis Prospective Payment System of 2011 includes all the services previously provided in the composite rate; however, the new fixed composite rate also includes all dialysis laboratories, all injectable medications, and all oral iron and vitamin D supplementation. Beginning in 2016, all ESRD-related oral medications including phosphorus binders and calcimimetics are included in the bundle. These services are no longer billed separately. The new bundled payment system also uses a pay-for-performance system in which providers may incur a financial penalty for underperformance in the areas of anemia management, ESA utilization, and urea clearance or urea reduction ratio. This provision to meet certain quality standards can penalize or provide a reduction of up to 2% in reimbursement.

CHAPTER 3

BASIC CHEMISTRY OF BODY FLUIDS AND ELECTROLYTES

Normal kidneys maintain a balance between body water and the substances dissolved in it within the narrow limits necessary for life. The kidneys also excrete the waste products of protein metabolism. Dialysis partially substitutes for these two important functions when the normal kidneys fail. Other functions of the kidney are discussed in Chapter 4. Fundamental to understanding the processes used by the kidneys, whether natural or artificial, is a basic knowledge of the chemistry involved and the measurements used.

METRIC SYSTEM

A solid review of the basic system of measurement is necessary because the metric system is used for the chemical and physical measurements related to body physiology. Length is expressed by the basic unit of meter. The basic unit of mass is the gram, and the liter is the basic unit of volume. Table 3.1 lists the common metric terms and their interrelationships.

The metric system is entirely decimal. Prefixes indicate smaller or larger units (Table 3.2). To relate the metric system to more familiar uses, the following approximations may be helpful:
- A man who is 6 ft, 4 inches tall is about 1.95 m in height.
- A dime is about 1 mm thick.
- A 154-lb person weighs 70 kg.

The following are commonly used conversion factors to change metric units to the English system of pounds, inches, and quarts.
- 1 meter (m) = 39.37 inches (in)
- 1 inch (in) = 2.54 centimeters (cm)
- 1 liter (L) = 1.057 quarts (US) (qt)
- 1 gallon (gal) = 3.785 liters (L)
- 1 kilogram (kg) = 2.2 pounds (lb)
- 1 ounce (oz) = 28.35 grams (g)
- 1 fluid ounce (fl oz) = 29.57 milliliters (mL)

Temperature is expressed in degrees Celsius. Zero degrees Celsius is the freezing point of water, and 100°C is its boiling point. The following table shows a comparison of some Celsius temperatures with the Fahrenheit scale:

	°F	°C
Boiling point of water	212	100
Normal body temperature	98.6	37
Freezing point of water	32	0

To convert Fahrenheit values to Celsius and Celsius values to Fahrenheit, use the following formulas:
Fahrenheit temperature = 9/5 (Celsius temperature) + 32
Celsius temperature = 5/9 (Fahrenheit temperature) − 32
An optional method to convert Fahrenheit values to Celsius and Celsius values to Fahrenheit is as follows:
To convert Fahrenheit to Celsius, subtract 32 and divide by 1.8.
To convert Celsius to Fahrenheit, multiply by 1.8 and add 32.

All physical things are composed of a finite number of kinds of matter. Matter is anything that possesses weight and occupies space or has mass. The basic kinds of matter are called elements. An element cannot be further divided without changing its chemical properties. There are 108 known elements. These may exist alone, in mixtures, or in chemical combinations (compounds). Some elements exist alone in their natural form as a solid, liquid, or gas. For instance, gold nuggets are pure, crystalline gold (Au). Metallic mercury (Hg) is a liquid under ordinary conditions. Helium (He) is a monatomic gas. The physical state depends on the melting or boiling point. Many elements do not exist in an uncombined state but exist only as compounds. Oxygen, as it exists in air, is not monatomic (O) but rather a compound of two oxygen atoms (O_2). Almost all hydrogen (H) exists in compounds, such as in water (H_2O).

WHAT IS A SOLUTION?

A solution is a homogeneous mixture of dissolved particles (solute) and a liquid (solvent). In physiologic solutions, the solvent is usually water. Physiologic saline contains 0.9 g of sodium chloride in 100 mL of water.

Table 3.1 Commonly Used Metric Units

QUANTITY	UNIT	ABBREVIATION	RELATIONSHIP OF UNITS
Length	Millimeter	mm	1 mm = 0.001 m
	Centimeter	cm	1 cm = 0.01 m
	Meter	m	1 m
	Kilometer	km	1 km = 1000 m
Area	Square centimeter	cm^2	1 cm^2 = 0.0001 m^2
	Square meter	m^2	1 m^2
	Square kilometer	km^2	1 km^2 = 1,000,000 m^2
Volume	Milliliter	mL	1 mL = 0.001 L
	Deciliter	dL	1 dL = 0.01 L
	Liter	L	1 L
	Cubic meter	m^3	1 m^3 = 1000 L
Mass	Milligram	mg	1 mg = 0.001 g
	Gram	g	1 g
	Kilogram	kg	1 kg = 1000 g

Table 3.2 Metric Decimal Prefixes

MULTIPLICATION FACTORS	PREFIX	ABBREVIATION
1		
$0.1 = 10^{-1}$	deci-	d
$0.01 = 10^{-2}$	centi-	c
$0.001 = 10^{-3}$	milli-	m
$0.000001 = 10^{-6}$	micro-	μ
$0.000000001 = 10^{-9}$	nano-	n
$0.000000000001 = 10^{-12}$	pico-	p

How Is the concentration of a Solution Measured?

Nonionized particles have been measured in terms of the weight of the solute per volume of the solvent. Blood glucose and urea are commonly measured as milligrams per 100 mL (mg/dL). For ionized particles, it is important to know the relative number of particles present and the contribution of their charge. These are measured more precisely by the use of molarity and normality and are usually expressed as mEq/L (milliequivalents per liter).

What Are SI Units?

The term *SI units* is the abbreviation of le Système Internationale d'Unités. This is an extension of the metric system that provides uniformity for the units of measurement and easy conversion. Since 1987, SI has been used to report data by most clinical laboratories in the United States. In this system, the amount of a substance is written as moles per liter rather than as mass, such as grams/liter (g/L) or milligrams/deciliter (mg/dL).

What Is an Electrolyte?

An electrolyte is a substance that dissolves in water to form ionized particles.

What Is an Ion?

An ion is a particle that has an electric charge. It may be a charged atom, such as a sodium ion, or a charged compound, such as a lactate ion. A positively charged ion is a cation, and a negatively charged compound is an anion.

What Is Conductivity?

Conductivity is the ability of a solution to conduct electric current. This is illustrated by an electrolytic cell. Fig. 3.1 shows such a cell: a container of solution with two electrodes. The electrodes are connected by wires through a battery and an ammeter; the ammeter measures the flow of current through the circuit. If the only communication between the electrodes is through very pure water, little or no current will flow because there is no way for electrons to pass through water.

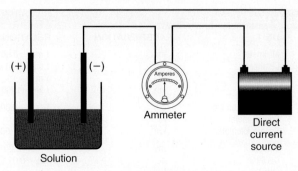

Fig. 3.1 An electrolytic cell.

If sodium chloride is added to water, current will flow. Sodium ions are attracted to the negative electrode (cathode), where each ion accepts an electron. At the same time, chloride ions are attracted to the positive electrode (anode), where each gives up an electron.

The ease with which electrons flow in a solution depends on the kind of electrolytes present and their concentration. Conductivity monitors are vital parts of dialysis fluid delivery systems that must produce solutions with a constant and precise solute content.

WHY IS CONDUCTIVITY AN IMPORTANT MEASUREMENT IN DIALYSIS?

Dialysate is produced by mixing a concentrated solution of electrolytes with very pure water. The correct proportion of the concentration of electrolytes and water is measured by the electrical conductivity of the solution. The proportion of electrolytes to water must be within certain limits to ensure patient safety. The conductivity of pure water is zero, whereas that of the dialysate depends on the amount of sodium in the solution. A dialysate solution containing too little sodium may cause water to shift into the patient's blood cells, resulting in hypotension, cramping, and hemolysis. Too much sodium in the dialysate may cause a high blood level of sodium that may make fluid leave the cells, which causes the blood cells to shrivel. This is known as crenation and may cause symptoms such as hypertension, profound thirst, and headache.

WHAT IS OSMOSIS?

Osmosis is the movement of fluid from an area of low solute concentration to an area of high solute concentration (Fig. 3.2). A strong electrolyte solution has reduced water concentration because some of the water has been replaced by the solute. If two solutions of different concentrations are separated by a membrane permeable only to water, water flows from the area of highest water concentration to the area of lowest water concentration. In other words, water flows from the area of lowest solute concentration to the area of highest solute concentration. Only water moves, not the solute.

WHAT IS DIFFUSION?

Diffusion is the movement of solutes from an area of higher solute concentration to an area of lower solute concentration so that both sides are equal (Fig. 3.3). Only the solutes move, not water.

Semipermeable membrane

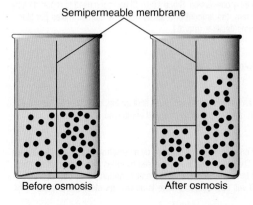

Before osmosis   After osmosis

Fig. 3.2 Osmosis is the process of movement of water through a semipermeable membrane from an area of low solute concentration to an area of high solute concentration. (From Lewis SM, Heitkemper MM, Dirksen SR: *Medical-surgical nursing,* ed. 9, St. Louis, 2013, Mosby.)

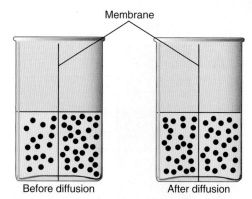

Fig. 3.3 Diffusion is the movement of molecules from an area of high concentration to an area of low concentration. Normal pH is maintained by a ratio of 1 part carbonic acid to 20 parts bicarbonate. (From Lewis SM, Heitkemper MM, Dirksen SR: *Medical-surgical nursing,* ed. 9, St. Louis, 2013, Mosby.)

Before diffusion   After diffusion

WHAT IS pH?

The measure of either the acidity or alkalinity of a substance is expressed as pH (Fig. 3.4). The term *pH* stands for the potential, or power, of hydrogen, and the pH value demonstrates the concentration of hydrogen ions in a solution. Solutions with a high concentration of hydrogen ions have a low pH, and solutions with a low concentration of hydrogen ions have a high pH. The normal hydrogen ion concentration in human extracellular fluid (ECF) ranges from 7.35 to 7.45. If a substance has a pH value less than 7, it is an acid. A substance that has a pH value greater than 7 is an alkali. If a substance has a pH value of 7, it is considered neutral. pH measures only the free hydrogen ions in solution. If some hydrogen ions are bound and not ionized, it does not affect the pH. pH is maintained by the action of buffers.

WHAT IS A BUFFER?

Buffers are substances that, in solution, maintain a constant hydrogen ion concentration despite the addition of either an acid or a base. Buffers minimize pH changes when an acid or a base is added to a solution. Bicarbonates, phosphates, amino acids, and proteins all act as buffers. Bicarbonate is the major plasma buffer.

WHY IS THE HYDROGEN ION CONCENTRATION IMPORTANT?

All metabolic processes of the body require a precise range of hydrogen ion concentration. If the hydrogen ion concentration exceeds that of pure water, the solution is acidic. If the hydrogen ion concentration is lower, the solution is basic, or alkaline. If the hydrogen ion concentration becomes too high or too low, massive metabolic derangement occurs. The hydrogen ion concentration compatible with life lies between 20 and 160 nmol/L (pH 7.8 to 6.8) (Fig. 3.5). Two body organs are involved in hydrogen ion regulation: the lungs and the kidneys. The lungs eliminate carbon dioxide (the major end product of metabolism) as rapidly as it is produced, and in doing so, regulate the partial pressure of carbon dioxide in the blood. The kidneys regulate blood pH by reabsorbing or excreting acids or bases. Kidney failure causes retention of hydrogen ions; this is called metabolic acidosis. See Chapter 5 for further discussion.

WHAT IS AN ACID, AND WHAT IS A BASE?

An acid is a substance that can donate a hydrogen ion, and a base is a substance that can accept a hydrogen ion. An acid may be called a proton donor, and a base may be called a proton receptor. Remember that the hydrogen atom consists of a positively charged nucleus, or proton, and a single negatively charged orbiting electron. The hydrogen ion (H^+) is a proton without an orbiting electron.

BODY WATER

HOW MUCH WATER DOES THE BODY CONTAIN?

Water is the major constituent of the body, and its volume varies with age, sex, and body fat. Water comprises 45% to 75% of the total body weight of an adult. The proportion varies inversely with the amount of body fat. A 70-kg man (154 lb) has about 42 L of total body water (60% of weight). Women have a lower proportion of body water. Infants and very young children have the highest proportion of body water (Fig. 3.6).

WHAT PURPOSE DOES THIS FLUID SERVE?

Body tissues are composed of living cells. Complex chemical processes within these cells produce energy in the form of heat, motion, and regeneration. Oxygen and nutrients are metabolized, and carbon dioxide and other wastes are produced. Water within the cell is the medium for these chemical processes.

Water also surrounds and bathes all cells, protecting them from the hazards of the external world. Water is the vehicle that transports nutrients from and wastes to the outside environment.

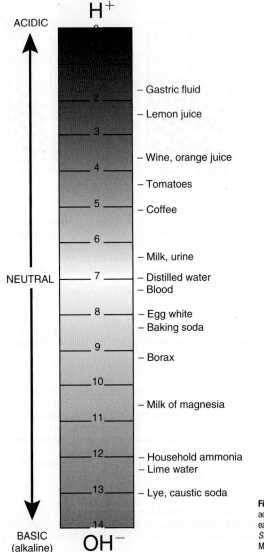

Fig. 3.4 The pH range on a logarithmic scale of 1 to 14. The actual concentration of hydrogen ions changes 10-fold with each pH unit on the scale. (From Thibodeau GA, Patton KT: *Structure and function of the body*, ed. 13, St. Louis, 2008, Mosby.)

Many conditions can disrupt the mechanisms that control fluid balance in the human body; therefore body fluid disorders are among the most commonly seen problems in patients seeking medical care.

How Is Water Distributed in the Body?

Total body water is the sum of all fluids within all compartments of the body. The total body water is distributed between two major compartments: the intracellular fluid (ICF) and ECF. Approximately two thirds (or 40% of the body weight) of the total amount of body water is contained in the ICF compartment, and one third (or 20% of the body weight) of the total amount of body water is contained in the ECF compartment. ECF can further be separated into interstitial (in the spaces between the cells and outside the blood vessels), intravascular (in blood plasma), and transcellular fluids (outside normal compartments), which include synovial, pericardial, intraocular, peritoneal, and other body fluids that do not interchange readily (Fig. 3.7).

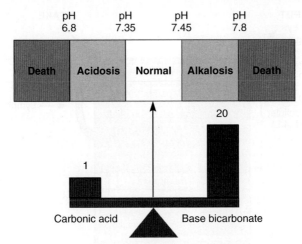

Fig. 3.5 The normal range of plasma pH is 7.35 to 7.45. Normal pH is maintained by a ratio of 1 part carbonic acid to 20 parts bicarbonate. (From Lewis SM, Heitkemper MM, Dirksen SR: *Medical-surgical nursing*, ed. 9, St. Louis, 2013, Mosby.)

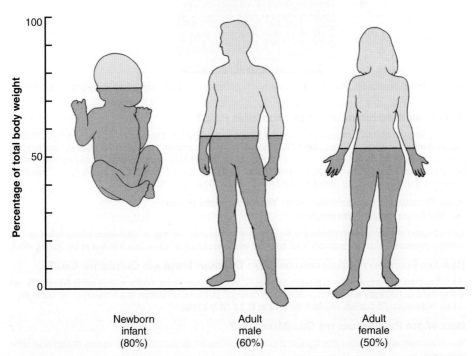

Fig. 3.6 Percentage of the total body weight composed of water. (From Thibodeau GA, Patton KT: *Structure and function of the body*, ed. 13, St. Louis, 2008, Mosby.)

WHAT ARE THE CONSTITUENTS OF THE INTRACELLULAR FLUID?

Intracellular fluid provides a medium for cells to function. The composition of ICF varies with the specific tissue. Muscle values are commonly used in these calculations. The concentration of potassium, the major intracellular cation, is 155 mEq/L; that of magnesium is 40 mEq/L; and that of sodium is only 10 mEq/L. Organic phosphates and protein are important anions; the total concentration of chloride and bicarbonate is only 10 mEq/L.

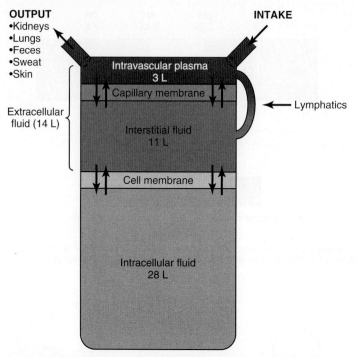

Fig. 3.7 Body fluid compartments. (From Hall JE: *Guyton and Hall's textbook of medical physiology,* ed. 12, Philadelphia, 2011, Saunders.)

WHAT IS THE COMPOSITION OF THE EXTRACELLULAR FLUID?

Plasma water and interstitial fluid are nearly the same. Sodium is the major cation found in ECF (135–145 mEq/L). Chloride and bicarbonate are the major anions. About 7% of the plasma volume comprises protein and lipid material that does not cross the capillary wall. The protein molecules are anionic; to maintain electrical neutrality, there are slightly fewer sodium and chloride ions in the plasma than in the interstitial fluid. Clinical calculations of electrolytes usually ignore these small differences and assume that the plasma electrolytes are representative of the total ECF.

WHAT DETERMINES THE DISTRIBUTION OF WATER BETWEEN PLASMA AND THE INTERSTITIAL COMPARTMENT?

The distribution of water between plasma and the interstitial compartment depends on the balance among colloid (protein and lipid) osmotic pressure, intracapillary blood pressure, and tissue turgor pressure. This is known as the Starling effect.

HOW ARE ELECTROLYTE CONCENTRATIONS KEPT DIFFERENT INSIDE AND OUTSIDE THE CELL?

The cell membrane is impermeable to proteins and organic phosphate complexes, confining them inside the cell. The cell wall contains metabolically active (energy-consuming) "pumps" that transport sodium ions from within the cell to the outside while moving potassium ions from the exterior to the cell's interior.

DOES WATER PASS ACROSS THE CELL MEMBRANE?

Yes, water moves quickly in either direction across the cell membrane to maintain total osmolar equality on both sides of the membrane.

ARE THERE NONELECTROLYTES IN BODY FLUIDS?

Yes. These include glucose, amino acids, and other nutrients and metabolic wastes such as urea. Their concentrations are relatively low compared with the electrolytes.

ARE UREA AND CREATININE ELECTROLYTES?

No. Both urea and creatinine are soluble in water, but they do not form charged particles.

Box 3.1 Normal Fluid Balance in an Adult	
INTAKE	
Fluids	1200 mL
Solid food	1000 mL
Water from oxidation	300 mL
	2500 mL
OUTPUT	
Insensible loss (skin and lungs)	900 mL
In feces	100 mL
Urine	1500 mL
	2500 mL

WHAT IS MEANT BY FLUID BALANCE?

A normal diet contains 500 to 1000 mL of water in the food itself. Approximately 300 to 500 mL of water is produced each day by food metabolism and tissue breakdown. Other fluids taken in, such as coffee, tea, juice, or other beverages, obviously represent water intake and average 1500 to 2000 mL/day.

Between 700 and 1000 mL of water is lost daily through evaporation from the lungs and insensible perspiration (Box 3.1). Vigorous activity or an increase in temperature causes additional losses (measurable in liters if the increase in environmental temperature is severe). A minimum of 400 mL of fluid or more must be excreted as urine each day to prevent the accumulation of metabolic wastes.

The electrolyte composition, pH, osmolality, and so on are precisely maintained in the body's internal fluid environment. The kidneys maintain this balance, called *homeostasis*. The kidneys conserve fluid or excrete excess as needed. When kidney failure occurs, meticulous attention to the balance of fluid intake and losses becomes a necessity.

CHAPTER 4

KIDNEY PHYSIOLOGY AND THE PATHOLOGY OF KIDNEY FAILURE

Before discussing the pathology of kidney failure, it is important to review the following functions performed by normal kidneys (Fig. 4.1):
- Elimination of metabolic wastes and other toxic materials
- Regulation of fluid volume
- Maintenance of electrolyte balance
- Regulation of blood pH
  In addition, the kidneys have several endocrine functions, including the following:
- Production of renin, which affects sodium, fluid volume, and blood pressure
- Formation of erythropoietin, which controls red blood cell (RBC) production in the bone marrow
  A normal kidney is also a receptor site for several hormones:
- Antidiuretic hormone (ADH), produced by the posterior pituitary, reduces the excretion of water.
- Aldosterone, produced by the adrenal cortex, promotes sodium retention and enhances the secretion of potassium and hydrogen ions.
- Parathyroid hormone (PTH) increases phosphorus and bicarbonate excretion and stimulates the conversion of vitamin D to the active 1,25-dihydroxycholecalciferol vitamin D_3 form.

It is important to note that other organs of excretion exist in the human body, but only the kidneys are able to precisely adjust the excretion or reabsorption of water and electrolytes to maintain homeostasis (Table 4.1).

KIDNEY PHYSIOLOGY

HOW IS BLOOD SUPPLIED TO THE KIDNEYS?

The kidneys are highly vascular organs that receive 20% to 25% of the resting cardiac output, which exceeds 1000 mL/min (Myers & Myers, 2019). Cardiac output is the volume of blood pumped per minute by each ventricle of the heart. Each kidney receives blood from a renal artery that originates from the abdominal aorta, and blood leaves the kidney through the renal vein. The renal artery branches out to form the afferent arterioles, which in turn form the glomerular capillaries of individual glomeruli. The glomerular capillaries then join to form the efferent arterioles, which in turn diffuse into the peritubular capillaries and the vasa recta (Fig. 4.2).

Blood flow to the kidney is dependent on hydration and cardiac output. Dehydration, blood loss, congestive heart failure, and myocardial infarction are examples of situations that would compromise blood flow to the kidney.

WHAT IS THE DIFFERENCE BETWEEN THE PERITUBULAR CAPILLARIES AND THE VASA RECTA?

The peritubular capillaries surround the proximal and distal convoluted tubules and allow tubular secretion and reabsorption to occur. The vasa recta capillaries and branches surround the loops of Henle of juxtamedullary nephrons and are located in the renal medulla. These play a major role in regulating the concentration of urine as it moves through the tubules.

WHAT IS A NEPHRON?

The nephron is the main functional unit of the kidney. There are more than 1 million such units in each of the two kidneys. Each nephron is a complex structure and has two main components: vascular and tubular. The vascular component consists of the afferent arteriole, glomerulus, efferent arteriole, and peritubular capillaries. The tubular component includes the Bowman capsule, proximal tubule, loop of Henle, and distal tubule. Nephrons do not regenerate; thus, they are not replenished if they become damaged. The glomerulus and Bowman capsule together are called the renal corpuscle.

The glomerulus consists of a network of thin-walled capillaries supplied by the afferent arteriole and is closely surrounded by a pear-shaped epithelial membrane called the Bowman capsule. The Bowman capsule opens into the proximal tubule, which forms a series of convolutions in the cortex of the kidney. The proximal tubule straightens out and then makes a U turn, known as the loop of Henle, in the medulla. The loop of Henle ascends, becomes adjacent to the glomerulus, and forms the distal convoluted tubule. The distal convoluted tubule finally joins other distal tubules to form a collecting duct to carry the freshly formed urine to the renal pelvis (Fig. 4.3). Each renal pelvis funnels the urine into its ureter, which connects with the urinary bladder. The urethra carries the urine from the bladder and allows it to be excreted from the body.

WHAT ARE THE PROCESSES INVOLVED IN URINE FORMATION?

Before understanding the process of urine formation, it is important to know the three specific steps involved in its formation. The first step is known as *glomerular filtration*. This step causes water and other dissolved substances to move

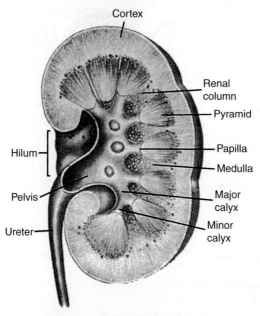

Fig. 4.1 Longitudinal section of a normal kidney.

Table 4.1	Organs of Excretion
ORGAN	**SUBSTANCES EXCRETED**
Kidneys	Water, electrolytes, nitrogenous wastes (urea, uric acid, creatinine)
Skin	Water, electrolytes, nitrogenous wastes
Lungs	Carbon dioxide, water
Intestines	Digestion wastes, bile pigments

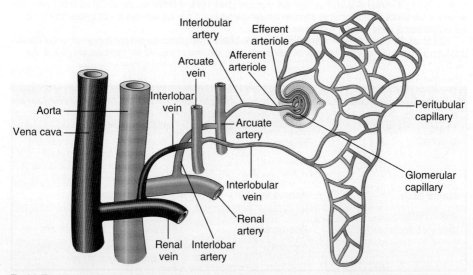

Fig. 4.2 The venous vessels of the kidney parallel the arterial vessels and are similarly named. (From Copstead LC, Banasik JL: *Pathophysiology,* ed. 4, St. Louis, 2010, Saunders.)

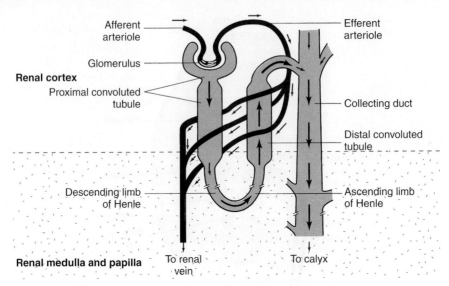

Fig. 4.3 Diagram of a nephron with the afferent arteriole, glomerulus, efferent arteriole, and collecting duct.

from the glomerulus into the Bowman's capsule or tubules. The second step is referred to as *tubular reabsorption*. In this step, water and other dissolved substances move from the tubules into the blood in the peritubular capillaries. The final process is *tubular secretion*, which involves the movement of selected substances from the blood in the peritubular capillaries back into the tubules. Table 4.2 presents the functions of the nephron and locations where the specific reabsorption and secretion of particular substances take place.

What Is the First Step in Urine Formation?

Blood enters the glomerulus through an afferent arteriole. Because of the blood pressure in the capillaries and because of their thin walls, filtration of blood is possible. The pressure in the glomerulus is greater than the pressure in the Bowman's capsule. This difference in pressure allows water and solutes to move from one space to the other (from the glomerulus into the Bowman's capsule). Water and dissolved solutes with a molecular weight of less than 68,000 Da (e.g., albumin) pass freely into the Bowman's capsule. This essentially protein-free fluid is the glomerular filtrate, and its rate of production is known as the glomerular filtration rate (GFR). The GFR is the amount of filtrate produced by the kidneys per minute. A man of average size produces about 180 L of filtrate per day or 125 mL/min. Ninety-nine percent of this filtrate is reabsorbed as it passes through the tubules. Table 4.3 identifies the total reabsorption into the bloodstream of some selected substances.

Glomerular filtration is dependent on sufficient blood circulation to the glomerulus and maintenance of normal filtration pressures. Filtration of molecules depends on their shape, size, and ionic charge. As the molecular weight and size

Table 4.2 Functions of Different Parts of the Nephron in Urine Formation		
PART OF NEPHRON	**FUNCTION IN URINE FORMATION**	**SUBSTANCES MOVED**
Glomerulus	Filtration	Water and solutes (e.g., sodium and other ions, glucose and other nutrients filtered from the glomeruli into the Bowman capsules)
Proximal tubule	Reabsorption	Water and solutes
Loop of Henle	Reabsorption	Sodium and chloride ions
Distal and collecting ducts	Reabsorption	Water, sodium, and chloride ions
	Secretion	Ammonia, potassium ions, hydrogen ions, and some drugs

From Thibodeau GA, Patton KT: *The human body in health & disease*, ed. 5, St. Louis, 2010, Mosby.

Table 4.3 Final Results of Tubular Reabsorption and Secretion of Selected Substances

SUBSTANCE	PERCENT REABSORBED
Water	99.2
Sodium	99.4
Potassium	86.1
Bicarbonate	100
Glucose	100
Urea	50
Insulin	0
Calcium	98.2
Creatinine	0

increase, the degree of filtration decreases. The glomerular basement membrane exerts a net negative charge. Substances carrying a negative charge will be repelled by the basement membrane, and their filtration will be prohibited.

WHAT HAPPENS TO THE FILTRATE AS IT MOVES THROUGH THE TUBULES?

The main functions of the tubules are reabsorption and secretion. Tubular reabsorption is the process that facilitates the return of the filtrate to the blood in the peritubular capillaries or vasa recta (Fig. 4.4). This process is very selective and dependent on the body's needs at the time. Materials that are reabsorbed into the bloodstream include ions such as sodium, potassium, chloride, bicarbonate, and calcium.

Of the 180 L of glomerular filtrate produced each day, approximately 2 L remains as the final urine. The rest of the water is reabsorbed along with glucose, amino acids, small proteins, and most electrolytes. The remaining filtrate becomes concentrated and begins to resemble the final urine as it progresses down the tubule. Final adjustments of the water-to-solute load occur in the distal tubule under the influence of ADH. The tubules conserve water and electrolytes by returning them to the blood. Hydrogen ions and metabolic wastes are excreted along with a volume of

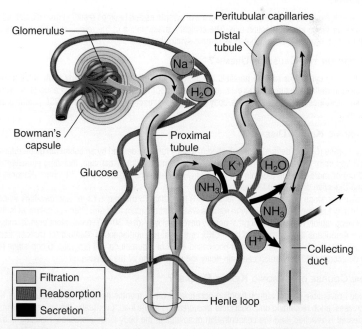

Fig. 4.4 The path of the filtrate as it moves through different parts of a nephron. (From Thibodeau GA, Patton KT: *Anatomy & physiology*, ed. 7, St. Louis, 2010, Mosby.)

water appropriate to the total body need. The majority of reabsorption occurs in the proximal tubule; however, some reabsorption also occurs across the distal tubule.

Tubular secretion adds materials from the blood to the filtrate. This process helps to remove toxic substances from the blood and to restore blood pH by excreting excessive hydrogen ions. Substances secreted into the tubules include potassium, hydrogen, ammonia, creatinine, and some drugs. This process accounts for a very small amount of the total sum of substances found in the filtrate.

KIDNEY FAILURE

WHAT HAPPENS WHEN THE KIDNEYS FAIL?

The normal urinary system maintains fluid volumes and the levels of many chemicals in the body. When the urinary system is not working properly, the normal blood composition is disrupted, and the patient experiences symptoms. Kidney failure may be acute or chronic. In both types of kidney failure, there is enough loss of nephron function to upset the normal steady state of the body's internal environment. The waste products of protein metabolism accumulate and will necessitate some kind of treatment.

This accumulation of waste products of protein metabolism is termed *azotemia,* indicating the retention of nitrogenous products (azote/azoto = nitrogen). Azotemia is a major component of the uremic syndrome.

WHAT IS UREA?

Urea is the waste product of protein metabolism and has a molecular weight of 60 Da. Urea is the most abundant organic waste and is freely filtered at the glomerulus. Most urea is produced during the breakdown of amino acids. The normal level of urea in the blood ranges from 8 to 25 mg/dL. Blood urea levels are influenced by many factors, which is why it is not the best indicator of kidney function or dysfunction. Increased levels may be seen with increased dietary consumption of protein, bleeding into the gastrointestinal tract, steroid use, dehydration, and any hypercatabolic state such as infection, fever, burns, trauma, or sepsis. Decreased levels may be seen with low dietary consumption of protein, liver disease, and overhydration.

WHAT IS CREATININE?

Creatinine is a protein produced by muscles and released into the blood. Muscle mass remains relatively constant day over day, so creatinine production does not change on a daily basis. Creatinine levels in the blood are determined by the rate at which creatinine is removed in the urine. Creatinine accumulates in the blood with diminished kidney performance. Thus, it is a good marker for assessing the function of the kidney.

WHAT IS UREMIA?

Uremia, or the uremic syndrome, encompasses a complex of symptoms and findings resulting from disordered biochemical processes that occur when kidney function fails. The clinical representation of the retention of compounds or toxins normally secreted in the urine is often labeled as uremic syndrome.

IS UREA RETENTION THE CAUSE OF UREMIA?

The severity of uremic symptoms roughly parallels the increase in blood urea. Urea clearly contributes to some of the symptoms, including malaise, lethargy, anorexia, and insomnia, but is not the primary toxin associated with uremia. Numerous other substances are retained in the body when kidney function fails. More than 200 potential uremic toxins have been identified.

WHAT IS CHRONIC KIDNEY DISEASE?

Chronic kidney disease (CKD) is defined as a reduction of kidney function defined by an estimated glomerular filtration rate (eGFR) below 60 mL/min/1.73 m^2 for more than 3 months evidence of kidney damage, including persistent albuminuria, defined as 30 mg or more of urine albumin per gram of urine creatinine for more than 3 months (National Institute of Diabetes and Digestive and Kidney Diseases, 2014).

Kidney failure or stage 5 CKD is defined as an eGFR less than 15 mL/min/1.73 m^2 and develops when the kidneys permanently lose most of their ability to remove waste and maintain fluid and chemical balances in the body. This process can develop rapidly (within 2–3 months) or may develop slowly (over 30–40 years). More than 30 million US adults or one in seven Americans are estimated to have CKD, and most are undiagnosed (Centers for Disease Control and Prevention [CDC], 2017). Not all patients with a decreased eGFR or albuminuria will progress to end-stage renal disease (ESRD). Early detection and intervention can help delay the progression of the disease.

WHAT IS THE COURSE OF CHRONIC KIDNEY DISEASE?

Progressive and irreversible loss of kidney function occurs over many months or years. As the number of functioning nephrons decreases, each remaining unit must clear an increasing solute load. Eventually, the limit to the amount of solute that can be cleared is reached, and the concentration of solutes in the body fluids increases, resulting in azotemia and clinical uremia. Fortunately, the slow rate of progression allows the body to adapt to some extent. The symptoms may be relatively mild proportionate to the chemical abnormalities.

How Is Chronic Kidney Disease Staged?

Chronic kidney disease is staged according to the patient's level of kidney function or GFR. The GFR varies according to age, gender, and body size; it tends to decline with age and decreases before the onset of kidney failure. Staging of CKD facilitates the application of clinical practice guidelines, clinical performance measures, and quality improvements to manage the disease at each level and thus preserve the residual kidney function as long as possible.

Identifying the presence and stage of CKD in an individual is not a substitute for accurate assessment of the cause of kidney disease, extent of kidney damage, level of kidney function, comorbid conditions, complications of decreased kidney function, or risks of loss of kidney function or cardiovascular disease.

What Are the Stages of Chronic Kidney Disease?

Chronic kidney disease can be expressed in a series of stages from 1 to 5. In 2015, the number of US residents receiving treatment for stage 5 CKD was nearly 500,000, and well over 200,000 were living with a kidney transplant. The number of new cases in the same year was 124,111, representing a 7.5% increase during the same year reflecting the aging and growing US population (United States Renal Data System, 2015).

The stage 5 CKD population represents only a small proportion of the total CKD population. Patients with stage 1 to 4 CKD far outnumber those who require maintenance dialysis or transplantation. The CDC estimate that more than 30 million people have CKD. Ninety-six percent of those in early stages (1 and 2) are not aware they have CKD, and 48% of those in later stage CKD (stage 4) are not aware of the disease (National Kidney Foundation [NKF], 2017).

The NKF gives the following examples of potential etiologies of CKD: diabetes mellitus (types 1 [T1DM] and 2 [T2DM]), systemic lupus erythematosus (SLE), human immunodeficiency virus (HIV) nephropathy, hepatitis B or C, hypertension, infection, stones, multiple myeloma, antibodies, and cystic diseases.

The NKF recommends that all individuals be assessed to determine whether they are at an increased risk of developing CKD. The evaluation should include assessment of serum creatinine levels, proteinuria, and the urinary sediment or a urine dipstick for white or RBCs. However, the best indicator of the level of kidney function is an estimate of the GFR. Certain factors have been identified to increase the progression of CKD to kidney failure; these include inadequately controlled diabetes and hypertension and repeated episodes of acute kidney injury (AKI), especially in older adults. The recommendations from the NKF focus on stages and not on disease etiology or pathology. The ultimate goal is to improve outcomes by maximizing opportunities for prevention (Box 4.1).

What Places a Person at Risk of Developing Chronic Kidney Disease?

The NKF has identified older age, family history, and ethnic descent (African American, American Indian, Latino, Asian, or Pacific Islander) as factors that increase susceptibility to kidney disease (Fig. 4.5). High levels of proteinuria, hypertension, poor glycemic control in patients with diabetes, and smoking are factors that can accelerate the progression of kidney disease. The most common causes of kidney failure in the United States are shown in Fig. 4.6. In most individuals, early-stage CKD is usually asymptomatic, necessitating blood and urine testing for diagnosis.

Early detection of proteinuria, a sensitive marker of kidney damage, allows timelier introduction of therapy to slow the progression of the disease. Early referral to a nephrologist, aggressive blood pressure control, and intensive blood glucose management in patients with diabetes may provide opportunities to delay the progression of CKD. Fig. 4.7 shows the risk of progression based on GFR and level or albumin creatinine ratio or level of proteinuria.

What Is the Goal of Treatment for Chronic Kidney Disease?

Not all patients progress through the stages in the same timeframe, but the goal is to delay the progression of the disease. Modifiable risk factors include blood pressure and diabetic control, weight control, hypercholesterolemia, nonsteroidal antiinflammatory drug usage, and cigarette smoking. Key measures to consider are making sure the etiology has been identified, implementing the appropriate treatment measure for the stage of CKD, monitoring patient symptoms, screening

---

Box 4.1 Stages of Chronic Kidney Disease

Within this framework, KDOQI classified CKD into five stages, as follows:

- Stage 1: kidney damage with GFR $\geq$90 mL/min/1.73 m^2
- Stage 2: kidney damage with GFR 60–89 mL/min/1.73 m^2
- Stage 3a: GFR 45–59 mL/min/1.73 m^2
- Stage 3b: GFR 30–44 mL/min/1.73 m^2
- Stage 4: GFR 15–29 mL/min/1.73 m^2
- Stage 5: GFR <15 mL/min/1.73 m^2 or kidney failure treated by dialysis or transplantation

GFR, Glomerular filtration rate; *KDOQI*, Kidney Disease Outcomes Quality Initiative.
From Fink HA, Ishani A, Taylor BC, et al: Chronic kidney disease stages 1–3: screening, monitoring, and treatment. Comparative Effectiveness Review No. 37. (Prepared by the Minnesota Evidence-based Practice Center under Contract No. HHSA 290-2007-10064-I.) AHRQ Publication No. 11(12)-EHC075-EF. Rockville, MD, 2012, Agency for Healthcare Research and Quality. https://effectivehealthcare.ahrq.gov/sites/default/files/pdf/kidney-disease-medicine_research.pdf.

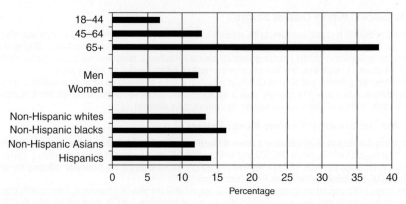

Fig. 4.5 Prevalence of chronic kidney disease (CKD) among US adults aged 18 years or older by sex and race or ethnicity.
- CKD is more common in people aged 65 years or older (38%) than in people aged 45 to 64 years (13%) or 18 to 44 years (7%).
- CKD is more common in women (15%) than men (12%).
- CKD is more common in non-Hispanic blacks (16%) than in non-Hispanic whites (13%) or non-Hispanic Asians (12%).
- About 14% of Hispanics have CKD.

(From Centers for Disease Control and Prevention: Chronic kidney disease in the United States, 2019. [n.d.]. Retrieved from https://www.cdc.gov/kidneydisease/publications-resources/2019-national-facts.html.)

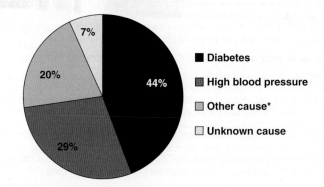

N=118,014 (all ages, 2014)
Source: US Renal Data System
*Includes glomerulonephritis and cystic kidney disease, among other causes.

Fig. 4.6 Primary causes of kidney failure. (Centers for Disease Control and Prevention. National Chronic Kidney Disease Fact Sheet, 2017. Atlanta, GA: US Department of Health and Human Services, Centers for Disease Control and Prevention; 2017.)

for complications, and educating the patient. As the GFR declines, the patient may experience the following complications: cardiovascular disease; imbalances of calcium, phosphorus, and vitamin D; hyperkalemia; metabolic acidosis; hypoalbuminemia; and hypertension. Symptoms may not emerge until a marked decline in GFR occurs.

WHAT IS MONITORED IN PATIENTS WITH CHRONIC KIDNEY DISEASE?

Patients with CKD stages 1 and 2 have minimal, if any, symptoms. The goals here are to control modifiable risk factors as mentioned earlier. The health care provider may monitor the GFR and level of albuminuria (Table 4.4). Patients with stages 3 and 4 CKD need to be monitored more closely for potential complications of a declining GFR. The patient at this time may be referred to a nephrologist to advise on measures to delay further progression and to monitor other complications of uremia when they surface. The nephrologist may evaluate for any medication dosage adjustments

				Persistent albuminuria categories: description and range		
				A1	**A2**	**A3**
				Normal to mildly increased	Moderately increased	Severely increased
				<30 mg/g <3 mg/mmol	30–300 mg/g 3–30 mg/mmol	>300 mg/g >30 mg/mmol
GFR categories (mL/min/ 1.73 m²): description and range	G1	Normal or high	≥90			
	G2	Mildly decreased	60-89			
	G3a	Mildly to moderately decreased	45-59			
	G3b	Moderately to severely decreased	30-44			
	G4	Severely decreased	15-29			
	G5	Kidney failure	<15			

Fig. 4.7 Risk of progression based on glomerular filtration rate and level or albumin creatinine ratio. *White* indicates low risk (if there are no other markers of kidney disease or no CKD); *Gray* indicates moderately increased risk; *Light blue* indicates high risk; and *Dark blue* indicates very high risk. (From Kidney Disease: Improving Global Outcomes CKD Work Group: KDIGO 2012 clinical practice guideline for the evaluation and management of chronic kidney disease. *Kidney International Supplements* 3(1):1–150, 2013.)

necessitated by a declining GFR, particularly for medications excreted by the kidneys. The nephrologist may make recommendations on diet (sodium, phosphorus, and protein restriction) as deemed appropriate for the patient. Mineral bone disease will be monitored and treated based on the patient's serum calcium, phosphorus, and PTH levels. Fibroblast growth factor (FGF-23) is a bone-derived hormone produced in response to hyperphosphatemia. FGF-23 works to decrease phosphorus levels by suppressing phosphate reabsorption in the tubules and decreasing the absorption of phosphorus from the intestines. FGF-23 has been associated with faster progression of CKD, cardiovascular disease, and premature death in patients with CKD, which underscores the need to maintain serum phosphorus levels as recommended by National Kidney Foundation-Dialysis Outcomes Quality Initiative (DOQI) guidelines of 2.7 to 4.6 mg/dL for CKD patients (Wolf, 2012). As GFR declines, treatment modality choices and dialysis access should be discussed. Fig. 4.8 shows a CKD monitoring algorithm.

WHAT IS END-STAGE RENAL DISEASE?

End-stage renal disease is the name formerly used for stage 5 CKD or when the patient requires maintenance dialysis for survival. In the course of CKD, renal insufficiency may often be managed for a considerable amount of time with diet, sodium restriction, phosphate control, blood pressure and blood glucose maintenance, and medication. As kidney function falls to 10% to 15% of normal, dialysis or transplantation becomes necessary for the patient to survive.

CHRONIC KIDNEY FAILURE AND CAUSES

Risk factors for CKD include diabetes, hypertension, obesity, and family history. Certain populations are at a greater risk for developing the disease:
- Women are more likely to be affected by CKD, but men are more likely to progress to ESRD.
- It is estimated 15% of Hispanics have CKD and are 35% more likely to progress to ESRD.
- Native American, Asians, and Pacific Islanders are more likely to develop CKD.
- African Americans are three times more likely to develop CKD than whites.
- Hispanics are 1.5 times more likely than non-Hispanics to develop ESRD.

Table 4.4 Preventing, Monitoring and Treatment of Chronic Kidney Disease Complications

TEST	RANGE OR GOAL	RELEVANCE AND ASSESSMENT
Urine albumin-to-creatinine ratio	Normal, 0–29 Albuminuria $\geq$30	Preferred measure for screening, assessing, and monitoring kidney damage and earliest sign of kidney disease. Elevation reflects risk for progression of CKD. May increase with strenuous exercise, fever, infection, dehydration, hyperglycemia, or congestive heart failure.
Blood pressure	<140/90 mm Hg	Control of blood pressure helps to delay progression of CKD and CVD. Most patients are prescribed an RAAS antagonist (i.e., ACE inhibitor or ARB). Serves as both renal and cardioprotective. May help to reduce albuminuria. Must monitor for hyperkalemia and enforce a low-sodium diet to increase effectiveness. Patients in stage 3 CKD are more likely to develop hypertension as the GFR declines.
Diabetes management	The ideal target HbA1c is ~7%, but this target is adjusted based on the needs of the patient.	Target HbA1c is adjusted based on the needs of the patient. The NKF KDOQI guidelines recommend (1) a target HbA1c of 7% to prevent or delay progression of the microvascular complications of diabetes, including CKD and (2) not treating patients with HbA1c <7% in patients at risk of hypoglycemia. We suggest that target HbA1c be extended to >7% in individuals with comorbidities or limited life expectancy and risk of hypoglycemia (NKF, 2012). Unintended improvement in HbA1c may indicate CKD progression.
Dietary management	Sodium Protein Phosphorus Potassium	Dietary guidelines are based on laboratory study results and physician recommendations. Dietitian consultation or referral as needed. Reduce sodium intake. Reduce protein intake if excessive to minimize stress on the kidneys. Reduce phosphorus and potassium intake if indicated.
CVD	LDL <100 mg/dL	Patients with CVD are at risk for CKD, and patients with CKD are at risk for CVD. Leading cause of mortality in CKD. They should follow a low-fat diet and increase physical activity.
Anemia	Normal hemoglobin, 11–12 g/dL	Monitor hemoglobin levels. Identify correctable causes of anemia. Oral iron supplements may be prescribed for mild iron deficiency. Patients in CKD stage 3 may begin to see a decrease in hemoglobin as GFR declines.
Mineral and bone disorder	Calcium Phosphorus PTH Vitamin D	Vitamin D may be reduced. Serum calcium may be reduced from decreased vitamin D. PTH may be elevated. Serum phosphorus may be increased or normal. May begin to see bone disease as early as stage 3 CKD.

ACE, Angiotensin-converting enzyme; *ARB,* angiotensin receptor blocker; *CKD,* chronic kidney disease; *CVD,* cardiovascular disease; *GFR,* glomerular filtration rate; *HbA1c,* hemoglobin A1c; *KDOQI,* Kidney Disease Outcomes Quality Initiative; *LDL,* low-density lipoprotein; *NKF,* National Kidney Foundation; *PTH,* parathyroid hormone; *RAAS,* renin–angiotensin–aldosterone system.

Modified from National Institutes of Health: *Making sense of CKD: a concise guide for managing chronic kidney disease in the primary care setting.* Washington, DC, 2014, National Institutes of Health and National Kidney Foundation: KDOQI Clinical Practice Guideline for Diabetes and CKD: 2012 update. *American Journal of Kidney Diseases* 60(5):850–886, 2012.

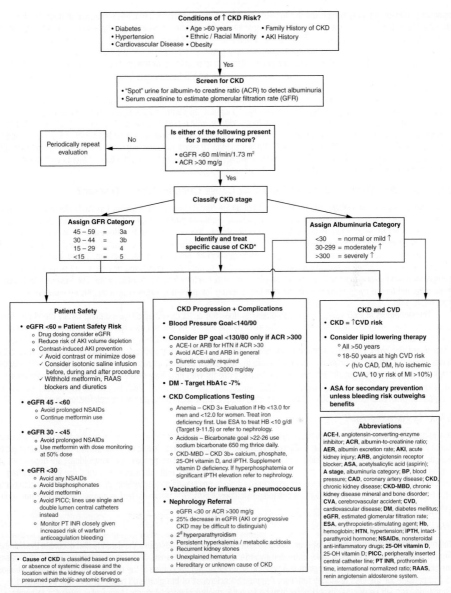

Fig. 4.8 How to manage your patients who have chronic kidney disease. (From National Kidney Foundation. Retrieved from https://www.kidney.org/sites/default/files/02-10-6800_ABG_PCPI_Algorithm2.pdf.)

WHAT ARE SOME GLOMERULAR CAUSES OF CHRONIC KIDNEY DISEASE?

Glomerular diseases damage the glomeruli and allow proteins and RBCs to leak into the urine. Glomerular diseases fall into two major categories: glomerulonephritis and glomerulosclerosis.

Glomerulonephritis is an inflammatory disease affecting the glomeruli of the kidney. It can either be a primary disease of the kidney or occur as a secondary complication of another disease, such as SLE, diabetes nephritis, or Goodpasture syndrome. The glomeruli become inflamed or damaged and allow RBCs and significant amounts of proteins to pass into the urine. Glomerulonephritis may be caused by streptococcal infection. The glomerular damage in streptococcal infection is not caused by the direct effects of the bacteria on the kidney but by the production of a large amount of antibodies that deposit in the glomeruli and cause the damage. As the immune system responds to infection, antigen–antibody complexes are formed. As these antigen–antibody complexes increase in number, they accumulate and block the glomeruli. The filtration capabilities of the glomeruli decline, and the affected individual begins to experience symptoms such as low serum albumin levels, hematuria, edema, hypertension, and decreased urine output.

Glomerulosclerosis describes the scarring or hardening of the blood vessels in the kidney. Systemic diseases such as lupus and diabetes mellitus cause the glomerular cells to produce scar tissue. The glomerular cells may produce growth factors that stimulate this scar tissue formation, or the growth factors may be transported to the glomerulus via circulating blood that enters the glomerulus.

Diabetic nephropathy can occur with both T1DM (insulin-dependent diabetes mellitus [IDDM]) and T2DM (non–insulin-dependent diabetes mellitus [NIDDM]). The glomerular basement membrane thickens with this nephropathy. Hyperglycemia increases the speed of blood flow to the kidney, which puts a strain on the glomeruli and elevates the intraglomerular blood pressure. As the glomeruli become damaged, their filtration capabilities become impaired. Diabetic nephropathy seldom develops in patients with T1DM of less than 10 years' duration and is more likely to occur in those with a disease tenure of 10 to 20 years. The treatment, complications, and specific care needs of patients with diabetic nephropathy are examined in Chapter 16.

ARE THERE ANY GENETIC DISEASES THAT CAN CAUSE CHRONIC KIDNEY DISEASE?

Polycystic kidney disease (PKD) is the most common of all life-threatening genetic diseases in the United States and may also lead to kidney failure. PKD demonstrates an autosomal dominant pattern of inheritance. This means that both sexes are equally likely to be affected. Because the gene is dominant, only one copy of the affected gene is needed for the disease to develop. Consequently, the likelihood of passing the affected gene to a son or daughter is one in two or 50%. PKD is a progressive disease that causes numerous cysts to develop anywhere along the nephron. These fluid-filled cysts replace the normal kidney tissue and begin to enlarge and compress the surrounding nephrons and renal vessels. The compressed renal tissue eventually becomes fibrotic and causes kidney function to deteriorate. The kidneys can become quite enlarged as the cysts grow in size and number, causing the patient to experience a significant increase in abdominal girth.

The symptoms of PKD vary among individuals, as does the onset of kidney disease among family members. Cyst development is seen in 50% of all affected individuals by the age of 18 years. Low back pain or flank pain is one of the most common symptoms of PKD. Urinary tract infections, hematuria, severe hypertension, and decreased kidney function are also seen. The cysts render the patient susceptible to infection because bacteria become imbedded around the cysts, making it difficult for antibiotics to penetrate to the kidneys or cysts. Nephrectomy may need to be performed when the kidneys become very painful or chronically infected. Patients with PKD may develop cysts elsewhere, such as in the ovaries, testes, pancreas, liver, or spleen. PKD can occur in both adults and children, but not all affected individuals progress to CKD. Approximately 50% of those affected require maintenance dialysis or transplantation while in their 60s.

WHAT IS AMYLOIDOSIS?

Amyloidosis is a disorder that causes the body's antibody-producing cells to produce abnormal protein fibers. These protein fibers join together and get deposited in various organs in the body. Elevated levels of these protein fibers accumulate in tissues and organs and may cause kidney failure when they accumulate. The symptoms of amyloidosis are dependent on the organ or body system affected. The heart, kidneys, nervous system, and gastrointestinal tract are the most often affected. The common symptoms of kidney amyloidosis include proteinuria and hypertension. Amyloidosis may also occur as a result of CKD and is known as dialysis-related amyloidosis (DRA). DRA may manifest as carpal tunnel syndrome, bone cysts, or pathological fractures.

WHAT IS NEPHROSCLEROSIS?

Nephrosclerosis is a term that translates as "hardening of the kidneys" and describes the damage that occurs to the kidneys from prolonged, severe hypertension. Untreated hypertension leads to sclerosis of the renal arterioles, which decreases the blood supply to nephrons. Some glomeruli become sclerotic during the course of the disease, resulting in hyperfiltration to compensate for the loss of kidney function. Progressive scleroses of the glomeruli occur as a result. Proteinuria, hematuria, and left ventricular hypertrophy may be found in nephrosclerosis patients. Aggressive attempts to control blood pressure are necessary to slow the decline of kidney function. Because hypertension is both a cause and complication of CKD, it is sometimes difficult to determine which came first.

WHAT ARE SOME INFECTIOUS CAUSES OF KIDNEY FAILURE?

Pyelonephritis is an infection of the kidney and renal pelvis. Bacteria spread most commonly by ascending from the lower urinary tract. Pyelonephritis usually does not progress to CKD unless there is an underlying urinary tract problem, for example, obstruction. Organisms that normally colonize the bowel, such as gram-negative bacilli and enterococci, are usually involved because they proliferate in the urine and then ascend to the kidneys. Kidney damage occurs as a result of the inflammation, fibrosis, and scarring caused by the infection.

Renal tuberculosis is an infection caused by *Mycobacterium tuberculosis.* The urinary tract is the second most common site for infection after the lungs. The kidneys become damaged by lesions that cause inflammation and caseation. The infection spreads throughout the kidney and destroys the kidney tissue. The kidneys become atrophied, scarred, and calcified.

Tuberculosis of the kidney usually occurs secondary to pulmonary disease. Renal tuberculosis may remain dormant for many years after pulmonary infection. The symptoms include increased urination, suprapubic pain, hematuria, and fever.

What Is Nephrotic Syndrome?

Nephrotic syndrome is not a specific kidney disease but a disorder that occurs when the glomeruli are damaged and protein leaks into the urine. Glomerulonephritis, diabetes mellitus, and lupus are examples of specific diseases that cause nephrotic syndrome. Other secondary conditions that may result in nephrotic syndrome include both viral and bacterial infections, such as streptococcal infection, mononucleosis, and hepatitis. Nephrotic syndrome depletes the volume of protein in the blood and thus causes fluids to shift into the tissues, resulting in edema. The loss of large volumes of protein into the urine also causes the urine to become very foamy. Treatment measures for nephrotic syndrome include decreasing the amount of salt in the diet to control edema, diuretics, cholesterol-reducing medication, blood thinners, and immune system–suppressing medications. Control of hypertension is very important.

Can a Person Develop Cancer of the Kidney?

Renal cell carcinoma or renal cell adenocarcinoma accounts for approximately 90% of renal malignancies. Renal cell carcinoma is found more frequently in men and has a high mortality rate when detected after metastasis. This disease usually affects only one kidney, although equal incidence is seen for both the right and left kidneys. Risk factors include tobacco use, analgesia abuse, and exposure to substances such as asbestos and cadmium. The tumor may arise in any part of the kidney and compress the kidney tissue, which inevitably causes tissue necrosis and diminished blood flow. Metastasis is often seen in the lungs, lymph nodes, liver, and bones. Patients most commonly exhibit hematuria followed by flank pain, weight loss, fever, and hypertension. A mass in the flank or abdomen is sometimes palpable.

What Is Renal Artery Stenosis?

Renal artery stenosis (RAS) is a condition that involves narrowing of the lumens of the arteries that supply blood to the kidneys. A major reduction in blood flow to the kidneys occurs, causing damage to the renal parenchyma. Decreased kidney perfusion leads to increased renin secretion, further damaging the kidneys. Atherosclerosis is the most common cause of RAS and significantly influences blood pressure and kidney function.

ACUTE KIDNEY INJURY AND CAUSES

How Is Acute Kidney Injury Defined?

Acute kidney injury is any sudden, severe impairment of kidney function. Onset is rapid, occurring over hours or a few days. Classically, oliguria (<400 mL of urine per 24 hours) is present. However, nearly half of the cases are of a nonoliguric variety, indicating that the patient's urine output is normal to near normal. Nonoliguric kidney failure is less fulminant and less difficult to manage than the oliguric form; dialysis is often not necessary. In 2004, an interdisciplinary group of nephrologists and critical care physicians formed to create the Acute Dialysis Quality Initiative (ADQI). Their goal was to achieve consensus on the definition of AKI and to propose uniform standards for diagnosing and staging AKI. The classification system defines three grades of increasing severity of AKI—risk, injury, and failure—and two outcome classes, loss and ESRD (represented by the acronym RIFLE [Risk, Injury, Failure, Loss, and End-Stage Renal Disease]). This system has been proposed for the classification of AKI in a number of clinical settings and is based on the changes in a patient's baseline serum creatinine levels, GFR, or urine output (Table 4.5).

Table 4.5 RIFLE Criteria for Acute Renal Failure Classification

	GFR CRITERIA	URINE OUTPUT CRITERIA
Risk	Serum Cr $>1.5\times$ of baseline	UO <0.5 mL/kg/hr $\times$ 6 hr
Injury	Serum Cr $>2\times$ of baseline	UO <0.5 mL/kg/hr for >12 hr
Failure	Serum Cr $>3\times$ of baseline *or* an increase of >0.5 mg/dL to a value of >4 mg/dL	UO <0.3 mL/kg/hr for >12 hr *or* Anuria >12 hr
Loss	Dialysis-dependent AKI >4 wk	
End-stage renal disease	Dialysis-dependent AKI >3 mo	

AKI, Acute kidney injury; *CR,* creatinine; *UO,* urine output.
RIFLE criteria for the diagnosis and classification of acute kidney injury (AKI). From Palevsky PM, Liu KD, Brophy PD, et al: KDOQI US Commentary on the 2012 KDIGO clinical practice guidelines for acute kidney injury. *American Journal of Kidney Diseases* 61(5): 649–672, 2013.

What Causes Acute Kidney Injury?

There are three categories of causes of AKI (also known as acute renal failure [ARF]): (1) prerenal, (2) intrarenal (intrinsic), and (3) postrenal (see Chapter 18, Box 18.1). These categories are identified on the basis of the location of the injury (Fig. 4.9).

Prerenal causes involve reduced blood flow to the kidney that is sufficient to impair function. The most common causes include low extracellular fluid volume (as in severe dehydration), heart failure, and blockage of the renal arteries. See Fig. 4.10 for additional causes of AKI.

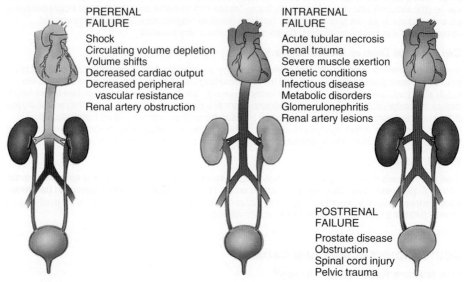

PRERENAL FAILURE

Shock
Circulating volume depletion
Volume shifts
Decreased cardiac output
Decreased peripheral
  vascular resistance
Renal artery obstruction

INTRARENAL FAILURE

Acute tubular necrosis
Renal trauma
Severe muscle exertion
Genetic conditions
Infectious disease
Metabolic disorders
Glomerulonephritis
Renal artery lesions

POSTRENAL FAILURE

Prostate disease
Obstruction
Spinal cord injury
Pelvic trauma

Fig. 4.9 Prerenal, intrarenal, and postrenal failure. (From Black JM, Hawks JH: *Medical-surgical nursing clinical management for positive outcomes,* ed. 8, St. Louis, 2009, Saunders.)

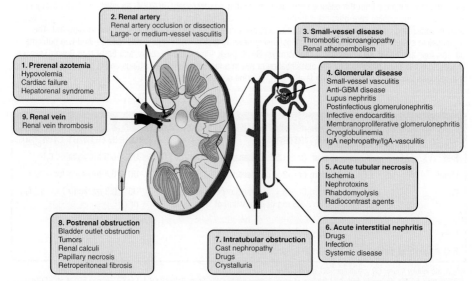

2. Renal artery
Renal artery occlusion or dissection
Large- or medium-vessel vasculitis

3. Small-vessel disease
Thrombotic microangiopathy
Renal atheroembolism

1. Prerenal azotemia
Hypovolemia
Cardiac failure
Hepatorenal syndrome

4. Glomerular disease
Small-vessel vasculitis
Anti-GBM disease
Lupus nephritis
Postinfectious glomerulonephritis
Infective endocarditis
Membranoproliferative glomerulonephritis
Cryoglobulinemia
IgA nephropathy/IgA-vasculitis

9. Renal vein
Renal vein thrombosis

5. Acute tubular necrosis
Ischemia
Nephrotoxins
Rhabdomyolysis
Radiocontrast agents

8. Postrenal obstruction
Bladder outlet obstruction
Tumors
Renal calculi
Papillary necrosis
Retroperitoneal fibrosis

7. Intratubular obstruction
Cast nephropathy
Drugs
Crystalluria

6. Acute interstitial nephritis
Drugs
Infection
Systemic disease

Fig. 4.10 Causes of acute kidney injury (AKI). AKI is classified into prerenal, renal, and postrenal causes. Renal causes of AKI should be considered under the different anatomic components of the kidney (vascular supply, glomerular, tubular, and interstitial disease). *GBM,* Glomerular basement membrane. (From Feehally J, Floege J, Tonelli M, Johnson RJ: *Comprehensive clinical nephrology,* Edinburgh, 2019, Elsevier.)

Postrenal causes involve blocked flow of urine leaving the kidney. The obstruction may be at the ureter, bladder, or urethral level.

Identification of prerenal and postrenal causes is important because they may often be corrected quickly, without causing residual damage to the kidneys.

Intrarenal AKI is caused by direct damage to the kidney tissue. This might occur during acute inflammation (rapidly progressive glomerulonephritis). Intrinsic AKI much more frequently results from severely compromised blood flow (hemorrhagic shock) or direct toxicity to kidney parenchymal cells; this may be caused by some antibiotics, myoglobin, or ethylene glycol. The result is acute tubular necrosis (ATN), which is the most common type of intrinsic AKI (Rahman, Fariha, & Smith, 2012). ATN is caused by injury to cells of the kidney tubules. Cell damage may be toxic (from chemicals or drugs) or ischemic (from severely reduced blood flow). Actual necrosis of cells does not always occur, but functional impairment is severe. Those most at risk for developing AKI are patients with underlying CKD. Older adults and those with diabetes are also at a greater risk of developing AKI because of undiagnosed reduced kidney function.

What Induces Acute Tubular Necrosis?

The most frequent causes of ATN include surgery, trauma, sepsis, cardiovascular collapse, and nephrotoxic injury. Multisystem failure with sepsis is a frequent cause of ATN and is associated with high mortality.

Nephrotoxins include hemoglobin (from hemolysis of RBCs) and myoglobin (from muscle breakdown or rhabdomyolysis) resulting from, for example, crush injury, heatstroke, and seizure. Many diagnostic and therapeutic agents, antibiotics (especially aminoglycosides), anesthetics, contrast media, cancer chemotherapy agents, and street drugs are toxic to the kidney in varying degrees.

What Is the Course of Acute Kidney Injury?

Acute renal failure from prerenal or postrenal causes reverses quickly when the precipitating factor is corrected. Most intrinsic kidney injury, or ATN, is recoverable. However, other effects of the injury or the medical or surgical catastrophe that precipitated kidney failure may continue. These, along with the complications of infection, sepsis, and hemorrhage, often have a very high mortality rate.

More information about AKI and its treatment can be found in Chapter 18.

CHAPTER 5

CLINICAL MANIFESTATIONS
OF CHRONIC KIDNEY DISEASE

The following features of a gradually developing uremic syndrome occur early: fatigue, impaired cognition, and pruritus. As all organ systems become involved, a broad complex of symptoms and findings evolves.

CARDIOVASCULAR SYSTEM

WHAT CARDIOVASCULAR ABNORMALITIES OCCUR WITH UREMIA?

Patients with chronic kidney disease (CKD) are a group of individuals at the highest risk of cardiovascular disease, and cardiovascular events are the major cause of death among dialysis patients. The risk of death from cardiovascular disease is 10 to 30 times higher in dialysis patients than in the general population. Adults with diabetes are two to four times more likely to die from heart disease than adults without diabetes (American Heart Association, 2018).

Hypertension is the most common cardiovascular complication seen in CKD and affects the majority of patients with CKD. More than 80% of patients with an estimated GFR (eGFR) less than 60 mL/min/1.73 m^2 have hypertension and uncontrolled hypertension predisposes a patient to end-stage kidney disease (ESKD) (Anderson & Agarwal, 2019). Hypertension causes CKD, and CKD causes hypertension, which can lead to other cardiovascular events such as heart attack and stroke. Some debate exists as to what the goal of the blood pressure should be in patients with CKD. Recommendations are based on stage of CKD as well as level of albuminuria.

Hypertension is associated with the progression of left ventricular hypertrophy (LVH), which places the patient at an increased risk of cardiovascular morbidity. Expanded extracellular fluid volume from fluid overload associated with sodium retention is the most prevalent cause. Many patients with CKD have increased plasma renin activity. Nephrectomy is an option to assist in the control of resistant hypertension but is rarely seen today with the current pharmacologic agents available for treatment.

Fluid volume and sodium regulation through diet, antihypertensive medications, and ultrafiltration help in the management of hypertension. Patients should be encouraged to exercise with their physician's approval, and they should be offered smoking cessation programs or literature.

Atherosclerosis is a major factor in morbidity and mortality. A defect in liver lipoprotein lipase is a possible cause of increased serum triglycerides. The risk of coronary artery disease, stroke, and peripheral arterial disease is increased.

Myocardial dysfunction presents as LVH resulting from hypertension, anemia, and atherosclerosis. With LVH, the left ventricle grows abnormally thick and interferes with the normal pumping action of the heart. The signs and symptoms of LVH depend on the cause but can include shortness of breath, chest pain, arrhythmias, dizziness, and congestive heart failure (CHF). The symptoms of LVH can be controlled or improved with the correction of hypertension and anemia, along with fluid volume control. Some patients experience no symptoms at all, but progression to cardiac failure is not unusual.

Coronary artery calcification may occur as a result of an imbalance in calcium phosphorus metabolism. Calcification of blood vessels, including the coronary arteries, which bring blood to the heart muscle, can place the patient at a risk of heart attack and stroke.

Congestive heart failure may be acute but is usually a chronic manifestation related to the retention of sodium and water. The symptoms of CHF include edema of the lower extremities, shortness of breath, and often fatigue, weakness, and an inability to perform physical activities. Weight gain from excess fluid is another common symptom.

Pericarditis is an acute or chronic inflammation of the pericardium and a cardiovascular complication seen in patients with CKD. Pericarditis may occur as a consequence of myocardial infarction or may be secondary to kidney injury (uremic pericarditis). The heart is surrounded by a double-membrane sac consisting of two layers of fibrous tissue. There is a small space between the two layers, which contains approximately 15 to 20 mL of fluid (Patton & Thibodeau, 2013). This pericardial fluid provides lubrication, allowing the layers of the pericardium to glide smoothly over one another during contraction of the heart without friction (Fig. 5.1). Uremic toxins, fluid overload, and bacterial or viral infections can all irritate the pericardial membrane, causing inflammation of the lining around the heart (the pericardium); this may trigger chest pain and fluid accumulation around the heart (pericardial effusion).

Patients often present with the classic triad of symptoms: chest pain, low-grade fever, and pericardial friction rub. Chest pain is intensified by deep inspiration, swallowing, and coughing and improves when sitting and leaning forward. Pericardial friction rub is harsh and leathery and heard best at the lower left sternal border during systole as the inflamed layers of the pericardial sac rub together. The friction rub is heard best when the patient is leaning forward. The pain often radiates to the shoulder, neck, back, and arms. Other symptoms include weakness, fatigue, increased white blood cell (WBC) count, and increased level of anxiety. Aggressive dialysis therapy (daily dialysis) with ultrafiltration to minimize uremic toxins and excess fluids is necessary. Heparin therapy during dialysis treatment is either decreased or withheld to minimize additional bleeding into the pericardial space. Antiinflammatory agents, both steroidal and nonsteroidal, may be prescribed to reduce inflammation and relieve pain.

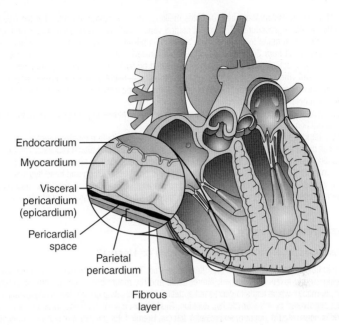

Endocardium
Myocardium
Visceral pericardium (epicardium)
Pericardial space
Parietal pericardium
Fibrous layer

Fig. 5.1 The pericardial sac is composed of two layers separated by a narrow fluid-filled space. The visceral pericardium (epicardium) is attached directly to the heart's surface, whereas the parietal pericardium forms the outer layer of the sac. (From Banasik J, Copstead-Kirkhorn LE: *Pathophysiology*, ed. 5, Philadelphia, 2014, Saunders.)

Pericardial effusion can develop when increased pericardial fluid, pus, or blood invades the pericardial space and interferes with the pumping action of the heart. Chest pain and elevated temperature will continue, but the pericardial friction rub may be absent on auscultation. Hypotension and shortness of breath may also be seen. The fluid is usually bloody; if the volume is large, tamponade may result.

Pericardial tamponade occurs when a large volume of fluid fills the pericardial space, compressing the cardiac muscle and heart chambers. Pericardial tamponade may have a slow or immediate onset and is associated with a high degree of mortality. Tamponade is a medical emergency and needs to be treated quickly. Treatment often includes removing the fluid in the pericardial space with a needle (pericardiocentesis). A pericardial window in which part of the pericardium is removed is sometimes necessary.

INTEGUMENTARY SYSTEM

WHAT INTEGUMENTARY CHANGES ARE SEEN WITH CHRONIC KIDNEY DISEASE?

The integumentary system is affected by the accumulated waste products associated with CKD. The skin is very dry, and patients complain of itching because of a decrease in the size and activity of the sweat and sebaceous glands. Brittle hair, nails, and skin are observed. Calcium may deposit in the skin, causing intractable pruritus, leading to excoriation of the skin from extreme itching. The skin color may appear tan-yellow or pale gray from the pallor of anemia coupled with the retention of urinary pigments called urochromes. Ecchymosis is commonly seen because of platelet dysfunction. Uremic frost refers to the whitish precipitates of urea crystals and salts that deposit on the skin, giving it a "frosty" appearance.

Uremic frost is a very late sign of CKD and is rarely seen today because most patients begin treatment in a timely manner. It is usually seen only in patients with advanced uremia that has been left untreated.

IMMUNE SYSTEM

WHY ARE INFECTIONS A PROBLEM?

Dialysis patients are at an increased risk of developing health care–associated infection. Bloodstream and other types of infections are a leading cause of death among hemodialysis patients. Data from the United States Renal Data System (USRDS) indicate that infections account for approximately 11% of all fatalities, with the majority resulting from septicemia (USRDS Annual Data Report, 2015).

Leukocyte abnormalities include a reduced WBC count in some patients. Granulocytes have a reduced response to infection and low bactericidal activity. In fact, infection is the second most common cause of death in dialyzed patients.

Susceptibility is enhanced by malnutrition, age, diabetes mellitus, immune system defects, and the frequency of cannulation and other invasive procedures. The use of central venous catheters is a major source of infection in dialysis patients, and efforts should be made to remove these as soon as possible and replace them with an internal vascular access such as a fistula. Data from 2014 indicate catheters (tunneled and nontunneled combined) were associated with 63% of bloodstream infections and 69.8% of access-related bloodstream infections in hemodialysis patients. Caution must be exercised when assessing body temperature because hypothermia is common, and responses to infection may not be accompanied by fever. Elevated uremic levels impair phagocytosis and suppress the inflammatory response as well as hypersensitivity reactions.

Urea has an antipyretic effect and causes subnormal body temperatures in patients. Poor nutrition plays a role in diminished WBC production.

Good nutrition, hand washing, and hygiene should be encouraged to help minimize infectious processes. It is recommended that all dialysis patients receive pneumococcal, influenza, and hepatitis B vaccines. The Centers for Disease Control and Prevention recommends that all dialysis care staff be assessed upon hire and annually at a minimum for competency in the following categories related to infection control practices: gloving and hand hygiene, catheter dressing change technique, vascular access technique, and safe injection and safe medication practices. Recommendations are also made to educate patients at least annually on proper hand hygiene and access care and assessment.

GASTROINTESTINAL SYSTEM

WHAT ARE SOME GASTROINTESTINAL MANIFESTATIONS OF UREMIA?

Patients with uremia have a poor appetite and are often nauseated. The nausea often diminishes after dialysis is initiated when the circulating uremic toxins are reduced. Altered taste and dry mouth are common. Patients often complain of a metallic taste in the mouth, which leads to decreased appetite. The circulating uremic toxins cause nausea and vomiting, which can also be aggravated by intradialytic hypotension. Gastrointestinal (GI) bleeding, which is often occult, is aggravated by medications (aspirin, heparin) and platelet defects. Uremic fetor, the smell of urine or ammonia on the breath from decomposing urea, is characteristic of patients with kidney disease. GI bleeding is seen from irritation of the GI mucosa resulting from the uremic environment and from capillary fragility as urea in the GI tract breaks down, releasing the irritant ammonia. Diarrhea may be seen from intestinal irritation or hyperkalemia.

Functional constipation is frequent in dialysis patients because of medications, fluid restrictions, a low-potassium and low-fiber diet, and decreased activity levels. Discretion must be used in the choice of laxatives because many products used to manage constipation contain magnesium, phosphorus, or potassium, all of which must be used in restricted amounts.

WHY IS PREVENTION OF CONSTIPATION IMPORTANT?

Because of a restricted diet (fruits and vegetables), limited fluid intake, and regular ingestion of phosphate binders (calcium based), patients with CKD tend to become constipated or develop fecal impactions. Functional constipation is more common in older dialysis patients. Such patients have a high incidence of diverticula of the colon. In addition, diverticulitis or perforation is not rare. Hematomas of the bowel and perforation caused by injudicious enemas have occurred. Cathartics and laxatives should be avoided. Stool softeners seem to work well, although they are often required in larger than usual doses. Patients should be encouraged to eat a high-fiber diet low in potassium and phosphorus, to adhere to a program of regular exercise, and to plan a regularly scheduled time for bowel movements to reduce the problem of constipation. Severe constipation may also cause hyperkalemia because stool potassium losses account for up to 40% of the total body potassium loss per day in dialysis patients (see Chapter 14).

ARE THERE ANY CONCERNS WITH THE ORAL CAVITY OR DENTITION?

Patients with CKD and those receiving maintenance dialysis are at a greater risk of periodontal disease and other oral cavity problems than the general population. Causes include restricted intake of fluids, leading to decreased salivary flow and dry mouth, a compromised immune system, diabetes mellitus, malnutrition, and impaired oral hygiene. All the oral manifestations predispose patients to oral infection, gingivitis, and periodontal disease. The inflammation caused by periodontitis can elevate C-reactive protein levels, increasing the risk of an atherosclerotic event.

It is important to include periodontal examination as part of the medical assessment and to ascertain whether the patient has access to dental care services. Dental health is important in patients with CKD both before and after transplantation. Patients who have received a transplant are at an increased risk for bacterial, viral, and fungal infections because of the suppressed immune system. Patients are often overwhelmed with their dialysis care and overlook their dental or oral health. The interdisciplinary team should activate the patient in his care and promote good oral health in the form of flossing, brushing, regular dental checkups, and evaluation and treatment of any oral cavity issues.

IS PEPTIC ULCER DISEASE COMMON IN DIALYSIS PATIENTS?

Some reports cite an increased incidence of peptic ulcer disease in dialysis patients; others do not. There are reports of higher than normal gastric acidity related to high blood levels of gastrin, which may be related to parathyroid overactivity.

Other studies indicate low gastric acidity related to increased urea and ammonia contents of gastric juices. The literature suggests that the incidence of ulcer disease in dialysis patients is about the same as that in the general nonuremic population.

DOES ASCITES OCCUR IN PATIENTS WITH CHRONIC KIDNEY DISEASE?

Ascites (massive fluid collection in the peritoneal cavity) is an infrequent problem that is very troublesome. Most cases are related to repeated fluid overload, poor nutrition, and cardiomyopathy. Although some patients overcome ascites, deterioration and death are frequent outcomes.

HEMATOLOGIC SYSTEM

WHAT ARE THE HEMATOLOGIC ABNORMALITIES?

Bleeding tendencies are seen as a result of a decrease in the quality and quantity of platelet production.

Anemia is the most common and severe hematologic defect. The hematocrit for men ranges from 46% to 52%; for women, this value ranges from 40% to 45%. People with uremia or those receiving maintenance dialysis are anemic and have considerably lower hematocrit values. Anemia from diminished erythropoietin secretion occurs and results in fatigue, pallor, shortness of breath, and chest pain. The hostile uremic environment decreases the survival of red blood cells (RBCs) from 120 to 70 days.

WHAT CAUSES ANEMIA?

The causes of anemia include (1) failure of production or inhibition of the action of erythropoietin, a hormone produced by the kidney that stimulates the bone marrow to produce RBCs; (2) a shortened life span of RBCs; (3) impaired intake of iron; (4) blood loss, including a tendency to bleed from the nose, gums, GI tract, uterus, or skin, caused by platelet abnormalities; (5) blood loss related to the dialysis procedure itself; (6) elevated levels of parathyroid hormone (PTH), which has a suppressive effect on erythropoiesis in the bone marrow; and (7) poor nutrition and diet.

HOW DOES DIALYSIS INFLUENCE ANEMIA?

Incomplete blood recovery after dialysis, dialyzer leaks, and frequent blood sampling contribute to anemia. A patient who is receiving adequate dialysis, is in a good nutritional state, and has adequate iron stores and intake usually stabilizes with a hematocrit between 20% and 30%. It is unusual for the hematocrit to go much higher except in people with polycystic kidney disease, in whom there may be a greater than normal production of erythropoietin. The measure of hemoglobin is most often used to detect, evaluate, and treat anemia in patients with CKD. The clinical practice recommendation from Kidney Disease Outcomes Quality Initiative (KDOQI) recommends in patients both on dialysis and nondialysis receiving erythropoiesis-stimulating agents (ESA) therapy to have a target hemoglobin in the range of 11.0 to 12.0 g/dL (National Kidney Foundation [NKF], 2007).

To minimize blood loss related to dialysis, particular care must be taken to (1) pretest dialyzers to prevent leaks, (2) monitor heparinization to prevent clotting, (3) return blood as completely as possible, (4) prevent damage to blood cells from incorrect pump occlusion or equipment malfunction, and (5) minimize the volume and number of blood samples drawn.

WHAT SYMPTOMS DOES ANEMIA PRODUCE IN PATIENTS WITH CHRONIC KIDNEY DISEASE?

In patients with CKD, anemia is usually present for many weeks or months, and patients become adjusted to it. As the hematocrit improves while patients are undergoing dialysis, they begin to feel better. These patients still have considerably fewer RBCs than normal and become dyspneic and tire easily. Other symptoms attributable to anemia include poor exercise tolerance, weakness, headaches, sexual dysfunction, anorexia, shortness of breath, chest pain, dizziness, pale skin, and inability to think clearly.

MUSCULOSKELETAL SYSTEM

HOW DO THE KIDNEYS KEEP THE BONES HEALTHY?

The kidneys keep the bones healthy by balancing the amount of calcium and phosphorus in the blood. Healthy kidneys produce a hormone called calcitriol, which enables the body to absorb calcium from the diet into the bloodstream. Vitamin D metabolism is profoundly impacted by all stages of CKD. Alterations begin as early as stage 3 CKD or earlier.

During the progression of kidney failure, the ability to excrete phosphate deteriorates. Phosphate ions accumulate in the body fluids and lead to a reciprocal decrease in serum calcium. The parathyroid glands seek to maintain a normal concentration of calcium in the body fluids and respond by increasing the production of PTH. This causes calcium to be resorbed from the bones, resulting in a loss of bone density and strength. In addition, the active form of vitamin D, which is needed for normal bone metabolism, is manufactured in the kidney and is deficient in patients with CKD. Dialysis does not fully correct disordered calcium–phosphorus metabolism, and progressive renal osteodystrophy (the term used for multiple bony manifestations) is a serious problem in many patients (Fig. 5.2). Dialysis patients have a higher incidence of hip fractures and bone loss. Calcium and phosphorus disorders, including renal osteodystrophy, vascular calcifications,

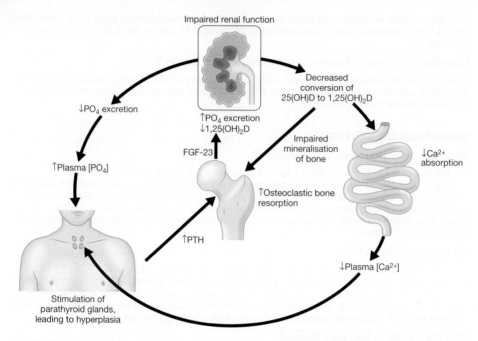

Fig. 5.2 Pathogenesis of renal osteodystrophy. *FGF,* Fibroblast growth factor; *PTH,* parathyroid hormone. (From Ralston SH, Penman ID, Strachan MW, Hobson RP: *Davidson's principles and practice of medicine,* ed. 23, Edinburgh, 2018, Elsevier.)

bone fractures, calciphylaxis, and even premature death, contribute to mortality and morbidity. Bone and mineral metabolism initiatives are common among dialysis providers to help manage this large clinical problem and include strict monitoring of the patient's laboratory values of calcium, phosphorus, and PTH. A coordinated interdisciplinary approach is required to help prevent bone disease and promote medication adherence in patients with CKD undergoing maintenance dialysis. Management of renal bone disease requires strict dietary control, adequate dialysis, and adherence to medication regimens, particularly with the use of phosphate binders with every meal and snack.

WHAT OTHER FACTORS ARE INVOLVED IN BONE DISORDERS?

Absorption of dietary calcium from the intestinal tract is decreased in CKD. There is resistance to the action of PTH, which normally enhances the resorption of calcium from bone. Chronic acidosis enhances calcium reabsorption from bones, further contributing to a loss of bone density. In addition, aluminum-containing phosphate-binding gels cause a form of renal bone disease. The aluminum in these gels is absorbed and deposited in bones, leading to a form of osteomalacia. Most of these aluminum-based binders are avoided.

WHAT ARE THE BONE CHANGES SEEN IN OSTEODYSTROPHY?

The bone changes seen in osteodystrophy include adynamic bone, osteomalacia, osteitis fibrosa, osteoporosis, osteosclerosis, and growth retardation (in children); metastatic calcification also occurs. Adynamic bone is a bone with little or no metabolic activity. Osteomalacia is deficient calcification of bones. Osteitis fibrosa is excessive destruction of bones by osteoclasts, with replacement by fibrous tissue. Osteoporosis is a deficiency of both the bone matrix and calcification, whereas osteosclerosis is an increase in bone density. The term *renal osteodystrophy* spans the totality of these various bone diseases in patients with uremia.

Metastatic calcification results when the product of serum calcium levels and phosphorus levels (measured in milligrams per deciliter) is 75 or greater. The 2003 KDOQI guidelines recommend maintenance of the calcium–phosphorus product at less than 55 mg^2/dL^2.

WHAT SYMPTOMS DOES OSTEODYSTROPHY CAUSE?

Many patients complain of sore, painful feet, back pain, and decreased mobility. Fractures, when they occur, are painful and heal poorly. Metastatic calcification causes precipitates to form in the soft tissues around joints. Itching may be intensified in the presence of a high calcium–phosphorus ratio. Skin ulcerations and gangrene of the tips of toes and fingers can occur. Aggravation of hypertension is frequent. Less apparent but more dangerous are diffuse deposits of calcium in the cardiac muscle and lung, which may lead to cardiovascular disease events. Cardiovascular morbidity and mortality can be predicted by the presence and severity of calcifications. CKD mineral bone disorders cause disability, decreased quality of life, increased hospitalizations, and death (NKF, 2007).

How Is Osteodystrophy Treated?

A priority system is necessary for the management of uremic osteodystrophy. The first objective is to maintain a low serum phosphorus level to prevent metastatic calcification and hyperparathyroidism. The serum phosphorus level depends on the intake, removal by dialysis, and binding of phosphate within the GI tract. Restriction of dietary protein intake also limits phosphate intake. A variety of agents are available to bind phosphate to prevent absorption from the GI tract. Agents containing aluminum should be avoided, and calcium-containing compounds should be used instead. Their activity depends on the surface area available for binding. The problem is determining the dose of phosphate binder that provides sufficient surface area throughout the day and is palatable enough for patient compliance. A periodic change in medication may make this more acceptable. Failure to bind phosphate adequately usually represents a failure of the patient to comply with the ordered phosphate binder regimen.

When serum phosphate is lowered to about 4 mg/dL and serum calcium is elevated to greater than 10 mg/dL, you will find a reduction in the parathyroid stimulation of osteoclasts that causes osteitis fibrosa. One must be cautious, however, to not reduce the PTH level too much. Adynamic bone disease occurs if the PTH level is decreased to normal. To help prevent secondary hyperparathyroidism for stage 5 CKD HD patients, the intact PTH concentrations should be 150 to 300 pg/mL according to KDOQI guidelines. Recent Kidney Disease Improving Global Outcomes (KDIGO) guidelines recommend maintaining PTH levels two- to ninefold the upper normal limit, which corresponds to a range of 130 to 600 pg/mL (Cozzolino, 2017). Elevation of serum calcium can be achieved in several ways. The usual concentration of diffusible calcium in dialysis fluids is well above that in the serum; thus, each dialysis provides a surge in calcium levels. Vitamin D may also be helpful in maintaining bone formation, apart from its role in the GI absorption of calcium. Finally, do not forget that alleviation of chronic acidosis of uremia is another objective of treatment. Some patients develop hypercalcemia on this regimen and require a lower calcium level in the dialysis bath.

Even if the treatment is successful in maintaining a low serum phosphorus level and high serum calcium level, some patients may experience persistent problems of renal osteodystrophy. Those with bone pain are likely to have a component of adynamic bone or osteomalacia. Those with fractures and high alkaline phosphatase levels may suffer to a large extent from osteitis fibrosa. Persistence of renal osteodystrophy with x-ray film changes consistent with hyperparathyroidism, high PTH levels, and high alkaline phosphatase levels may warrant either a four-gland removal or subtotal parathyroidectomy. Bone biopsy may be considered for patients who need further assessment of the cause of clinical symptoms and biochemical abnormalities.

What Is Calciphylaxis?

Calciphylaxis is a rare but potentially life-threatening complication that may occur in patients with CKD undergoing maintenance dialysis. The causes of calciphylaxis are poorly understood, but this complication usually results from several comorbid factors. Hypercalcemia, hyperphosphatemia, and hyperparathyroidism all seem to be contributing factors in this condition.

When serum phosphorus and serum calcium levels become elevated simultaneously, insoluble calcium phosphate crystals develop. You will see this occur when the calcium–phosphorus product exceeds 70 mg/100 dL, although this level is not required for patients to develop calciphylaxis. These calcium phosphate crystals deposit in the soft tissues of the body, including the lungs, joints, heart valves, cornea, and skin. Soft tissue calcifications usually affect the trunk and lower extremities but can also occur in the breast, thigh, abdomen, shoulder, or buttocks. Calciphylaxis usually begins as painful, purplish skin lesions that later form nodules. These nodules ulcerate and finally form eschar with underlying tissue necrosis. Blood flow to the tissue is diminished, and the area eventually becomes necrotic. These lesions are difficult to heal and often become infected. Calciphylaxis is associated with a high mortality rate, after ulcerations develop, with death usually occurring from sepsis from infected wounds or skin lesions. Treatment measures include hyperbaric therapy, debridement, wound care, and antibiotic therapy. Sodium thiosulfate (STS) given intravenously may be used as a chelation agent and treatment option. Other treatment measures revolve around lowering of the serum calcium and phosphate levels. Prompt identification and treatment of this condition may help to diminish the morbidity and mortality associated with this disease.

What Joint Disorders Occur as a Result of Chronic Kidney Disease?

Uric acid levels are frequently elevated in patients with CKD. Hyperuricemia may be associated with a goutlike involvement of one or more joints. Occasionally, there is a true gouty attack, but most episodes are of pseudogout. Dialysis amyloidosis (DA) may also be seen in maintenance dialysis patients.

What Is Pseudogout?

Pseudogout is an acute inflammation, usually involving a single area at or near a joint. The back of the hand or wrist, finger joints, and shoulders are common locations. Pain comes on abruptly followed rapidly by tenderness, swelling, and limitation of motion. This lasts for 3 to 5 days or longer unless treated.

How Can Pseudogout Be Treated?

Colchicine or one of the nonsteroidal antiinflammatory agents often relieves distress in 24 to 36 hours.

ARE THERE RESIDUAL EFFECTS OF PSEUDOGOUT?

Soft tissue swelling may persist for several weeks. Areas of metastatic calcification at the site are sometimes seen on x-ray examination.

IS THERE ANY PREVENTIVE TREATMENT FOR PSEUDOGOUT?

Frequent dialyses usually keep the uric acid below serious levels. If a very high level of uric acid persists, use of allopurinol may be considered.

WHAT IS DIALYSIS AMYLOIDOSIS?

Amyloid is a peculiar form of protein that precipitates in various body tissues. There are many different kinds of amyloid, including amyloid composed of β_2-microglobulin that is unique to dialysis patients. This protein is normally excreted by the kidneys but is poorly dialyzed and therefore accumulates in the blood of patients with CKD. This protein then deposits in the joints and periarticular structures of the shoulders, hands, wrist, neck, and other areas, causing pain and limitations of motion. If progressive, DA can be extremely debilitating.

WHO IS SUSCEPTIBLE TO DIALYSIS AMYLOIDOSIS?

Patients undergoing dialysis for long periods (>3 years) are prone to DA. The majority of patients undergoing dialysis for more than 10 years have DA. Patients dialyzed with high-flux synthetic membranes are less likely to experience this complication.

WHAT IS CARPAL TUNNEL SYNDROME?

Carpal tunnel syndrome (CTS) in dialysis patients is the compression of the median nerve at the wrist by the carpal tunnel sheath, which has been thickened by the deposition of amyloid. CTS causes pain, numbness, and tingling of the thumb and first two digits. Pain medications, nonsteroidal antiinflammatory drugs, and deep therapeutic ultrasound may ease joint symptoms. Kidney transplantation usually causes rapid disappearance of symptoms.

NEUROLOGIC SYSTEM

WHAT NEUROLOGIC CHANGES OCCUR WITH UREMIA?

Fatigue, slow mental processes, anxiety, depression, and agitation are common with uremia. Seizures occur if azotemia increases rapidly. Sleep disturbances in the form of insomnia, restless leg movements, and sleep apnea are major concerns. Restless leg syndrome (RLS) causes the individual to have an uncontrollable urge to move the extremities in response to unpleasant sensations. The lower extremities are most often affected, and the discomfort usually occurs when the patient is at rest. Movement helps to alleviate the symptoms. Symptoms occur most often in the evening and begin to diminish in the early morning. The causes of RLS are not precisely defined but might be associated with anemia. Electroencephalographic (EEG) changes (increased slow-wave activity) occur and are related to an increased PTH level. The calcium and aluminum contents of the brain tissue are increased.

WHAT IS THE POTENTIAL FOR INSOMNIA IN THIS PATIENT POPULATION?

Inability to sleep or fitful sleeping during the usual hours of rest is a common problem among dialysis patients. Both physiologic and psychologic factors account for the insomnia experienced by patients with CKD. Often patients sleep throughout the dialysis procedure, and it may be that the need for sleep at other times is reduced. Other patients seem to have a pathological inability to rest soundly. Higher levels of stress, anxiety, and depression, as well as fluid and electrolyte, and acid–base changes are all associated risk factors for the presence of insomnia (Park & Ramar, 2017). Response to sedatives and tranquilizers is usually poor, and the risk of dependency is considerable. No adverse effects from the lack of sleep have been seen, and it is suspected that the problem is most often one of fitful or interrupted sleep, which is interpreted as "no sleep." Sleep apnea is more common in dialysis patients than in the general population. The reason for this is unclear, but formal sleep studies may be useful for selected patients.

WHAT IS DIALYSIS DEMENTIA?

Dialysis dementia is a rare syndrome, and it was first described in 1972. It may appear after a few months or after several years in patients who are seemingly adequately dialyzed and doing well. There is a peculiar complex of garbled speech, asymmetric muscle jerking, mental deterioration, and seizures, along with characteristic EEG changes. A number of studies have implicated aluminum accumulation as a cause, primarily from administered aluminum hydroxide. With the use of calcium-containing phosphate binders in place of aluminum hydroxide, this syndrome has largely disappeared. A number of factors may contribute to the cognitive changes seen in patients with CKD (Fig. 5.3). Screening for cognitive impairment, particularly in older adults, may be beneficial to identify a baseline and monitor for changes over time. An evaluation of patient safety, ability to perform activities of daily living, and compliance with treatment regimen will need follow-up and evaluation as symptoms persist.

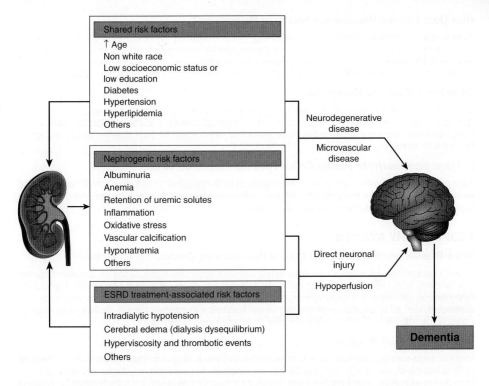

Fig. 5.3 Proposed mechanisms of chronic cognitive impairment in chronic kidney disease. *ESRD,* End-stage renal disease. (Modified from Kurella Tamura M, Yaffe K: Dementia and cognitive impairment in ESRD: diagnostic and therapeutic strategies. *Kidney International* 79(1):14–22, 2011.)

What Is Uremic Neuropathy?

Neuropathy indicates deterioration of nerve function. It may develop gradually as kidney failure progresses or may appear suddenly after infection or an episode of fluid overload. Peripheral neuropathy may present as burning feet, twitching, restless legs, reduced vibratory sensation, and decreased reflexes. Slowed nerve conduction velocity, which is present in most dialysis patients, contributes to the neuropathic symptoms. Motor neuropathy or myopathy may present as weakness of the proximal muscles of the arms and legs. Changes usually begin at the toes and progress upward. The upper extremities may be involved but less often than the lower extremities.

Is Neuropathy Common?

Neuropathy, in the subclinical or clinical form, has been reported in up to 80% of patients with CKD. It is often seen when dialysis begins, possibly because that is when a careful search is done. Clinically significant neuropathy is less common with earlier institution of dialysis.

Can Neuropathy Be Detected Before Symptoms Appear?

Nerve conduction velocity measurements are used to detect and quantitate the progression or improvement of neuropathy. Most patients with moderately advanced uremia have some delay in nerve conduction, often long before symptoms appear.

The test, although not difficult, is subject to many variables that make its reproducibility questionable and small changes difficult to evaluate. Another consideration is that this diagnostic evaluation is not always covered by the patient's insurance.

Is Neuropathy Relieved by Dialysis?

If dialysis is begun early, when only prolongation of the conduction time is demonstrable, frequent dialysis may prevent worsening. More severe nerve damage responds very slowly to dialysis. If the amount and frequency of dialysis are inadequate, neuropathy may develop or, if already present, will worsen.

How Does Dialysis Prescription Relate to Neuropathy?

When adequate dialysis is prescribed and delivered (Kt/V$_{urea}$[a] $\geq$ 1.2, with a protein catabolic rate of 1 g/kg/day), neuropathy is rarely seen. If it does develop, it strongly suggests that the patient is underdialyzed, and urea kinetic modeling should be performed to assess this. Even if the modeling parameters fall within an acceptable range, worsening neuropathy requires intensification of the dialysis procedure (larger dialyzer, more time, and higher blood and dialysate flow rates).

What Is the Cause of Neuropathy?

The cause of neuropathy is not known. The pathological changes in the nerves are similar to those seen in some cases of diabetes mellitus, in certain vitamin deficiency states, and in chronic alcoholism. A number of authorities believe that neuropathy results from accumulated medium- to large-size toxic metabolites in the body. However, specific toxic agents have not been identified.

Is There Involvement of Nerves Other Than the Peripheral Nerves?

A few patients develop deafness for which no other cause can be demonstrated. Other dialysis patients have developed gastric atony or bowel dysfunction resembling the autonomic disturbances seen in some individuals with diabetes. Impotence may also be related to uremic toxin accumulation.

RESPIRATORY SYSTEM

What Respiratory Problems Are Seen in Patients with Chronic Kidney Disease?

Pulmonary edema from excess fluid accumulation and left ventricular dysfunction may occur and are seen more frequently in patients with acute kidney injury. Dialysis and kidney transplant patients appear to be at a higher risk of developing tuberculosis, in part related to immunosuppression along with socioeconomic, demographic, and comorbid factors (Romanowski et al, 2016). Kussmaul respiration may be seen in patients with metabolic acidosis. The body compensates by increasing the rate and depth of respiration in an effort to excrete excess carbon dioxide.

What Is Metabolic Acidosis?

Metabolic acidosis is a condition that occurs when excess hydrogen ions build up in the blood. Initially, buffers in the blood combine with the excess hydrogen ions, and there are no symptoms. As the number of hydrogen ions increases, fewer buffers are available to bind with these ions. The pH of the blood then decreases, and patients respond physically to help eliminate the excess hydrogen ions. Under normal conditions, the kidneys would eliminate more hydrogen ions in the urine to compensate.

REPRODUCTIVE SYSTEM

Does Chronic Dialysis Contribute to Menstrual Dysfunction?

Women commonly experience cessation of menstruation as part of the uremic syndrome and by the time they require maintenance dialysis. It is uncommon but possible for a woman with ESRD to become pregnant. Fertility declines as the GFR declines, and many women are counseled against becoming pregnant. Although fertility issues are common for women with CKD, advancements in pregnancy care for patients on dialysis have made it more feasible and less of a risk (Tangren, Nadel, & Hladunewish, 2018). Most are amenorrheic or have oligomenorrhea of an anovulatory nature. Hypermenorrhagia may develop in some women after the initiation of dialysis, requiring treatment for the large blood losses. To prevent unnecessary (undesirable) blood loss, patients should be instructed to report any abnormal or excessive menstrual flow. Early detection of the problem may eliminate the need for surgical intervention.

A significant proportion of women receiving maintenance dialysis are troubled by galactorrhea. Endocrine studies suggest a defect at the hypothalamic–pituitary level such that the hormonal feedback mechanisms do not function normally.

What About Infertility?

Infertility is very common in both male and female patients on maintenance dialysis. Studies indicate poor sperm formation in most men. The exact mechanism is less clear in women, but, as indicated previously, is presumed to be endocrine in nature.

What Other Sexual Problems Have Been Associated with Chronic Dialysis?

Sexual dysfunction is a very real problem for most maintenance dialysis patients. Reduction of libido and impotence in men are common as uremia develops. Various sociologic and psychological studies, depending largely on questionnaire responses, have suggested that total or partial impotence is a problem in 60% of men receiving maintenance dialysis. However, another study suggests that 50% to 70% of the impotence among male dialysis patients has an organic basis,

---

[a]Kt/V$_{urea}$ is a way to measure the dialysis dose. The measurement takes into account the dialyzer efficiency (K), the treatment time (t), and the total volume of urea in the body (V$_{urea}$).

although it remains unknown whether this is neuropathic, endocrine, or vascular. In addition, medication (particularly antihypertensive agents) must always be considered as a potential cause of impotence. The reproductive problems described previously are often relieved after the correction of anemia with ESAs.

METABOLIC DISTURBANCES

Uremia is associated with abnormal metabolism of glucose, lipids, and protein.

How Does Chronic Kidney Disease Affect Glucose Metabolism?

Patients with CKD without diabetes have abnormal glucose metabolism. Cellular sensitivity to insulin is reduced. After a glucose load, the peak blood sugar is near normal, but the rate of decline is slow.

When stage 5 CKD is the result of type 1 diabetes mellitus, peripheral cellular resistance to insulin is especially severe. Violent swings between hypoglycemia and hyperglycemia are frequent. Total insulin needs decrease to some extent after the patient begins dialysis, but wide swings in blood glucose and problems with insulin dosage continue because of the decreased ability of the kidneys to metabolize insulin and the consequent increase in the half-life of insulin. A decrease in the filtration and excretion of glucose can lead to hyperglycemia with CKD requiring strict glycemic monitoring.

In the United States, most diabetic CKD cases are the result of type 2 diabetes. Such patients are usually obese and resistant to insulin. Most diabetic symptoms are improved by weight reduction and increased activity. Many patients respond to oral hypoglycemic agents.

Does Chronic Kidney Disease Affect Lipid Metabolism?

Type 4 hyperlipoproteinemia is common. The elevated very-low-density lipoproteins (VLDLs) are somewhat different from the normal VLDLs and may be a result of reduced hepatic lipoprotein lipase activity, possibly related to insulin resistance. Carnitine deficiency has also been suggested to play a role.

How Is Protein Metabolism Affected By Chronic Kidney Disease?

Protein calorie malnutrition is common. The loss of lean tissue mass is masked by an increase in body water with occult edema. Serum albumin levels tend to be low because of poor protein intake, although impaired hepatic synthesis may play a part. Several nonessential amino acids are elevated, and certain essential polypeptides are decreased.

What Other Endocrine Abnormalities Occur with Uremia?

Additional endocrine abnormalities include changes in insulin production and effects and PTH perturbations. Most other endocrine activities are also affected by uremia. These include the following:

- Plasma norepinephrine levels are increased; epinephrine levels are inconsistent.
- Cortisol levels are near normal, with a normal response to adrenocorticotropic hormone (ACTH). Aldosterone levels are increased.
- Both glucagon and gastrin values are elevated. This results from a loss of renal metabolic clearance.
- Hypothyroidism is more frequent in patients with CKD than in the general population. Euthyroid individuals on dialysis have low total thyroxine (T4) and triiodothyronine (T3) values and reduced free T3, but free T4 is normal. Conversion of T4 to T3 in peripheral tissue is reduced. Thyroid-binding globulin is low. Thyroid-stimulating hormone (TSH) is mostly normal, but the response to thyroid-releasing hormone is reduced.
- Besides ACTH and TSH, the anterior pituitary produces four other hormones that are affected by uremia. Growth hormone and prolactin levels are increased and poorly regulated. There are both increased production and decreased elimination. No systemic effect has been attributed to the elevation of either hormone.

Follicle-stimulating hormone (FSH) and luteinizing hormone (LH) play critical roles in the pituitary–gonadal axis in both sexes. The abnormal production of estrogen and progesterone or testosterone by the gonads in uremia adversely influences the feedback mechanisms to the pituitary gland. LH levels are elevated in both men and women. FSH values are normal or minimally increased in both sexes. The end effects include testicular atrophy, low sperm count, and impotence in men and dysmenorrhea or amenorrhea in women. Infertility is usual in both men and women. There is accumulating evidence that patients receiving ESA therapy have fewer sexual problems of this type. Much of these data are subjective. A number of objective studies support reductions in the levels of prolactin and growth hormone after administration of erythropoietin, but the mechanism is not clear. It is also unclear whether the effects that have been noted are the result of the correction of anemia or some specific effect of erythropoietin.

CHAPTER 6

DIALYZERS, DIALYSATE, AND DELIVERY SYSTEMS

The dialyzer is a selective filter for removing toxic or unwanted solutes from the blood. The filtration process uses a semipermeable membrane between the blood flowing on one side and the dialysis fluid, called the dialysate, flowing on the opposite side. The delivery system prepares a dialysate of the correct chemical composition and then delivers it at the proper temperature and other parameters to the dialyzer.

All dialyzers consist of a series of parallel flow paths designed to provide a large surface area between the blood and the membrane and between the membrane and the dialysate. There are two basic flow path geometries: (1) rectangular cross section, seen in parallel-plate dialyzers, and (2) circular cross section, seen in hollow-fiber dialyzers. Virtually all hemodialyzers in clinical use today are the hollow-fiber type; however, for historical purposes, the parallel-plate and coil dialyzers will be discussed.

COIL DIALYZERS

WHAT ARE THE CHARACTERISTICS OF COIL DIALYZERS?

Coil dialyzers consist of a cellulose acetate membrane tightly wrapped around a plastic or metal coil and encased in a rigid plastic housing. The coil dialyzer was the first type of dialyzer sold commercially and mass produced, and it is known as the dialyzer of the 1950s. The priming volume of the coil dialyzer was very large, ultrafiltration was unpredictable, and blood leaks were quite common.

PARALLEL-PLATE DIALYZERS

WHAT ARE THE CHARACTERISTICS OF PARALLEL-PLATE DIALYZERS?

Parallel-plate dialyzers are assembled in layers, like a sandwich. Sheets of membrane are placed between supporting plates, which have ridges, grooves, or crosshatches to support the membrane and allow the flow of the dialysate along it. Blood flows through the sheets of the membrane. The contained volume of blood is small, and heparin requirements are also usually small. A disadvantage of parallel-plate dialyzers is that they are compliant. This means that the volume of blood that they hold increases as the transmembrane pressure (TMP) increases. Another disadvantage of parallel-plate dialyzers is that they are not well suited for reuse.

HOLLOW-FIBER DIALYZERS

The hollow-fiber artificial kidney (HFAK) is by far the most commonly used dialyzer. HFAKs are available in a wide variety of sizes and membranes.

WHAT SERVES AS THE SEMIPERMEABLE MEMBRANE IN THE HOLLOW-FIBER ARTIFICIAL KIDNEY?

Tiny hollow fibers of about 150 to 250 μm in diameter are used. Blood flows through these tens of thousands of hollow fibers. The fibers are formed from a variety of materials, both cellulosic and synthetic. The wall thickness may be as little as 7 μm, although some synthetics have wall thicknesses of 50 μm or more (Fig. 6.1).

WHAT ARE THE ADVANTAGES OF HOLLOW-FIBER DIALYZERS?

The contained blood volume is very low in relation to the dialyzer's surface area because of the dialyzer's flow geometry. Resistance to blood flow is low because of the large number of blood passages. Hollow-fiber dialyzers are not compliant; therefore, their shape or the volume they hold does not change under a high TMP. Ultrafiltration can be precisely controlled. They are well adapted to reuse, although dialyzer reprocessing is rarely used today.

WHAT ARE THE DISADVANTAGES OF HOLLOW-FIBER DIALYZERS?

Meticulous deaeration (removal of air or gas) of the fiber bundle is required before beginning a dialysis procedure. Otherwise, the fibers may air lock and not admit blood or cause clotting of the dialyzer after the treatment has been initiated. There may be uneven distribution of blood at the inflow header space, with reduced perfusion of some of the center fibers. Hollow-fiber dialyzers may be sterilized with ethylene oxide (ETO). Residual toxic products of ETO sterilization retained in the potting material of the headers can cause adverse patient reactions. Patients may require higher heparin doses to prevent the hollow fibers from clotting.

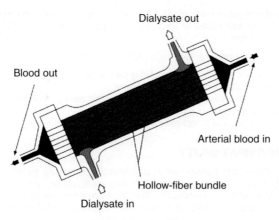

Fig. 6.1 Hollow-fiber dialyzer.

ARE THERE OTHER WAYS TO STERILIZE HOLLOW-FIBER DIALYZERS?

Yes. Some producers use gamma irradiation. Other manufacturers use steam sterilization. Both methods are effective. Electron beam, or e-beam, is a newer method of factory sterilization of hollow-fiber dialyzers. Electron-beam sterilization involves the use of high-energy electrons to process dialyzers. The DNA chains of the microorganisms become disrupted and are inactivated, which produces a sterile dialyzer. The electron beam does not use chemicals or radioactive materials during the sterilization process and may be a good alternative for patients who are sensitive to ETO.

MEMBRANES FOR HEMODIALYSIS

The membranes used in hemodialysis are of two basic types: (1) organic cellulose derivatives and (2) synthetic membranes.

Willem Kolff used cellulose sausage casings for the first successful clinical dialysis. Cellulosic membranes continue to be used in many dialyzers. Synthetic membranes were developed in the search of a membrane with increased permeability and decreased immunoreactivity. The development of volume-controlled ultrafiltration equipment for hemodialysis made the use of these high hydraulic permeability membranes practical. They in turn have made high-flux hemodialysis, hemofiltration, and continuous renal replacement therapy viable options in renal treatment.

WHAT IS THE NATURE OF A CELLULOSIC MEMBRANE?

Cellulose ($C_6H_{10}O_5$) is a complex carbohydrate polymer that forms the structural material of plants. Commercial cellulose is obtained from wood products and cotton. Treatment with heat and chemicals produces a thin liquid substance, which is coagulated and formed into sheets or pressed through dies or molds as hollow fibers. Different kinds of processing result in membranes of varying thicknesses, water-absorptive qualities, and permeabilities.

WHAT ACCOUNTS FOR THE PERMEABILITY OF CELLULOSIC MEMBRANES?

Electron microscopy shows that the fibers of cellulosic membranes swell when wet, forming a tortuous maze. The "pores" are actually twisting, irregular tunnels that force water or a solute molecule to travel a distance several times the thickness of the membrane to pass through.

WHAT ARE SOME CELLULOSIC MEMBRANES NOW USED IN HEMODIALYSIS?

Cuprophan has been widely used. The cellulose is treated with ammonia and copper oxide during manufacture; cuprammonium rayon and Hemophan are modifications. Saponified cellulose ester, cellulose acetate, and triacetate are other widely used cellulosic materials.

WHAT ARE THE ADVANTAGES AND DISADVANTAGES OF CELLULOSIC MEMBRANES?

One distinct advantage of cellulosic membranes is the fact that they have been used for many years, and therefore their transport characteristics are well known. They are also relatively inexpensive. However, all cellulosic membranes have some degree of bioincompatibility with blood. This poses a number of problems, which are discussed later in this chapter.

WHAT ARE THE FEATURES OF SYNTHETIC MEMBRANES?

Synthetic membranes are thermoplastics. They have a thin, smooth luminal surface supported by a spongelike wall structure. Those used for hemodialysis include polyacrylonitrile (PAN), polysulfone (PS), polyamide, and polymethyl methacrylate (PMMA), among others. Convective transfer accounts for their overall mass transport. Greater removal of medium- and large-sized molecules is observed with these membranes. All have ultrafiltration coefficients of 20 to 70 mL/hr/mm Hg or more. They are well adapted for reuse. Synthetic membranes have much fewer bioincompatibility problems than cellulosic membranes.

What Are the Negative Aspects of Synthetic Membranes?

Synthetic membranes have several negative aspects, including the following:
- They are expensive in comparison with cellulosic membranes.
- Automated ultrafiltration control is required because of the very high water permeability.
- Adsorption of proteins to the membrane surface can be a problem.
- The high permeability creates a risk of backfiltration from the dialysate to the blood.

MEMBRANE BIOCOMPATIBILITY

Each time blood comes in contact with a foreign surface, an inflammatory response is elicited. This response is used to gauge the biocompatibility of a hemodialysis membrane. When there are an intense reaction and a high level of inflammation, the membrane is said to be bioincompatible. When the response and inflammation are mild, the membrane is classified as biocompatible. The level of membrane biocompatibility may be associated with both short- and long-term consequences.

What Is Complement Activation?

The complement system is a series of plasma proteins that react sequentially to cause a variety of biological events. This system works with the immune system to defend the body from substances that the body determines to be "nonself." When blood encounters a hemodialysis membrane, the response elicited is similar to the one that occurs when the body's immune system is challenged by bacteria.

What Are Some of the Intradialytic Manifestations of Complement Activation?

The first clinical manifestation to be associated with complement activation is leukopenia. Immediately after starting hemodialysis using a cellulosic membrane, patients' white blood cell (WBC) or "leukocyte" counts drop sharply. This begins to correct after about 15 minutes. By the end of a 4-hour dialysis, the WBC count returns to the initial level or is perhaps slightly higher because of a compensatory response by the bone marrow. This leukopenia is transient but may be important in patients with compromised cardiac or pulmonary systems. C5a, an end product of the complement cascade, activates WBCs. When WBCs are activated, they become "sticky." These cells aggregate, or clump, and are sequestered in the first capillary bed they encounter, usually the lungs. The clumps of WBCs reduce pulmonary capillary perfusion and reduce the patient's ability to efficiently exchange oxygen and carbon dioxide between the blood and alveolar air. This may manifest as intradialytic hypoxemia. Other intradialytic problems possibly associated with complement activation include chest pain, back pain, coagulation abnormalities, low-grade systemic inflammation, and, in severe cases, anaphylaxis. Activation of complement peaks at 15 minutes and can last as long as 90 minutes. The amount of complement generated relates to the type and surface area of the membrane being used.

Which Membranes Induce the Highest Levels of Complement Activation?

Cellulose and cellulose-based membranes induce more complement activation than synthetic membranes (Table 6.1). The chemical composition of the cellulosic surface is similar to that of the cell wall of bacteria: both are chains of polysaccharide structures. The body responds to blood-cellulose contact in much the same way as it does to bacterial invasion. Free hydroxyl groups on the membrane surface are likely the primary source of the intense complement activation. Chemical alterations to buffer the free hydroxyl groups are used to create "modified cellulosic membranes," such as cellulose acetate and Hemophan. In cellulose acetate membranes, some of the surface hydroxyls are linked with acetyl groups. Hemophan membranes are buffered by amino groups attached to the reactive sites. Both these modifications reduce the amount of complement generated; however, these membranes are still less effective than synthetic membranes in minimizing complement production.

Why Do Synthetic Membranes Induce Less Complement Activation Than Cellulosic Membranes?

Being synthetic, these membranes lack the reactive sites found on cellulosic membranes; thus, the amount of complement activation generated during hemodialysis is less than that with cellulosic membranes.

What Are Some of the Long-Term Considerations When Selecting a Membrane for Hemodialysis?

Long-term use of bioincompatible membranes may be associated with an increased incidence of infection and malignancy and with impaired nutritional status. Patients dialyzed using cellulosic membranes have a higher incidence of β_2-amyloid disease (β_2AD) than those dialyzed using synthetic membranes; however, the occurrence of dialysis related amyloidosis has decreased with the more frequent use of high flux dialyzers (Nissenson & Fine, 2017). The increased risk of infection and malignancy is thought to be due to repeated attacks on the patient's immune system. When a patient's blood

Table 6.1 Dialysis Membrane Properties

MEMBRANE	MEMBRANE NAME (EXAMPLE)	HIGH OR LOW FLUX	BIOCOMPATIBILITY
Cellulose	Cuprophane	Low	Low
Semisynthetic Cellulose			
Cellulose diacetate	Cellulose acetate	High and low	Intermediate
Cellulose triacetate	Cellulose triacetate	High	Good
Diethylaminoethyl-substituted cellulose	Hemophane	High	Intermediate
Synthetic Polymers			
Polymethylmethacrylate	PMMA	High	Good
Polyacrylonitrile methacrylate copolymer	PAN	High	Good
Polyacrylonitrile methallyl sulfonate copolymer	PAN/AN-69	High	Good
Polyamide	Polyflux	High and low	Good
Polycarbonate-polyether	Gambrane	High	Good
Ethylene vinyl alcohol copolymer	EVAL	High	Good
Polysulfone	Polysulfone	High and low	Good

From Feehally J: Types of dialyzers. In *Comprehensive clinical nephrology*, ed. 6, St. Louis, 2018, Elsevier.

is repeatedly exposed to bioincompatible surfaces, the body responds as though under attack. The immune system kicks in, complement is generated, and the inflammatory response is triggered. There can be tissue damage, and future stimuli may elicit only a limited response, thus predisposing the individual to infection and potential malignancy.

Malnutrition is a major contributor to the morbidity and mortality of hemodialysis patients. Even with adequate protein intake, malnutrition is a problem and seems to relate to an accelerated catabolic process, most evident on dialysis days. A catabolic effect associated with bioincompatible membranes has been documented and may lead to systemic inflammation, leading to protein energy wasting (Ikizler & Deger, 2017). β_2AD is important in long-term morbidity. Clinical manifestations include arthropathies, bone lesions and pathological fractures, soft tissue swelling, and carpal tunnel syndrome.

DOES BIOCOMPATIBILITY OF THE MEMBRANE AFFECT PATIENTS WITH ACUTE RENAL FAILURE?

This is not clear. There is a consensus that the more compatible membranes do contribute to better recovery and survival. Less complement activation, less WBC activation, and less inflammation associated with more biocompatible membranes are believed to be responsible.

DIALYZER REUSE

Dialyzer reprocessing is the process of cleaning and sterilizing a previously used dialyzer for reuse in the same patient. "Reuse" refers to the clinical use of a reprocessed dialyzer. Dialyzer reuse was practiced safely and effectively for many years but is rarely used in the United States at this time. The United States Renal Data System no longer reports information on the number of dialysis centers performing reuse because it is performed so rarely. Dialyzer reuse is, however, practiced in other parts of the world, especially those with limited resources (accessed 2018). Strict standards must be followed to reprocess and reuse dialyzers; these standards are set by the Association for the Advancement of Medical Instrumentation (AAMI) Standards and Recommended Practices.

WHAT ARE THE ADVANTAGES OF REUSE?

Fundamentally, with reuse, the average cost per dialysis is substantially reduced. The "first-use syndrome," an infrequent phenomenon of chest or back pain, nausea, and malaise occurring in the first half hour of a run with a new cellulose dialyzer, is absent or rare with reused dialyzers. A decrease in the generation of biomedical waste is also an advantage of dialyzer reuse.

WHAT ARE THE DISADVANTAGES OF REUSE?

Processing, testing, identification, and storage of reused units require space and personnel time. Consumption of high-quality water is greatly increased. Sterilizing agents, particularly formaldehyde, are hazardous to personnel and patients. Quality control of manual processing is difficult to ensure. Automated systems minimize these problems but at a high initial cost. The risk of bacterial contamination to the patient and the potential for transmission of infectious agents are other disadvantages of dialyzer reuse.

Are There Guidelines for Reuse Procedures?

The guidelines for reuse procedures were defined by the AAMI and subsequently given the force of law by the US Food and Drug Administration. The Centers for Medicare & Medicaid Services Conditions for Coverage for End-Stage Renal Disease require facilities that practice dialyzer reuse to meet the AAMI guidelines for dialyzer reprocessing. (See Chapter 9 for more on the reuse of dialyzers.)

DELIVERY SYSTEMS

The delivery system prepares and delivers the dialysate to the dialyzer unit. Most systems provide the dialysate for a single patient; others have the capacity to supply several dialyzer stations simultaneously.

What Is the Solution Delivery System?

The Solution Delivery System is a method of delivering the solutions used for making the dialysate to the machine. Bicarbonate from a mixing tank and acid from a storage tank are transferred to an overhead holding tank called the "head" tank. The solutions are then gravity fed to a solution distribution system and then fed to the patient care area to be delivered through a series of pipes to the machines.

What Are the Functions of the Dialysate?

The dialysate carries away the waste materials and fluid removed from the blood by the dialysis procedure, prevents the removal of essential electrolytes while helping to normalize electrolyte levels, and averts excess water removal during the procedure. The dialysate also functions to correct the acid–base balance of the patient. These functions are achieved by making the chemical composition of the dialysate correspond as nearly as possible to that of normal plasma water.

What Chemicals Are Used?

There are usually five compounds involved in a dialysate: sodium chloride, sodium bicarbonate or sodium acetate, calcium chloride, potassium chloride, and magnesium chloride. Glucose may be included in some formulations.

How Are the Chemicals Made Into a Dialysate?

Manufacturers provide dialysis concentrates in containers of various sizes. The sodium chloride content is near saturation, and the other constituents are in proportion to their final concentration in the dialysate. Some equipment is present on site for making the concentrate from dry chemicals, which reduces transportation costs.

How Is the Bicarbonate-Based Dialysate Prepared?

Bicarbonate dialysate is prepared by mixing water prepared and treated by AAMI standards, with an acid concentrate and bicarbonate concentrate. Calcium and magnesium will not remain in solution with bicarbonate because of the low hydrogen ion content, and calcium carbonate has a tendency to precipitate when mixed with an acid concentrate. To solve this, two separate concentrates are used. The proportioning (delivery) system is more complex because it must mix and monitor three liquids instead of only two.

A variety of mixing and delivery systems are available for preparing concentrate for hemodialysis. Manual mixing is done in smaller dialysis units with few stations as well as in the acute care setting. Bicarbonate powder is added to a jug filled with processed water and mixed for use at an individual patient station. In larger scale dialysis units, large tanks of dialysate are prepared with an automated mixing device. Finally, refilled cartridges or bags containing the bicarbonate powder can be used directly on the dialysis machine (Desai, 2015). One such bicarbonate delivery is known as the "Bi*b*ag," a receptacle consisting of a disposable bag filled with bicarbonate powder. The Bi*b*ag is attached to the dialysis machine and mixes into a saturated solution. It is then proportioned to achieve the ordered prescription for the patient. This online delivery of bicarbonate provides a hygienic bicarbonate delivery and takes up less storage space for home hemodialysis patients (Fresenius Medical Care, 2014).

What Chemicals Are Present in the Bicarbonate Concentrates?

The "A" (indicating acidified) concentrate contains most of the sodium; all of the calcium, magnesium, and potassium; chloride; and a small amount of acetic acid to maintain the pH low enough to keep the calcium and magnesium in solution when mixed into the dialysate.

The "B" (bicarbonate) concentrate contains sodium bicarbonate. Some systems include part of the sodium chloride as well as the B concentrate; this increases the total conductivity, making it easier to monitor the concentrate. Table 6.2 shows the tabular formula used for a volume–volume type of dilution.

In the proportioning system, the B concentrate is usually diluted partially with water. A concentrate is then proportioned into the mixture just before it goes to the dialyzer. In the closed system, carbon dioxide cannot bubble off,

Table 6.2 Tabular Formula for a Volume-Volume Type of Dilution

COMPONENT	mEq/L in Final Dilution						
	Na^+	K^+	Ca^{++}	Mg^{++}	Cl^-	HCO_3^-	CH_3COO^-
Concentrate B	59				20	39	
Concentrate A	81	2	3.5	0.7	87.2		4
Final	140	2	3.5	0.7	107.2	35	

the reaction between sodium bicarbonate and acetic acid cannot proceed to completion, and the hydrogen ion content keeps the calcium in solution.

WHAT ARE THE POTENTIAL PROBLEMS WITH THE BICARBONATE DIALYSATE?

Liquid B concentrate is not stable; some manufacturers add a small amount of a special polymer as a stabilizer. Others provide dry sodium bicarbonate as a powder to be mixed at the facility. The mixing process requires care to ensure that much of the carbon dioxide formed during the procedure is not lost from solution; the concentrate must be used within 24 hours of mixing or per facility guidelines.

Bicarbonate concentrate is very susceptible to bacterial contamination and proliferation. The stabilized solution should be used within the manufacturer's designated timeframe. All containers for mixing, holding, or dispensing the B concentrate must be scrupulously sanitized at regular intervals. Contamination must be avoided. One manufacturer uses a delivery system that accepts a closed container of dry bicarbonate on a special holder. Warm water passes through the column, producing a saturated solution of bicarbonate that is proportioned with water and then with the A concentrate by a conductivity-controlled feedback system.

There are many formulations of the A concentrate to tailor the final dialysate sodium, potassium, calcium, and magnesium concentrations to the dialysis prescription. Each brand of delivery system has unique proportioning and mixing ratios. Extreme care must be exercised to ensure that the concentrates selected are correct for the delivery system being used.

WHAT HAPPENS IF THE BICARBONATE CONCENTRATE IS OVERMIXED?

Care must be taken so as not to overmix the bicarbonate concentrate because vigorous mixing may result in a loss of carbon dioxide from the solution. This will increase the pH of the solution and potentiate the precipitation of calcium and magnesium carbonate in the fluid pathway. This can cause the patient to experience a drop in serum calcium as the calcium level in the dialysate is lowered. A timer should be used to prevent overmixing of the dialysate concentrate.

WHAT KIND OF WATER IS USED TO PREPARE THE DIALYSATE?

The water used to prepare the dialysate must meet the AAMI standards for chemical content and for bacterial and pyrogen content. In most instances, this involves complex and expensive treatment of the feed water. Chapter 8 discusses the various processes involved in achieving "dialysis-quality water."

The current AAMI standards for the product water used to prepare the dialysate suggest that the microbial count must be lower than 100 colony-forming units (CFU)/mL and the endotoxin level must be less than 0.25 endotoxin units (EU)/mL, with respective action levels of 50 CFU/mL and 0.125 EU/mL (AAM/AAMI, 2008).

WHAT IS THE LIMULUS AMEBOCYTE LYSATE TEST?

The limulus amebocyte lysate (LAL) test is used to detect and quantify bacterial endotoxins. It is an assay for endotoxin that uses a protein extract from the *Limulus* or horseshoe crab. The result is reported in nanograms per milliliter or in endotoxin units (1 ng/mL = 5 EU/mL).

WHY IS DIALYSATE VERIFICATION AND MONITORING SO IMPORTANT?

Serious patient reactions and deaths have resulted from dialysate preparation errors or equipment malfunction. The dialysate must be verified for each dialysis. Each delivery system should have a function check daily.

WHAT METHODS ARE USED TO CHECK THE DIALYSATE COMPOSITION?

The most common test of the dialysate is total conductivity. This does not measure specific ions but the overall conductivity contributed by all ions (hence, it is a secondary test). Conductivity meters must be calibrated carefully to the "normal" or "safe" range for each type of concentrate used. If two or more dialysate formulas are used, the safe range for each must be clearly identified because each has a different ionic concentration. Most manufacturers indicate on the label of the concentrate containers the conductivity of their dialysate when it is properly mixed.

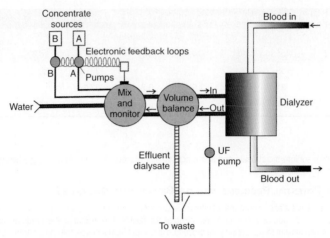

Fig. 6.2 Prototype of an electronic proportioning system for a bicarbonate dialysate with volumetric ultrafiltration (UF) control.

How Do Proportioning Systems Correctly Mix the Dialysate?

A liquid concentrate is required to correctly mix the dialysate. Several systems for mixing correct proportions of the concentrate and water have been used, but those most widely used use microprocessor circuitry to control the speed of the proportioning pumps for continuous conductivity and for monitoring other parameters downstream of the mixing area (Fig. 6.2). The speed of the pumps and thus the volumes of the concentrates added are precisely controlled by the electronic feedback circuit to ensure that the dialysis fluid is properly mixed.

What Are the Disadvantages of Proportioning Systems?

These very complex, highly sophisticated, microprocessor-controlled electronic and hydraulic devices are quite expensive. Many functions are preprogrammed and may not be readily changed. Sensors and monitoring devices must be fail-safe and redundant. Troubleshooting is often difficult, and factory-based service personnel may be needed for repairs.

How Is Dialysate Temperature Controlled?

The heater or heat exchanger is controlled by one or more sensors and a microcontroller circuit. Fluid temperature should be maintained within 0.5 °C of the set point. There should be a separate sensor, independent of the heat control, for online monitoring, with visual and audible alarms for any out-of-limit state. Accuracy should be checked regularly with a certified glass thermometer. Many chronic kidney disease patients have a core body temperature of 36° to 36.5 °C. Added heat in excess of replacement causes a vasodilatory response, which may be detrimental at a time when the normal vasoconstrictive response to the reduced volemia from ultrafiltration is acting to minimize hypotension. Fluid temperature greater than 41 °C causes hemolysis of red blood cells, which can continue for several hours. Additional information on hemolysis can be found in Chapter 13.

Why Are Deaeration Devices Necessary?

Water contains considerable amounts of dissolved air and microbubbles. When it is warmed, the dissolved air comes out of solution as expanding microbubbles. These have a negative effect on temperature and conductivity sensors and on flowmeters. Bubbles can reduce the dialysate–membrane contact in hollow-fiber dialyzers.

Most deaeration devices use warmers along with negative pressure to bring the dissolved gases out of solution. An air trap or coalescing filter then captures the gases and vents them to the outside.

What Problems Are Associated with Dialysate Flowmeters?

A solute film tends to build up with time and reduce accuracy. Calibration of the flowmeter or flow controller should be part of the routine servicing of the machine. At the bedside, actual flow can be quickly determined by a timed, measured outflow collection from the drain hose. Ultrafiltration control should be temporarily set to zero during the measurement.

What Is the Importance of the Dialysate Pressure Monitors?

Ultrafiltration is now controlled almost exclusively by volumetric or flowmetric controls. The dialysate pressure monitors serve as a check on ultrafiltration control and TMP. The manufacturer's directions must be followed carefully when adjusting and calibrating these monitors.

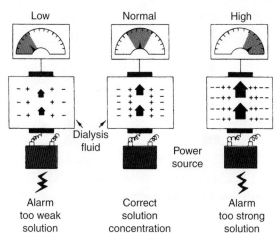

Fig. 6.3 Conductivity monitor.

How Is Dialysate Concentration Controlled and Monitored?

The most suitable apparatus to control and monitor dialysate concentration is the conductivity monitor (Fig. 6.3), which must be temperature compensated. Normal accuracy ranges from ±1% to 3%. The conductivity sensor is essentially an electrolytic cell, as described in Chapter 3. The electrodes of continually operating monitors are eroded by electrolytic action, with a gradual loss of sensitivity over time. Most delivery systems use at least dual conductivity sensors, the readings of which must match. A confirmation test with a handheld conductivity meter should be routine before the start of each patient treatment. If the conductivity is out of safe limits during the dialysis treatment, an alarm will sound, and the dialysate flow will stop. Before any adjustment of the conductivity monitors, a primary test, such as the laboratory measurement of sodium or chloride, should be done to verify the actual composition of the dialysate at the time.

Is Dialysate pH Monitored?

There should be some type of pH verification with an independent method before the start of each patient treatment. The approved AAMI pH range is 6.9 to 7.6. There should be audible and visual alarms for any out-of-limit state. Sensors for pH drift with the passage of time and must be recalibrated by the manufacturer's personnel.

How Is Blood Flow Rate Measured?

Blood is moved through the dialyzer by peristaltic rollers that work by progressively compressing special segments of blood tubing against a semicircular housing. Most blood pumps have speed indicators calibrated to show flow according to the speed of rotation. The internal diameter of the pumping segments of the tubing in use must match that for which the pump indicator has been calibrated. Variations in tubing, pressure conditions in the blood circuit, and a lack of linearity across the indicator scale cause discrepancies of ±10% to 15% between the indicated and actual blood flow.

  The calibration of each pump should be verified regularly under standard conditions, with the same brand and lot of tubing used clinically. Water at 37 °C should be pumped from a container through the tubing, which is partially clamped to approximate the negative pressure between the needle and the inflow side of the pump during dialysis. The outflow should be collected in a graduated cylinder for 3 to 5 minutes. The volume (milliliters) divided by time (minutes) gives the flow rate. A record of each calibration should be kept on the machine and in the central file.

How Do Blood Leak Detectors Work?

Blood should remain in the patient's bloodlines at all times and should not cross into the dialysate. Blood leak detectors are a safely feature of all dialysis machines to detect when blood has breached the dialyzer. Blood leak detectors are situated in the effluent dialysate line (Fig. 6.4). A beam of light is directed through a column of dialysate onto a photoelectric cell. A change in translucence and light scattered in the dialysate reduces the light received by the photocell, stopping the blood pump and activating visible and audible alarms. The AAMI recommends that blood leak detectors in the dialysis machine should activate an alarm if blood escapes through the membrane at a rate of 0.35 mL/min or more (AAMI, 2008).

  Particulate matter and air bubbles are frequent sources of false alarms. If a blood leak is not easily confirmed visually, the dialysate should be checked with an approved blood leak test strip. If standard maintenance procedures do not eliminate the problem, the manufacturer's representative should correct or replace the unit.

How Do Air Bubbles in Blood Detectors Behave?

Whenever a pump is used to propel blood through the extracorporeal circuit, some degree of negative pressure is created at the intake side. Air may be sucked into the line at connections that are not absolutely tight (such as at the needle hub),

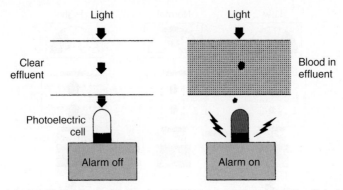

Fig. 6.4 Blood leak detector. (Modified from Nosé Y: *Manual on artificial organs*, vol. 1: *The artificial kidney,* St. Louis, 1969, Mosby.)

through needle punctures or breaks in the tubing, venous needle displacement, or from empty fluid containers attached at the infusion sidearm. These potential air sources are especially important because the pumping speed is increased in an effort to achieve high blood flow rates. Air in blood can obstruct the fibers of HFAKs and, if the quantity is sufficient, air may pass the venous bubble trap and cause a massive air embolism in the patient.

A commonly used detector employs an ultrasonic beam to identify air, foam, and microbubbles in blood (Fig. 6.5). The air detector is seated between the patient's venous limb and the dialyzer ensuring the return of blood to the patient is free of air. Sound travels more quickly through fluid than through air; thus, even minuscule bubbles slow the sonic beam and result in an alarm. Sonic detectors may be armed while the bloodlines contain only saline because they do not respond to light or light changes in the surrounding environment.

Most air and foam detectors have no external sensitivity adjustment. There should be a low-level alarm, clearly discernible from a distance, to indicate the disarmed status. No patient should be permitted to undergo dialysis with the air and foam detector in the disarmed state.

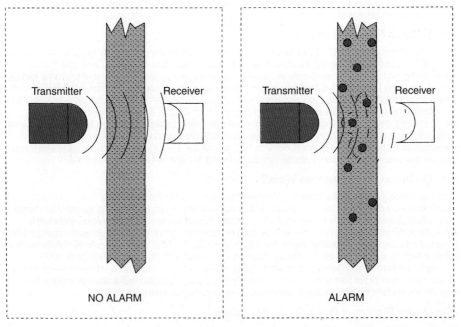

Fig. 6.5 Sonic air/foam detector.

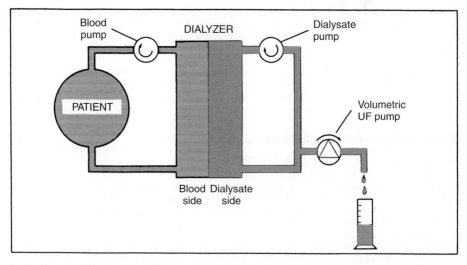

Fig. 6.6 Volumetric ultrafiltration (UF) control. (Redrawn from Vlchek DL: Staying tuned in to the high-tech world. Part II: dialysis delivery systems. *Dialysis Transplantation* 18, Aug 1989.)

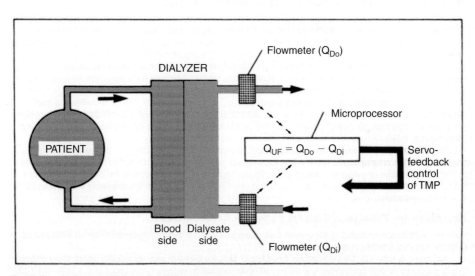

Fig. 6.7 Servo feedback ultrafiltration control. *TMP,* Transmembrane pressure. (Redrawn from Vlchek DL: Staying tuned in to the high-tech world. Part II: dialysis delivery systems. *Dialysis Transplantation* 18, Aug 1989.)

How Do Ultrafiltration Controls Work?

These devices exactly match the outflow dialysate volume with the inflow volume in addition to a precisely measured extra effluent volume representing the desired (programmed) ultrafiltrate. There are two basic types of ultrafiltration controllers: volumetric and flowmetric (Figs. 6.6 and 6.7).

How Do Volumetric Ultrafiltration Devices Operate?

The most common volumetric system uses two diaphragm chambers to balance the inflow and outflow dialysate. Although one side of the first chamber is being filled with fresh dialysate, its diaphragm is forcing out an equal volume of used fluid from the other side. Simultaneously, in the second chamber, one side is being filled with spent fluid from the dialyzer while the opposite side is ejecting an equal volume of fresh dialysate to the dialyzer. When the diaphragms have deflected across the width of the chambers, the valves are reversed so that the side that was emptying now gets filled and vice versa. The volume of ultrafiltrate is removed from the outflow dialysate channel by a metering pump before the outflow volume is matched to the inflow, thus removing the desired amount of ultrafiltrate from the patient. Because the volumes in and out of the controller are precisely equalized, whatever pressure (negative or positive) is necessary will be created for the removal of the measured ultrafiltrate volume by the dialyzer.

How Does the Flowmetric Ultrafiltrate Control System Work?

In a flowmetric system, there are one or two very accurate flowmeters in both the inflow and the outflow dialysate pathways to measure the flow of fluid passing through these pathways. The speed of the dialysate pump in the outflow path is varied by an electronic control module so that the volume through the outflow meter is exactly equal to the volume through the inflow meter plus the programmed amount of ultrafiltrate.

HIGH-EFFICIENCY AND HIGH-FLUX DIALYSIS

What Equipment is Needed for High-Efficiency Dialysis?

High-efficiency dialysis has the following four requirements:
- A highly permeable (high-efficiency) cellulosic membrane (e.g., ultrathin Cuprophan, Hemophan, cellulose acetate ester) or synthetic membrane with a surface area of $1.5\,m^2$ or more and a high mass transfer coefficient
- A reliable blood flow rate of 350 mL/min or more; a dialysate flow rate of 500 mL/min or more
- A bicarbonate dialysate delivery system
- An ultrafiltration control system
  The combination of a large area of membrane of high mass transfer capability with high blood flow rate and dialysate flow rate produces increased small molecule transfer. Intermediate- and large-sized solute transfer rates are enhanced by the increased area and permeability.

What Are the System Requirements for High-Flux Dialysis?

As with high-efficiency dialysis, in the high-flux system, it is important to maintain a high blood flow rate, high dialysate flow rate, and precision control of the ultrafiltration volume. High-flux dialyzers use synthetic membranes of very high permeability, with convective transfer providing a major share of solute transport (see Chapter 7). These dialyzers have ultrafiltration coefficients of 20 to 100 mL/hr/mm Hg or more. The ultrafiltration coefficient (K_{uf}) of a dialyzer expresses the volume of fluid transferred across the membrane. High-flux dialyzers have an ultrafiltration coefficient (K_{uf}) of more than 15 mL/hr/mm/Hg. The measure of a dialyzer's ability to clear solutes and urea in particular is referred to as coefficient of urea (KoA). The KoA represents the maximum clearance of the dialyzer in millimeters per minute for a given solute. The KoA is proportional to the surface area of the dialyzer membrane (Hoque & Fakir, 2011). You will see a much greater volume of urea clearance with these dialyzers. In addition to urea removal, high-flux membranes are more highly permeable to larger molecules such as vitamin B_{12} and $\beta2$ microglobulin and some medications such as vancomycin (Skorecki et al, 2016).

The ultrafiltration controller precisely manages net fluid removal. However, in doing so, it generates a dialysate pressure profile that creates reverse filtration from the dialysate to the blood in the distal portion of the dialyzer. A problem of blood contamination by pyrogenic material and endotoxin fragments is created because the high-flux membranes readily pass particles of 2000 to 10,000 Da. The LAL test (see Glossary and earlier in this chapter) is used to monitor the dialysate for endotoxins.

How Might the Problem of Reverse Filtration Be Countered?

Bacterial multiplication continues as the dialysis fluid courses through the dialyzer; pyrogenic materials increase and cross the high-flux membrane during backfiltration.

Addition of a molecular filter or ultrafilter (see Chapter 8) to the dialysate path immediately ahead of the dialyzer may be necessary for high-flux dialysis. A 50,000- to 100,000-Da ultrafilter will reject intact endotoxins; a 1000- to 10,000-Da ultrafilter will be necessary if endotoxin fragments are the problem. Some manufacturers have a provision for ultrafilters in their delivery systems. For an ultrapure dialysate, the bacterial count should be less than 0.1 CFU/mL, and the endotoxin level should be less than 0.03 EU/mL.

PRINCIPLES OF HEMODIALYSIS

CHAPTER 7

HISTORICAL BACKGROUND

Thomas Graham, a London chemist, reported the principles of the semipermeable membrane in 1861 and gave the process of selective diffusion the name *dialysis.* In 1913 Abel, Rowntree, and Turner devised an apparatus for the dialysis of blood using a number of collodion tubes through which blood flowed while a saline solution bathed the outsides of the tubes (Fig. 7.1). This device was used successfully to treat animals with uremia. Kolff and Berk later developed the first clinically successful artificial kidney but not before the introduction of heparin for anticoagulation and the availability of cellulose in the form of cellophane tubing. They used a rotating drum of wooden slats around which a spiral of cellophane tubing was wrapped. The lower portion of the drum was immersed in a bath of dialysis fluid while the blood was propelled along the tubing by rotating the drum. In 1948, Skeggs and Leonards designed a parallel-plate dialyzer; the first disposable dialyzer was the Travenol twin-coil unit, marketed in 1956. Gambro began the production of disposable parallel-plate devices around 1965, and hollow-fiber artificial kidneys were developed in the United States at the same time.

SOLUTE TRANSFER

WHAT DOES HEMODIALYSIS MEAN?

Hemo, of course, means blood. *Dialysis* connotes a separation or filtration process. Metabolic wastes or toxins are filtered from the blood by a semipermeable membrane and carried away by the dialysis fluid. The goals of hemodialysis are to manage uremia, fluid overload, waste products, and electrolyte imbalances that occur as a result of chronic kidney disease.

WHAT WASTE PRODUCTS ARE REMOVED BY DIALYSIS?

A large number of substances accumulate in uremia (see Chapter 4). The molecular size of many of these substances is less than 500 daltons (Da). A dalton is a unit of mass and is sometimes called atomic mass unit (amu). Particles with size less than 500 Da diffuse readily across cellulosic membranes. Particles in the range of 500 to 2000 Da, sometimes called middle molecules, diffuse poorly across such membranes. Polypeptides in this size range have been suspected of causing some uremic symptoms, although this has never been proven. Molecules larger than 3000 Da are not generally regarded as toxic, with the exception of β_2-microglobulin (11,800 Da) and its relation to amyloidosis, bone disease, and anemia. See Table 7.1 for the molecular weights of some common substances.

WHAT FACTORS AFFECT THE DIFFUSION OR REMOVAL OF TOXINS IN DIALYSIS?

- *Dialysate temperature:* The higher the temperature, the greater the solute removal.
- *Dialysate flow rate:* The greater the dialysate flow rate, the greater the removal of solutes.
- *Blood flow rate:* The greater the blood flow rate, the greater the removal of solutes.
- *Molecular weight of solutes:* The smaller the molecular weight, the greater the removal of solutes.
- *Concentration gradient:* The greater the concentration gradient, the greater the amount of diffusion.
- *Membrane permeability:* The more permeable the membrane, the greater the removal of solutes.

WHAT IS A SEMIPERMEABLE MEMBRANE?

A semipermeable membrane is a selective membrane that acts as a sieve. The semipermeable membrane used in dialysis allows the passage of some substances and fluid but not all. It may be thought of as having submicroscopic openings or pores. Solute particles larger than these openings cannot pass through and are retained. Particles small enough to pass through do so at a rate inverse to their size: very small particles traverse more rapidly than those somewhat larger.

HOW DOES THE SEMIPERMEABLE MEMBRANE FUNCTION IN HEMODIALYSIS?

The patient's blood is passed through a compartment formed by the semipermeable membrane. The dialysis fluid surrounds this compartment. Red blood cells (erythrocytes), white blood cells (leukocytes), platelets, and most plasma proteins are too large to pass through the pores of the semipermeable membrane. Water and small particles, such as electrolytes, cross by diffusion (Fig. 7.2), as do urea (60 Da), creatinine (113 Da), and glucose (184 Da).

WHAT IS DIFFUSION?

Diffusion, or conductive transport, may be defined as the movement of solutes from an area of higher solute concentration to an area of lower solute concentration. Molecules in solution are in constant motion and seek to spread uniformly throughout the solution. The rate of spread depends on the concentration, size, and electric charge of the particles. Diffusion of particles across a semipermeable membrane is the basis of dialysis. Diffusion occurs until equilibrium is reached (Fig. 7.3).

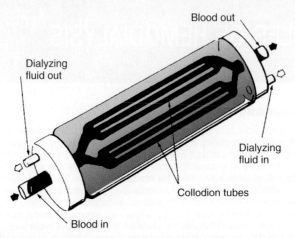

Fig. 7.1 Vividiffusion apparatus of Abel, Rowntree, and Turner. (Adapted from Nosé Y: *Manual on artificial organs,* vol. 1: *The artificial kidney,* St. Louis, 1969, Mosby.)

Table 7.1 Molecular Weights of Some Common Substances

SUBSTANCE	MOLECULAR WEIGHT (DA)	SUBSTANCE	MOLECULAR WEIGHT (DA)
Acetylsalicylic acid (aspirin)	180	Hemoglobin	68,800
Albumin	68,000	Insulin	5500
β_2-Microglobulin	11,600	Myoglobin	17,000
Cholesterol	386	Sodium	23
Creatinine	113	Urea	60
Dextrose	198	Vancomycin	1486
Glucose	180	Water	18

Modified from Hall JE: *Guyton and Hall: Textbook of medical physiology,* ed. 13 (pp. 335–346), Philadelphia, 2016, Elsevier.

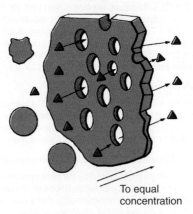

To equal concentration

Fig. 7.2 Semipermeable membrane.

WHY ARE ALL SOLUTES AND WATER IN BLOOD NOT REMOVED BY THE DIALYZER?

The dialysis fluid is an electrolyte solution similar in composition to normal plasma water. Water molecules cross the membrane in both directions, as do electrolytes and other small particles. Only if the concentration of a particular kind of particle is greater on one side than on the other will there be a net flow from the side of higher concentration to the side of

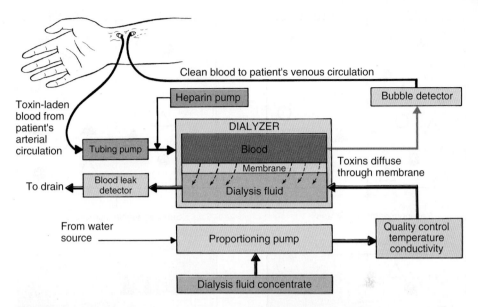

Fig. 7.3 Typical hemodialysis system. Toxin-laden blood from the patient diffuses across the membrane within the dialyzer into the dialysis fluid. Clean blood is returned to the patient. (From Black JM, Hawks JH, Keene AM: *Medical-surgical nursing: Clinical management for positive outcomes,* ed. 7, Philadelphia, 2005, Saunders.)

lower concentration. Solutes and waste products of a small molecular size diffuse from the blood side (high concentration) to the dialysate side (low concentration). This is the concentration gradient, which simply means a difference in concentration. A concentration gradient is necessary to accomplish solute removal in dialysis (Fig. 7.4).

ARE MEMBRANES PERMEABLE TO MEDIUM- AND LARGE-SIZED MOLECULES?

Several synthetic materials are used for high-flux dialysis. These include polyacrylonitrile (PAN), polycarbonate, polysulfone, polyamide, polymethyl methacrylate (PMMA), and other membrane materials.

WHAT IS MEANT BY MASS TRANSFER RATE OR SOLUTE FLUX?

Artificial kidneys, or dialyzers, are designed to remove metabolic wastes from the body, restore water and electrolyte balance, and correct acid–base disturbances. The dialysis process involves the transport of unwanted or excess solute and excess water from the blood across a semipermeable membrane. The engineering term for such transport is mass transfer, and the rate of movement is the mass transfer rate or solute flux.

WHAT FACTORS AFFECT THE MASS TRANSFER RATE?

At a constant temperature, flux is governed by the solute concentration gradient and the physical characteristics of the dialyzer. The latter include the effective membrane surface area, membrane permeability, blood and fluid flow rates, and flow geometry. The mass transfer rate varies continually throughout the course of a clinical dialysis procedure.

WHAT IS MEANT BY FLOW GEOMETRY?

Flow geometry refers to the direction of flow of the blood and dialysate. Countercurrent flow occurs when the blood and dialysate flow in opposite directions, creating an optimal concentration gradient. Concurrent flow occurs when the blood and dialysate both flow in the same direction, creating a much smaller and thus less desirable concentration gradient for dialysis to take place.

TRANSPORT

WHAT IS MEANT BY DIFFUSIVE TRANSPORT?

As noted, solute particles diffuse through the dialysis membrane from the side of higher concentration to the side of lower concentration. This movement is termed *diffusive transport* or, less commonly, *conductive transport.*

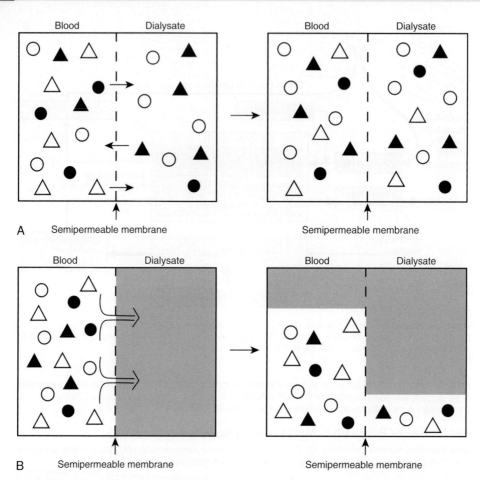

Fig. 7.4 Diffusion across a semipermeable membrane. Solutes with a higher concentration in the blood compartment (potassium is indicated by the *solid circle*, and uremic toxins are indicated by the *open triangle*) diffuse freely across the membrane because of the concentration gradient. Solutes with a similar concentration in both compartments (sodium chloride is indicated by the *open circles*) will have little movement across the membrane. (From Himmelfarb J, Ikizler TA: Chronic kidney disease, dialysis, and transplantation: A companion to Brenner and Rector's The Kidney, ed. 11, Philadelphia, 2019, Elsevier.)

WHAT DETERMINES THE RATE OF DIFFUSIVE TRANSPORT?

The rate of transfer depends on the following:
- The concentration gradient across the membrane for each solute
- The surface area of the membrane. The greater the area, the more solute moved per unit of time.
- The mass transfer coefficient for the solute of interest for the particular membrane. The mass transfer coefficient increases for thinner or more porous membranes. It is also affected by the flow rates of both the blood and dialysis fluid (Fig. 7.5).

WHAT IS THE SIEVING COEFFICIENT?

The amount of solute convected across a membrane in proportion to the quantity of ultrafiltrated fluid depends on the ratio of the pore size to the particle size. If the pore size to particle size ratio is high, there is no restriction on solute transfer, and the sieving coefficient is said to be 1. If none of the particles can be squeezed through, the sieving coefficient is zero.

WHAT IS CONVECTIVE TRANSPORT?

When water moves across a membrane because of a pressure gradient (ultrafiltration), there is a friction effect on solute molecules. Low-molecular-weight molecules or particles can be swept through the membrane along with the ultrafiltrate. This associated solute movement is termed *convective transport* (from the Latin word *convectus*, meaning "carried together") or solute drag.

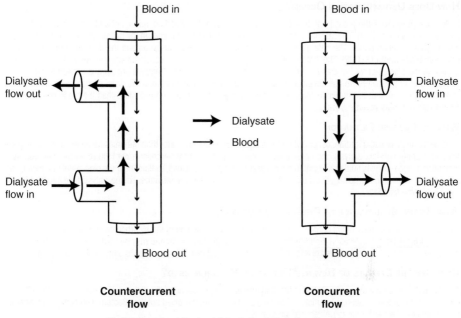

Fig. 7.5 Examples of blood and dialysate flow in the hollow-fiber dialyzer.

WHAT IS THE IMPORTANCE OF CONVECTIVE TRANSPORT?

Solute particles larger than 500 Da may have a low sieving coefficient; however, because of their low diffusive transport, the convective component becomes a major fraction of their total transfer. Convective transport is of prime importance in high-flux hemodialysis and in the techniques of continuous arteriovenous hemofiltration, hemodialysis, and diafiltration.

WHAT IS MEANT BY CLEARANCE?

Clearance is an empirical measure indicating a calculated volume of blood that is completely cleared of a substance in a given time. Clearance is expressed in milliliters per minute (mL/min). It is a theoretical, not a real, volume.

Controlled fluid removal at dialysis is essential. Ultrafiltration occurs in hemodialysis when the fluid is removed under pressure. Most current dialyzers use elements of both positive blood compartment pressure and negative fluid compartment pressure (Fig. 7.6).

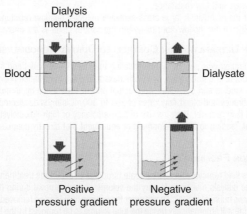

Fig. 7.6 Ultrafiltration.

How Does Ultrafiltration Occur?

Hydrostatic pressure is the pressure that forces plasma fluid out of the blood compartment and into the dialysate compartment of the dialyzer. The rate of fluid removal is influenced by the difference in the hydrostatic pressure of the blood and dialysate compartments. The difference in the hydrostatic pressure of the blood and the dialysate represents the transmembrane pressure (TMP). The TMP reflects both positive and negative pressures in the dialyzer. Positive pressure is applied to the blood side of the dialyzer, which pushes the plasma fluid out. Negative pressure is applied to the dialysate side of the dialyzer to pull the plasma fluid out of the blood compartment to the dialysate compartment. It is very important to ensure that the dialysate compartment never exerts a pressure more positive than the blood compartment. This is referred to as *reverse filtration.*

What Is Reverse Filtration?

Reverse filtration, or backfiltration, occurs when the dialysate pressure is greater than the pressure on the blood side of the dialyzer. During high-flux dialysis, the ultrafiltration control system prevents excessive net fluid removal. This process generates a blood-dialysis fluid profile within the dialyzer that is positive (blood-to-fluid) near the blood inlet but may, under some circumstances, become negative (fluid-to-blood) toward the outlet. The movement of the dialysis fluid into the blood is termed *reverse filtration.*

What Is the Significance of Reverse Filtration?

The water used in the preparation of the dialysis fluid is not sterile. Addition of the bicarbonate concentrate encourages and supports bacterial proliferation. Endotoxins and breakdown products form and may be carried across the high-flux membrane into the bloodstream when reverse filtration occurs. Pyrogen reactions as well as other adverse effects may occur.

How Can the Effects of Reverse Filtration Be Countered?

A molecular filter (ultrafilter) can be placed in the fluid delivery line just ahead of the dialyzer. This device uses ultrafiltration membranes to remove suspended particles of molecular size but not dissolved solutes. Bacteria and pyrogen or pyrogen fragments are rejected by the ultrafilter (see Chapter 8).

What Is the Relationship Between the Hydrostatic Pressure and the Ultrafiltration Rate?

For a particular dialyzer, at any given TMP, a certain amount of fluid will be removed per unit of time at specific blood and fluid flow rates. During the investigational phase of a new dialyzer, an average ultrafiltration rate per mm Hg TMP is calculated. This is the ultrafiltration coefficient (k_{UF}), and it is unique to each dialyzer. The k_{UF} is expressed as milliliters per hour (mL/hr) of fluid removed for each mm Hg. The higher the k_{UF}, the greater the amount of fluid that can be removed with less pressure applied to the semipermeable membrane. (See Chapter 13 for information on how to calculate the TMP for a patient treatment.)

What Affects Resistance in the Blood Circuit?

The two major components affecting resistance in the blood circuit are (1) the viscosity of the blood and (2) the geometry of the blood pathway.

Viscosity is largely a matter of hematocrit. The viscosity of blood at 30% hematocrit is approximately 2.3 to 2.5 centipoise, about 2 to 2.5 times that of water.

Several aspects are important to the geometry of the blood pathway:

- *Length of the pathway:* Hollow-fiber dialyzers have low resistance because of the short (15- to 50-cm) pathways.
- *Number of pathways:* With a large number of pathways, the divided resistance is lower. Hollow-fiber dialyzers have several thousand pathways and low resistance.
- *Cross-sectional area of the pathway:* A large cross-sectional pathway has low resistance; a small cross-sectional pathway has high resistance. For hollow-fiber dialyzers, the control factor is the internal radius of the fiber.

How Is the Amount of Ultrafiltration Controlled During Hemodialysis?

In the past, control of ultrafiltration was sought by manipulating the TMP. Blood outlet and fluid inlet pressures, which are critical variables in the control of ultrafiltration, are often inexact. The k_{UF} information provided by the manufacturer is most often based on in vitro studies and may differ from actual patient experience by as much as $\pm 30\%$. Even with conventional cellulosic membranes and blood flow rates of 200 to 300 mL/min, wide discrepancies may occur between planned and actual fluid removal. With the use of high-efficiency or high-flux dialysis, precision in ultrafiltration management became crucial, leading to the development of equipment that directly controls ultrafiltration on a minute-to-minute basis.

What Is Ultrafiltration Profiling?

Normal ultrafiltration provides fluid removal at a constant rate throughout the dialysis treatment. Ultrafiltration profiling is a technology available on some dialysis machines to vary the volume of fluid removal during the course of the dialysis treatment. Normally, the dialysis nurse or technician will enter the volume of fluid to be removed or the patient's goal for that dialysis treatment. The machine will automatically divide the total volume to be removed by the length of the treatment. With ultrafiltration profiling, fluid removal is varied according to the profile chosen. For example, if you are dialyzing a patient who routinely becomes hypotensive at the end of the treatment, the machine may be set to remove the greatest volume of fluid in the first half of the treatment, when most of the fluid is available to be removed. The rate of removal will then be decreased for the remainder of the treatment when there is less fluid available to refill the vascular space and the patient may avoid a hypotensive episode. Other profiles are available and can be selected according to the types of symptoms the patient experiences before, during, and after dialysis. All the profiles will remove the required total volume during the patient's treatment but at different intervals and rates, thus increasing treatment tolerance and decreasing the complications related to fluid removal.

WHAT SHIFTS OCCUR BETWEEN THE INTRACELLULAR AND EXTRACELLULAR FLUID COMPARTMENTS DURING HEMODIALYSIS?

The removal of accumulated body water from the patient is achieved with ultrafiltration. The ultrafiltrate from the circulating blood volume or vascular compartment is first removed, and the vascular compartment is then refilled with fluid from the extravascular compartment. When ultrafiltration occurs too rapidly, the rate of removal may exceed the repletion rate from the extravascular space, and hypovolemia and hypotension will occur. Inadequate refilling, that is, moving fluid from the tissues back into the vascular space during the dialysis treatment, is suspected to be a major cause of hemodialysis-related hypotension.

Infusion of hypertonic saline will increase osmolality in both the vascular and extravascular spaces. This in turn attracts fluid from the much larger intracellular pool and avoids the hypovolemia that causes low blood pressure.

WHAT IS SODIUM MODELING?

Sodium modeling or sodium variation is a tool that may be used to minimize some of the complications associated with hemodialysis treatment. The specific treatment complications that can be prevented with the use of this therapy are dialysis-associated hypotension and cramping. An understanding of how these complications occur is essential to understand this technology. As the hemodialysis patient is ultrafiltrated, the plasma fluid is removed from the intravascular space. With rapid dialysis, the intravascular space is depleted of fluid, and the "refill" from the extravascular space does not occur sufficiently quickly. When the plasma volume is depleted or decreased, hypotension results. Cramping in the extremities may occur because perfusion is also compromised by a decreased vascular volume. Hypoalbuminemia and right-sided heart failure may also contribute to delayed vascular refilling.

The sodium variation system helps maximize the refilling of the vascular space during ultrafiltration. This procedure involves the development of a computer model of sodium and water movement between compartments during dialysis. The sodium content of the dialysis fluid is varied during the procedure according to the preprogrammed plan. The sodium concentration of the dialysate being delivered to the dialyzer is increased to a level higher than the sodium concentration in the blood. The sodium in the dialysate is ramped up to approximately 150 to 160 mEq/L early in the course of the treatment and is ramped down over the course of the treatment to approximately 140 mEq/L. This may be done in either of two ways: (1) addition of a special sodium chloride (NaCl) concentrate to the dialysis fluid by an infusion pump or, more commonly, (2) varying the proportion of the usual concentrate as the treatment progresses, thus changing the final sodium concentration. For example, a commonly used proportioning yields a dialysis fluid sodium level of 140 mEq/L; a 10% increase in the amount of concentrate as it is mixed increases the final fluid sodium level to 154 mEq/L, with only minor quantitative changes in the concentrations of other electrolytes, such as potassium and calcium. The sodium level can be raised to as high as 160 mEq/L. The sodium level is slowly returned to normal by the end of the dialysis treatment with no adverse effects; however, attention must be paid to monitoring the development of postdialytic hypernatremia. The patient would complain of increased thirst or present with hypertension or increased interdialytic weight gain from intradialytic sodium loading. For this reason, the use of sodium modeling has been discouraged as a method to support intradialytic blood pressure and prevent other intradialytic complications associated with fluid removal. Other preventative measures or means of managing intradialytic symptoms such as lowering the dialysate temperature, holding blood pressure medications pretreatment, extending treatment times, or more frequent assessment of target weight should be considered.

OTHER TECHNOLOGIES CAN BE USED TO ASSIST IN OPTIMAL FLUID REMOVAL DURING DIALYSIS?

The Crit-Line Monitor (CLM) is a fluid management tool that can allow clinicians to safely and effectively ultrafiltrate patients to their appropriate ideal or dry weight. This technology allows monitoring of the patient's plasma refill rate. The patient's plasma refill rate can be compared with the ultrafiltration rate of the machine. If fluid removal or ultrafiltration is greater than the volume the patient can shift into the intravascular space, the clinician can intervene before the patient becomes hypovolemic or has a hypotensive episode. The clinician can also determine if the rate of fluid removal will help the patient achieve their dry weight for that treatment. The CLM noninvasively measures blood volume changes, oxygen saturation, and hematocrit. See Chapter 13 for additional information on the CLM.

HOW IS THE ACID–BASE BALANCE ACHIEVED DURING HEMODIALYSIS?

When continuous fluid proportioning systems were introduced in 1963, bicarbonate could not be used in the concentrate because it would cause the calcium and magnesium to precipitate. Sodium acetate, which the body metabolizes to bicarbonate, was substituted to avoid the precipitation problem. Acetate-based concentrates became the standard for many years. They had several disadvantages, particularly the effects of cardiovascular instability that commonly occurred during the dialysis treatment.

The introduction of short, rapid dialysis and high-flux dialysis made the return to bicarbonate-based fluids mandatory for these procedures. The bicarbonate dialysate is now the standard of practice at most facilities. One of the goals of hemodialysis is to correct the metabolic acidosis associated with kidney failure. The use of bicarbonate as a buffer during hemodialysis corrects acidosis by adding base and removing acid. During the dialysis treatment, bicarbonate is transferred from the dialysate to the blood. Diffusion of bicarbonate helps the patient to achieve the acid–base balance by buffering the hydrogen ions.

How Is Bicarbonate Used in Dialysis Fluid Production?

The concentrate to be used is packaged in two parts. The "acid concentrate" contains chemicals other than sodium bicarbonate, plus a small amount of acid. The "bicarbonate concentrate" contains sodium bicarbonate and some sodium chloride (necessary to increase the conductivity for monitoring purposes). Three streams of fluid are blended by the proportioning equipment, for example: water (34 parts), acid concentrate (1 part), and bicarbonate concentrate (1.8 parts).

Different types of equipment use concentrates of different compositions and different mixing proportions. Each proportioning ratio requires its own particular acid and bicarbonate concentrates. Use of an incorrect concentrate can lead to a dialysate preparation of the correct conductivity but incorrect composition. Accidental use of a mismatched concentrate is a potentially fatal error. The 2008 End-Stage Renal Disease Conditions for Coverage suggest restricting the use of all machines in a facility to one proportioning ratio. If different ratios are used in the same facility, the supplies for the different ratios must be segregated and labeled clearly to avoid mismatch. In addition, all staff should be aware and understand that there is more than one ratio in the facility.

CHAPTER 8

WATER TREATMENT

Water is a complex and incompletely understood chemical compound. The purest form of water is freshly formed rain as it leaves the clouds. This is also a very high-energy form of water. In the journey from the rain cloud to the final delivery tap, much of this energy is expended in acquiring various impurities as solutes or suspensions.

Improved dialysis technology has made high-purity water that is critical for dialysis fluid preparation a reality. The water used to prepare dialysate must be highly processed and continuously monitored to ensure patient safely. Organic materials or trace elements, even in small amounts, can be detrimental to a dialysis patient because of the massive exposure to dialysate. Fortunately, the science of water purification has made parallel advances. Enhanced membranes for reverse osmosis (RO), ultrafiltration (UF) devices to screen out endotoxins as well as bacteria, and improved monitoring systems are being applied in the renal community.

WHAT IMPURITIES MAY BE PRESENT IN TAP WATER?

Three categories of contaminating substances can cause patient injury or equipment malfunction: (1) chemical solutes, (2) bacteria or bacterial products, and (3) particulate matter. Of these, chemical and bacterial contaminants may be directly harmful to patients undergoing dialysis.

HOW DO IMPURITIES GET INTO WATER?

Falling rainwater passing through the air contacts carbon dioxide and sulfur dioxide, forming carbonic and sulfuric acid in a weak solution. Upon hitting the ground, this water encounters limestone and other minerals and forms calcium bicarbonate and sulfate, magnesium carbonate, and other salts. Other sources of contamination include pollution, surface water, particles leaching from the soil, rocks, and pesticides. Calcium carbonate is the most prevalent impurity in tap water and accounts for most of its hardness.

WHAT OTHER INORGANIC CHEMICALS MAY BE PRESENT IN TAP WATER?

Sodium, chloride, iron, aluminum, nitrate, manganese, copper, zinc, iodide, and fluoride are common ionic constituents. The types of minerals present in the geographic area and the time for which the water is in contact with them determine the content.

Trace elements that may be present include arsenic, silver, strontium, selenium, chromium, lead, cadmium, cyanide, barium, and tin, among others.

ARE THESE CHEMICALS HARMFUL?

Both acute and chronic problems may occur with exposure to water contaminants (Table 8.1). Nitrates and chloramines may cause methemoglobinemia, in which red cell hemoglobin cannot transport oxygen. Excess copper may cause hemolysis. Manganese can be toxic, and iron may possibly be toxic. Fluoride can contribute to cardiac abnormalities and is believed to aggravate uremic bone disease; it does accumulate in bone and is toxic to enzyme systems. Tin has been found in significantly higher quantities in the tissues of dialyzed uremic patients than in nonuremic individuals. Aluminum accumulates and is related to dialysis dementia syndrome, as well as to a form of anemia and osteodystrophy. Zinc causes gastrointestinal (GI) upset and may produce anemia. In areas of radioactivity, the presence of strontium-90 (^{90}Sr) may pose a danger.

ARE THERE OTHER MATERIALS IN TAP WATER?

Nonionic organic compounds, particularly nitrogenous matter such as proteins and polypeptides, phenols, indoles, and aldehydes, may be present. Solid particles of iron, sand, and silica are common. Suspended materials, including mud, algae, plankton, bacteria, viruses, pyrogenic matter, and dissolved gases (ammonia, carbon dioxide, and chlorine), are often present. The content of these materials as well as ionic impurities vary with the water source, season, and distribution system.

Some water supplies have identifiable amounts of pesticides or herbicides, such as chlordane, dichlorodiphenyltrichloroethane (DDT), aldrin, lindane, and 2,4,4'-trichlorobiphenyl.

Most water supplies contain various kinds of bacteria. Many are not detected by routine testing for coliform organisms. Such organisms include *Flavobacterium, Achromobacter, Serratia,* and *Pseudomonas* spp. and several atypical mycobacteria.

Table 8.1 Toxic Effects of Water Contaminants

TOXIC EFFECT OR SYMPTOM	CONTAMINANT
Anemia	Aluminum, chloramine, copper, zinc
Bone disease	Aluminum, fluoride
Hemolysis	Chloramine, copper, fluoride, nitrates
Hypertension	Calcium, magnesium, sodium
Hypotension	Bacteria, endotoxins, nitrate
Metabolic acidosis	Low pH, sulfate
Muscle weakness	Calcium, magnesium
Nausea and vomiting	Calcium, copper, low pH, magnesium, nitrate, sulfate, zinc
Neurologic changes (encephalopathy, headache, seizure, confusion)	Aluminum, sodium, zinc

IF THE WATER SUPPLY MEETS THE REQUIREMENTS OF THE SAFE DRINKING WATER ACT AND ENVIRONMENTAL PROTECTION AGENCY STANDARDS, IS IT SAFE FOR DIALYSIS?

No. Contaminants in the water used to make the dialysis fluid may enter the patient's bloodstream through the dialysis membrane. In addition, most dialysis procedures use bicarbonate as the buffer. Some delivery systems, in the bicarbonate mode, will not function properly if the pH is outside the range of 6.5 to 7.8. The pH of untreated tap water may be extremely acidic or extremely alkaline. It is essential for the water, dialysate, and equipment used for hemodialysis treatment to meet the quality standards found in the Association for the Advancement of Medical Instrumentation (AAMI) publication *Dialysate for Hemodialysis* (ANSI/AAMI RD52:2004). The standards for dialysis outlined by AAMI have been adopted as part of the Conditions for Coverage (CfCs), mandated by the Federal Regulations of the Centers for Medicare & Medicaid Services (CMS).

WHY IS SPECIAL WATER TREATMENT NECESSARY TO MAKE THE DIALYSIS FLUID?

During hemodialysis, the amount of water that contacts the patient's blood is more than 25 times the amount consumed by drinking. A hemodialysis patient is exposed to approximately 300 to 600 L of water depending on her or his dialysis prescription, and a patient on nocturnal dialysis is exposed to 590 to 860 L a week (Coulliette & Arduino, 2013). A substance present in water at a level of only one quarter of its upper limit of safety for drinking purposes may enter the body in 10 to 25 times the amount during hemodialysis. Ingested water is processed by the GI tract before reaching the bloodstream. This selective membrane can alter the rate at which foreign substances are absorbed from ingested water. In a dialysis system, the dialysis membrane cannot select ions to be absorbed or rejected, and these ions pass via diffusion. Substances that are harmless in drinking water may be toxic in water used for hemodialysis.

WHAT METHODS ARE USED TO TREAT WATER FOR USE IN HEMODIALYSIS?

- Filtration
- Activated carbon filters (adsorption)
- Water softeners
- RO
- Deionization (DI) (ion exchange)
- Ultraviolet (UV) light exposure

WHAT IS ACCOMPLISHED BY FILTRATION?

Suspended particles (mud, sand, rust, and algae) are removed by mechanical filtration through a wound filament or membrane cartridge or by tanks containing granular material that can be backflushed. These effectively filter particles down to about 5 mm in size. Submicron filters are available to screen out particles as small as 0.5 mm. The smaller the size of the filter, the more efficient it is in filtering substances.

WHAT TYPES OF FILTERS ARE USED?

The use of multimedia depth filters (i.e., sand filters) is a very economical and efficient way to remove suspended particles by filtering water through sand or coal. Cartridge filters remove particulate matter by filtering water through a very stiff or rigid device. An ultrafilter is a very thin and delicate filter that removes much smaller solutes, such as endotoxins. Ultrafilters are highly effective for the removal of fine particles, bacteria, endotoxins, and other pyrogenic matter, as well as high-molecular-weight organic molecules.

WHAT IS THE SILT DENSITY INDEX?

The silt density index (SDI) is an indicator of the colloid and suspended particulate matter present in tap water. The measuring device indicates the pressure drop over time as the tap water crosses a 0.45-mm membrane filter. The more suspended materials present, the slower the water passes. An SDI of less than 5 is optimal for the feed water for most RO systems.

WHAT IS THE ACTION OF THE CARBON TANK?

Chlorine and chloramines are standard treatment additives in most US municipal water treatment plants. Chlorine and chloramine are added to kill bacteria in water; however, they can also destroy red blood cells. The carbon tank contains granular activated carbon (GAC), which removes chlorine and chloramines from water by adsorption. Chlorine and chloramines are toxic to blood, and patient exposure to these organics can be extremely harmful. Carbon filters or tanks also remove organic matter and odor-producing materials by the same method. Adsorption is a physical process that does not involve a chemical reaction; it is simply the process by which liquids, gases, or suspended materials cling to a surface, such as activated carbon. The carbon tank will not remove electrolytes, such as calcium or sodium.

Two carbon tanks are required and should be plumbed in series, with water passing directly from the first tank (worker tank) into the second tank (polisher tank) (Fig. 8.1). A sample port should be present after each tank to test for chlorine and chloramines. The water immediately leaving the first tank should be sampled for chlorine and chloramines with an approved testing method. If the sample shows that the water coming out of the first tank contains chloramine in excess of the limit of 0.1 ppm, a second sample should be obtained from the water leaving the second tank. If the sample from the second testing port is within limits, operations can continue for 72 hours until a replacement bed is installed. Testing of the water should continue at an increased frequency to ensure that there is no further chlorine breakthrough. Dialysis treatments should be suspended if the sample from the second tank contains chlorine levels greater than the

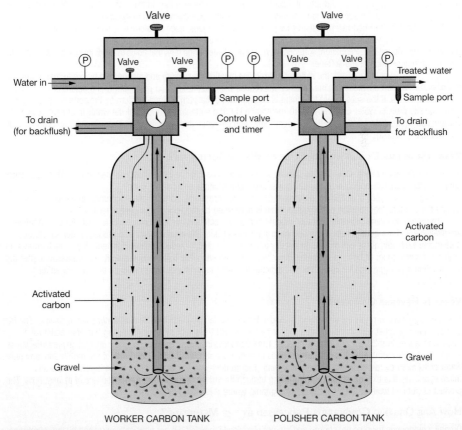

Fig. 8.1 Carbon tanks. (From Bieber S: Water treatment. In Nissenson AR, Fine RN, eds: *Handbook of dialysis therapy*, Philadelphia, 2017, Elsevier, pp. 123–143.)

allowable limit. Before testing, the water system should operate for a minimum of 15 minutes in the normal operating mode so that you have a sample that represents the current status of your water. You would not want to test a sample that has been exposed to the carbon bed for a prolonged period of time. The maximum allowable level for free chlorine is 0.5 mg/L (ppm), and the maximum allowable level for total chlorine (free chlorine + chloramine) is 0.1 mg/L (ppm). Chlorine and chloramine testing should be done at the beginning of each treatment day, before the beginning of each patient shift, or every 4 hours, whichever is shorter. Proper documentation of the results is critical. Empty bed contact time (EBCT) is the amount of time it takes for water to flow through the carbon tanks. The AAMI standard (RD62:2006) and End-Stage Renal Disease CfCs require an EBCT equal to or exceeding 10 minutes (minimum of 5 minutes of exposure in each tank).

The first tank (worker tank) removes virtually all of the chlorine, and the second tank (polisher tank) acts as a standby or backup in the event of failure of the first tank to effectively remove all of the chlorine and chloramines. The tanks must be backwashed nightly to redistribute the carbon and to expose more surface area for more effective adsorption. The polishing tank has a low flow through it and little chlorine present, making it a good location for bacterial growth. Rotating the polishing tank and the working tank will help minimize the growth of organisms and extend the life of the tanks.

There are two common types of carbon tanks: (1) portable exchange and (2) backwashable permanent tanks. Portable exchange tanks are "changed out" on a cycle developed by the facility. The vendor then replaces them with "new charcoal"–filled tanks. Permanent tanks are equipped with a control unit that allows them to be backwashed at the facility's discretion. The vendor or the facility replaces the carbon at intervals. If the carbon tanks are rebedded at the facility, care must be taken to follow the local waste management guidelines as well as the manufacturer's recommendations for personal protective equipment. Backwashing does not regenerate the carbon beds. Because carbon has a finite surface area, backwashing redistributes the carbon to expose any unused surface area.

What Is the Action of a Water Softener?

A water softener is a device located after the carbon tanks that exchanges ions in the water. Water hardness is caused primarily by calcium and magnesium ions. A water softener exchanges calcium and magnesium ions for sodium ions on a milliequivalent-for-milliequivalent basis. Other positively charged ions, such as aluminum, iron, and manganese, are also removed by the water softener. For each calcium ion removed, two sodium ions are added. The sodium is later removed by the RO system. Permanent softeners have a concentrated brine tank that holds the sodium chloride and controls the on-site regeneration of the softener.

If the feed water is very hard, the softener will remove most of the calcium and magnesium before further treatment. If a deionizer is used downstream, the softener will reduce the divalent ion load presented to the deionizer resin bed and prolong its life. If the subsequent treatment is RO, removal of calcium and magnesium by the softener may result in higher quality product water and a longer RO membrane life. If a softener is not part of the water treatment system, calcium could potentially build up on the RO membranes and decrease their effectiveness. Calcium build-up is sometimes referred to as "scaling."

What Problems Occur with the Use of Water Softeners?

If the raw water is very hard, considerable sodium is substituted in exchange for calcium and magnesium. Municipal water supplies often vary seasonally or even during a single day if multiple sources are used.

There are two types of softeners: portable exchange and permanent. Portable exchange units are provided ready for use by the vendor. Regeneration of the media resin is performed by the vendor at a central facility.

There are no online monitors that will indicate "hard" or "soft" water, but commercial test kits for total hardness are available and are quite reliable. The degree of hardness of both the source water and product water should be determined each day, at the end of a treatment day at a minimum, and recorded in a water softener log. Total hardness, in grains per gallon (gpg) or ppm, is measured after the water softener. The total hardness limit when measured after the water softener is 1 gpg or 17.2 ppm. This will indicate the need for a regeneration cycle, as well as any softener malfunction.

What Is Reverse Osmosis?

Reverse osmosis is currently the ultimate in UF and is the most effective method of treating water used in dialysis. The RO process removes most contaminants left in water by the pre-RO treatment systems, including bacterial endotoxins, metal ions, aqueous salts, and other contaminants. The RO process involves movement of water under high pressure across a semipermeable membrane. The dissolved solutes or contaminants collect on the feed side of the membrane, and pure water collects on the product side of the membrane. The product water is virtually free of dissolved solutes and microorganisms. It is expected that the water going through the membrane will have a rejection rate of at least 80%. The product or purified water is then sent to a holding tank, where it is stored before use.

How Are Organic Compounds Processed by the Membrane?

Organic compounds have no net charge and are not electrically repelled but are physically screened by the membrane. Almost all particles of a molecular weight greater than 200 Da are rejected. This includes bacteria, viruses, and pyrogens.

What Types of Membranes Are Used for Reverse Osmosis?

Membranes for RO use must be (1) freely permeable to water, (2) highly impermeable to solutes, and (3) able to tolerate very high operating pressures. Desirable characteristics include tolerance to a wide range of pH values and temperatures and resistance to attack by bacteria and chemicals such as chlorine.

Membranes in general use include (1) cellulose, (2) aromatic polyamide, (3) thin-film composites, and (4) high-flux, chlorine-resistant polysulfone.

1. Cellulose acetate membranes have high water permeability but poor rejection of low-molecular-weight contaminants. The range of pH tolerance is limited; the membranes degrade at temperatures greater than 35°C (95°F) and are vulnerable to bacteria. They are relatively inexpensive.
2. Polyamide membranes have a wide range of pH tolerance and are more resistant to bacterial action and hydrolysis than cellulosic membranes. They are very susceptible to degradation by free chlorine.
3. Thin-film composites are expensive. The supporting layer is usually a porous polysulfone. Fixed to this is a thin, dense, solute-rejecting surface film such as polyfurane cyanurate or a polyamide. Composite membranes have better water flux and better solute rejection than cellulose acetate. They are less subject to compaction and bacterial action.
4. Chlorine-resistant polysulfone membranes have a very long service life. They tolerate a wide range of pH values and temperatures. Water flux is high. They differ from other membranes in that if divalent ions are present in the feed water, rejection of monovalent ions is greatly reduced. Therefore, it is essential that the feed water be softened or deionized before entering the RO unit.

What Configuration of Reverse Osmosis Modules Is Used?

The module design must include features such as a large membrane surface area, tolerance for very high pressure (up to 500 psi), good flow characteristics, and a low pressure drop. The configurations in use for hemodialysis water include (1) the spiral-wound or spiral-wrap (Fig. 8.2) and (2) hollow-fiber modules.

Spiral-wound units consist of two layers of membrane with a fabric material fastened between them, like a sandwich. The fabric material is the product carrier. The membrane-sandwich sheet, along with a plastic mesh separator, is wrapped in a spiral around a central perforated tube in a manner somewhat similar to that of an old-style coil dialyzer. The feed water under high pressure enters one end of the unit and flows along the channels provided by the plastic mesh; some water is forced by the hydraulic pressure through the membrane. The central fabric conducts this filtered water to the central tube, from which it emerges as the product water.

In hollow-fiber units, the membrane is formed as capillary fibers with an inside diameter of 80 to 250 mm. Several thousand of these fibers are bundled inside a high-pressure cylinder. Pressurized feed water surrounds and permeates the hollow fibers, forming the product water inside the capillary lumina. The small internal diameter of the hollow fibers can contribute to plugging and reduced permeate flow.

What Are the Special Advantages of Reverse Osmosis Over Other Types of Water Treatment?

Reverse osmosis has several advantages, including the following:
- Bacteria, viruses, and pyrogenic materials are rejected by the intact membrane. In this respect, RO water approaches distilled water in quality.
- Available units are relatively compact and require little space. They are well suited for home dialysis.
- In terms of average use the membrane has a life of a little more than 1 to 5 years before replacement is necessary.
- Periodic complete disinfection of the RO system is required.

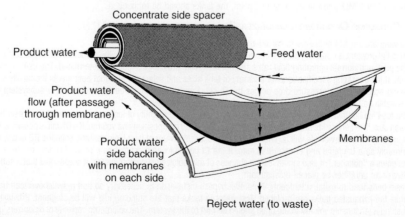

Fig. 8.2 Spiral-wrap reverse osmosis module.

WHAT ARE THE DISADVANTAGES OF REVERSE OSMOSIS SYSTEMS?

The disadvantages of RO systems include the following:
- The membranes have a limited service life. For instance:
- Cellulose acetate membranes have limited pH tolerance. They degrade at temperatures greater than 35°C (95°F). They are vulnerable to bacteria. They eventually hydrolyze.
- Polyamide membranes are intolerant of temperatures greater than 35°C (95°F). They have poor tolerance for free chlorine.
- Thin-film composites are intolerant to chlorine.
- High-flux polysulfones require softening or DI of the feed water to function properly.
- As with hemodialysis membranes, leaks are possible. Continual monitoring of the product water flow rate and conductivity is necessary.
- The product water volume is 25% to 75% of the feed water volume and is sometimes referred to as the percent recovery. The remaining 25% to 75% goes to waste, varying according to the type of central RO system in use.
- The membrane must be kept continually wet throughout its entire life. The flow cannot simply be stopped and the unit filled with water; bacterial growth, hydrolysis of the membrane, and pyrogen production are likely to result. When not in operation, the unit should be held in a sterilant-filled state.
- Chloramines (oxidant compounds formed from the reaction between the chlorine and ammonia used as bactericidal agents in some city water supplies) are nonionic and diffuse freely across the RO membrane. Anemia resulting from chloramines has occurred in some dialysis patients. A carbon filter should always be used ahead of an RO system to remove any chloramine.
- To meet peak flow needs in large hemodialysis facilities, a reservoir or holding tanks for processed water from the RO unit may be necessary. The water is recirculated in a continuous loop from the RO unit to the tanks and back to prevent stagnation. The tanks and plumbing are sites for potential microbial growth and endotoxin formation. Tank design is important in minimizing contamination. A steeply rounded or conical tank bottom with the drain port at the extreme low point ensures complete emptying. The reentry port should be near the top and should use a special nozzle to spray the underside of the cover. This prevents water droplets from forming on the cover, and the cascade of water down the sides prevents the collection of stagnant water. The top should have a microbial filter in the air vent. This design also provides excellent sterilant contact during chemical disinfection and complete flushing away of the sterilant at "rinse-out." Chlorine or iodine may also be metered into the system between the RO unit and the tanks to control the growth of organisms (Fig. 8.3).

WHAT IS DEIONIZATION?

Deionization refers to the removal of ionized minerals and salts from a solution, in this case the feed water. Positively charged ions (cations) are exchanged by the resin beads for hydrogen ions, and negatively charged ions (anions) are exchanged to form hydroxide ions (Fig. 8.4). The hydrogen (H^+) and hydroxide ions ($OH-$) formed as a result combine to create water molecules. Deionizers produce water of high ionic purity, but they do not remove bacteria or pyrogens. Indeed, deionizers often make the quality of water worse in terms of the bacterial and endotoxin content; the resin bed provides an environment conducive to bacterial proliferation. It is essential to follow DI equipment with submicron filtration or a UF unit (Fig. 8.5).

HOW IS WATER QUALITY MONITORED WITH THE USE OF A DEIONIZER?

It is imperative that some type of monitor be installed to ensure the chemical quality of the product water. Deionizer water quality values are expressed in resistivity units. The AAMI guidelines state that product water should not have a resistance below 1 MΩ (megohm/cm); at that point, the tanks should be exchanged.

WHAT PROBLEMS OCCUR WITH DEIONIZERS?

The following are several problems to consider in the case of deionizers:
- An initial problem is obtaining the maximum flow rate needed. As with softeners, the proper size of the DI set is critical. The peak and normal operating flow rates and operating line pressures should be determined. The user should then look at the operating specifications for a variety of tank sizes and select the size that best meets the facility's needs, taking account of the pressure drop across the DI set. Pressure indicators before and after this subsystem are advisable so that the difference in pressure can be easily determined.
- The total ion content of the feed water is a problem; only a finite quantity of ions can be removed by a resin bed of a given size. The service life of a deionizer depends on the water composition and volume. If a DI unit is positioned ahead of an RO unit, its service life will be short. It will be processing water of high ionic content while the RO unit will serve primarily as a bacterial and endotoxin screen. If the DI unit is located downstream of the RO device, the DI unit becomes a "polisher." It also increases the chances of microbiological contamination. It is essential that a submicron filter or an ultrafilter be placed downstream.
- Resin beds tend to exhaust suddenly. A parallel bypass installation is necessary so that a switchover can be made while the exhausted tanks are replaced. The water in tanks that are standing idle will be stagnant. Provision for flushing a reasonable volume to the drain should be part of the system. The volumetric capacity of deionizers (gallons of water passing through the tanks) is rated in gpg of total dissolved solids (TDS), expressed as calcium carbonate.

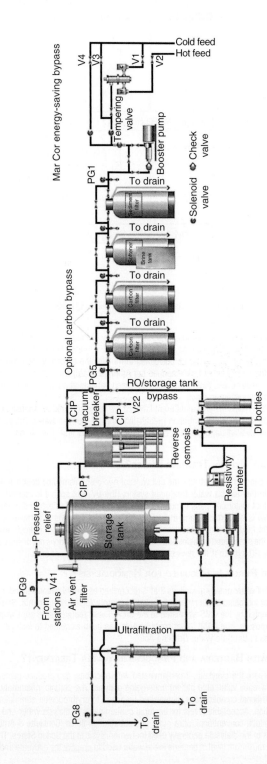

Fig. 8.3 Recirculating loop water treatment system with a holding tank. *CIP*, Clean In Place; *DI*, Deionization; *PG*, Pressure Gauge; *RO*, Reverse Osmosis; *V*, Valve. (Courtesy Mar Cor Services, Harleysville, PA.)

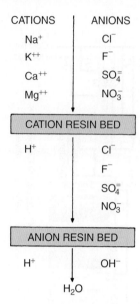

CATIONS	ANIONS
Na$^+$	Cl$^-$
K^{++}	F$^-$
Ca^{++}	SO$_4^=$
Mg^{++}	NO$_3^-$

CATION RESIN BED

H$^+$	Cl$^-$
	F$^-$
	SO$_4^=$
	NO$_3^-$

ANION RESIN BED

H$^+$	OH$^-$

$$H_2O$$

Fig. 8.4 Schematic diagram of a two-bed deionizing system.

(Note: One gpg approximates 17.1 mg/L CaCO$_3$.) The rated capacity of the deionizer divided by the TDS of the feed water will give an approximation of the volume of water that may be treated before the unit exhausts. Online continuous readout resistivity meters should be positioned to monitor the effluent water. When the resistance degrades to 1 MΩ/cm, the tanks should be exchanged (an AAMI standard). DI systems must have a method to ensure that water with resistance less than 1 MΩ does not reach patients at any time. All DI systems must have an automatic divert to drain the system in place.

• Usually the anion and cation resins exhaust at different times. If the tanks are used to exhaustion, previously removed ions may be released, possibly at a concentration greater than that of the feed water. The water may become extremely acidic or extremely alkaline, depending on which resin exhausts first. This situation may be hazardous to patients or equipment.

How Is Ultraviolet Light Used in Treating Water?

Ultraviolet light is a form of radiation that penetrates the cell walls of microorganisms and destroys them by altering their deoxyribonucleic acid (DNA). In the dialysis water treatment system, the UV light source is housed in a clear protective quartz sleeve. It is placed so that water can pass through a flow chamber where it is exposed to intense UV radiation. It is important that the water flow is not turbulent and that the water is free of suspended particles. UV light passes more easily through clear translucent fluids. Cloudy liquids make penetration of UV light more difficult and can potentially allow microbes to hide behind the suspended particles and not be eliminated. UV light does not destroy endotoxins and must be followed by an ultrafilter or RO system if the device is located in the pre-treatment area.

What Degree of Water Purity Is Required for Hemodialysis?

The AAMI has developed a set of water quality guidelines that is recognized as the US national standard. The standard now applies not only to chemical or inorganic contaminants but also to microbiologic contaminants. Some of the standards and regulations have been adopted by the CMS as related to the CfCs. These requirements are shown in Table 8.2 along with the adverse effects of exposure. The AAMI list of contaminants has been expanded to include antimony, beryllium, and thallium following changes in the Safe Water Drinking Act.

What Problems Exist with Bacteria and Pyrogens in Water Treatment?

Dialysate or water used to prepare the dialysate, if contaminated with microbes, can produce bacteremia and an inflammatory response in an already vulnerable patient undergoing dialysis. The chronic inflammation can contribute to cardiovascular disease, nutritional complications, diminished response to erythropoietin-stimulating agents, and a decline in residual renal function. Acceptable levels for bacterial contaminants in dialysis water and dialysate vary as determined by the type of product: conventional, ultra-pure, and substitution fluids (Coulliette & Arduino, 2013). "Conventional dialysate" refers to the dialysate generally used for hemodialysis in the United States. The CMS CfCs require conventional dialysis to have a maximum level of bacteria in the water used to prepare the dialysate and reprocess dialyzers

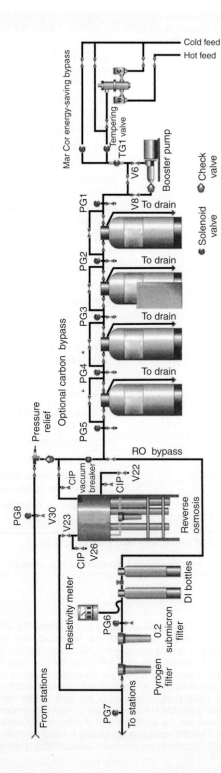

Fig. 8.5 Direct feed water treatment system to produce ultrapure water. *CIP*, Clean In Place; *DI*, Deionization; *PG*, Pressure Gauge; *RO*, Reverse Osmosis; *V*, Valve. (Courtesy Mar Cor Services, Harleysville, PA.)

Table 8.2 AAMI Water Quality Guidelines[a]

	AAMI SUGGESTED MAXIMUM LEVEL (MG/L)	ADVERSE EFFECTS FROM EXPOSURE[b]
Aluminum	0.01	Anemia, bone disease, neurological changes, "Dialysis Dementia"
Antimony	0.006	*Nausea/vomiting*
Arsenic, lead, silver	0.005 each	Cancer, skin changes, damage to central nervous system, brain and kidneys
Bacteria	<200 CFU/mL	Hypotension, nausea/vomiting
Beryllium	0.004	Bone damage
Cadmium	0.001	*Nausea/vomiting, diarrhea, salivation, sensory disturbances,* kidney/liver/bone damage
Calcium	2 (0.1 mEq/L)	*Nausea/vomiting, headache, muscle weakness, tachycardia, hypertension,* abnormal bone mineralization, soft tissue calcifications, pancreatitis
Chloramines	0.1	*Hemolysis, chest pain, arrhythmias, nausea/vomiting*
Chlorine	0.5	*Hemolysis, chest pain, arrhythmias, nausea/vomiting*
Chromium	0.014	Liver damage
Copper, barium, zinc	0.1 each	*Chills, flushing, headaches, projectile vomiting, hypotension,* anemia, liver damage, pancreatitis
Endotoxin	<2 EU/mL	Hypotension, nausea/vomiting
Fluoride	0.2	*Chest pain, nausea/vomiting, hypotension,* headache, bone disease
Magnesium	4 (0.3 mEq/L)	Nausea/vomiting
Mercury	0.0002	Kidney damage
Nitrate (N)	2.0	*Hemolysis, hypotension, nausea/vomiting, weakness, confusion*
Potassium	8 (0.2 mEq/L)	Nausea, nerve impulse interference
Selenium	0.09	*Fatigue, irritability, hair/nail loss,* kidney/liver damage
Sodium	70 (3.0 mEq/L)	*Increased thirst, nausea, headache, hypertension, pulmonary edema, seizures, coma*
Sulfate	100	Metabolic acidosis, nausea/vomiting
Thallium	0.002	Liver/kidney damage

[a]The physician has the ultimate responsibility of determining the quality of water used for dialysis.
[b]Acute symptoms are shown in italics.
From Vlchek DL, Burrows-Hudson S: *Quality assurance guidelines for hemodialysis devices*, Washington, DC, February 1991, U.S. Department of Health & Human Services, U.S. Food and Drug Administration; U.S. Environmental Protection Agency: *Drinking water contaminants*, 2001.

must be less than 200 colony-forming units (CFU)/mL with an action level of 50 CFU/mL, but AAMI recommends a maximum bacteria level less than 100 CFU/ml and an action level of 50 CFU/mL. One should follow the standards established by the individual provider, whether those standards be as outlined by the CMS or AAMI. The CMS CfCs established conventional dialysate as the minimum requirement for dialysis fluids. New membranes are much more porous to water, solutes, and suspended matter. Transmembrane movement is bidirectional relative to the pressure and solute concentration gradients. In most instances, proper prefilters with an RO unit or DI with submicron postfiltration will meet the standard. Bacteria proliferate on filter surfaces, carbon tanks, softener and DI resin beds, and the feed water surface of the RO membrane. Cleansing with an approved disinfectant to minimize bacterial growth in all components of the water treatment system must be done monthly at a minimum. The disinfectant must of course be thoroughly rinsed from the system before the water is used for patients. Chemical sterilization kills bacteria but does not destroy them and actually fixes some of the protein and polysaccharide components and endotoxins. Copious rinsing is needed to wash this debris away from the collecting surfaces.

A majority of facilities use bicarbonate-containing concentrates in their fluid-proportioning systems. Many facilities use dialyzers with high-flux membranes, along with controlled UF devices.

When stored, the bicarbonate concentrate supports the proliferation of endotoxin-forming microorganisms. Whether these originate from the water used to prepare the concentrate or from the bicarbonate powder, it is likely that more strict microbial and endotoxin limits will be necessary. For high-flux dialysis, where backfiltration poses a problem, delivery of a sterile, pyrogen-free fluid from the proportioning system to the dialyzer may become necessary.

How May Microbiological Contaminants Be Further Reduced?

The following means are most commonly used to reduce microbiological contaminants:
- Submicron (0.05-mm) filters stop the passage of bacteria and viruses. Such filters must be replaced frequently and are expensive. They do not exclude all pyrogenic matter.
- UF rejects bacteria and endotoxins effectively. The initial installation is relatively expensive, but operation is economical. Sanitization is simple, and service life is good.

How Is Ultrafiltration Used to Remove Bacteria and Endotoxins?

Ultrafiltration membranes have an effective pore size of more than 0.001 mm. Pores of this size do not retard the movement of osmotically active solutes; hence, compared with RO membranes, less hydraulic pressure is needed for the transmembrane movement of water.

Ultrafiltration membranes are often called molecular filters; they filter suspended particles of molecular size rather than dissolved substances. The larger particles do not have the osmotic effect of dissolved solutes. There is little osmotic backpressure compared with RO membranes and hence less need for high hydraulic pressure. However, these molecular filters reject bacteria, endotoxins, and endotoxin fragments that are thousands of daltons in size. Ultrafilters that exclude particles of 50,000 to 100,000 Da are available; in fact, an even tighter membrane excluding particles of 1000 to 10,000 Da is available.

Ultrafiltration devices may be placed ahead of RO units to prevent bacterial growth or accumulation of particulate material on the feed water surface of the RO membrane. When used as the final step before delivery of the product water to the proportioning system, UF will ensure its microbiological quality.

What Tests Are Done to Maintain the Water Treatment Systems?

Bacterial Culturing

Bacterial culturing is performed to detect the presence of bacteria in water. Colony counts are typically read at 24 and 48 hours. Bacterial cultures are also performed on the dialysate. The maximum level of endotoxin in the water used to prepare the dialysate and reprocess the dialyzers must not exceed the CMS standard of less than 2 endotoxin units (EU)/mL. Testing is performed monthly. If a problem with bacteria is identified by positive cultures, testing should be conducted weekly until the problem is resolved.

Conductivity

Conductivity is verified in the feed and product water to ensure that they contain the proper amount of ions. It can be measured with a pHoenix meter (which also measures pH and temperature). Conductivity may also be measured with a handheld meter, such as the Myron-L.

Resistivity

Resistivity determines the efficiency of removal of ions from the water processed in a deionizer. Water with high resistivity will have low conductivity because of the low amount of ions in the solution.

Hardness Test

This test detects the presence of calcium and magnesium in the water.

Total Dissolved Solids

Total dissolved solids is the sum of all ions in a solution and verifies the effectiveness of the RO membranes. This can be checked with a handheld meter. The results are expressed in ppm.

The CMS CfCs require technicians who perform monitoring and testing of the water treatment system to undergo a training program approved by the medical director and governing body.

What Microbiological Standards Apply to Dialyzer Reuse?

The microbiological standards that apply to dialyzer reuse are defined in the *AAMI Recommended Practice for Reuse of Dialyzers* (RD47). The CMS rules published in 2008 endorse the recommendations made by the AAMI in 2004. The water used in reprocessing should have a bacterial count of less than 200 CFU/mL or an endotoxin level of less than 2 EU/mL. This also may be made stricter because of problems with bicarbonate and high-flux dialyzers. The required action level for the total microbial count in water is 50 CFU/mL, with an action level for endotoxins of 1 EU/mL (Coulliette & Arduino, 2013).

What Kind of Water Processing Is Best for Individual Dialysis Units?

The kind of water processing depends on the quality of the available tap water and its solute content. The feed water should be analyzed for chemical and bacteriological content on a regular basis and should meet the Environmental Protection Agency drinking water standards. The product water, the final purified water used to prepare the dialysis fluid, should meet the AAMI and other applicable standards. The components of a system that meets these requirements may include the following:

- Initial sediment filter(s)
- Resin-type softener (water hardness checked once at the end of each day)
- Activated carbon filters (two in series)
- RO unit (with continuous conductivity and resistivity monitoring of inflow and outflow water)
- DI unit (continuous resistivity monitoring of outflow, plus monthly bacteriological and limulus tests and chemical analysis)

A complete system of this type will provide maximum purity water, approaching a resistance of 18 MΩ/cm. Thorough investigation is necessary to reach the desired purity of water in the most economic manner. Ongoing monitoring is essential to ensure its maintenance.

What Cost Factors Are Involved in Establishing an Adequate Water Treatment System?

Before setting a dollar figure on how much to spend, the facility should consult a knowledgeable designer of dialysis facility water treatment systems and a reliable supplier and installer. The facility's needs, current and future, should be determined. Consideration should be given to each of the following factors:

- Quality of the feed water
- Peak volume needs
- Desired quality of the product water
- Expertise of the technical staff
- Cost of the feed water
- Compliance with standards
- Type(s) of therapy to be delivered
- Ease of operation
- Maintenance requirements

The components listed should be included only to achieve a particular goal, with the final objective of meeting or exceeding the recommended standards for conventional or ultra-pure dialysate. If the source water is of very low mineral content, it may be possible to achieve 1-MΩ/cm product water by RO or DI alone after appropriate filtration. It is always mandatory to have activated carbon tanks. Only the minimum number of components necessary should be used to meet or exceed the recommended standards.

Preparation of bicarbonate dialysate and high-flux dialysis may necessitate more stringent microbial control than is required by the current AAMI standards and CMS CfCs.

Who Determines the Type of Purification System and Quality of Water Used for Dialysis?

The medical director has the ultimate responsibility of ensuring the quality of water used for dialysis. If standards are not met, the medical director may be cited as the negligent party. This person must have oversight and must validate this responsibility by meeting the interdisciplinary team on a monthly basis at the Quality Assessment and Process Improvement meeting. All documentation of water quality testing, including bacterial and endotoxin studies, must be reviewed and signed off by the medical director (CMS, 2014).

DIALYZER PREPARATION AND REPROCESSING

CHAPTER 9

DIALYZER PREPARATION

Each dialyzer has its own specific characteristics and preparation procedure for patient use. Manufacturers' instructions are updated frequently as alterations are made or improved techniques are developed. It is very important to read the package inserts frequently to ensure adherence to the current recommendations. Always check and follow the manufacturer's instructions for use (IFU).

WHAT ARE THE ESSENTIAL PARAMETERS WHEN A DIALYZER IS PREPARED FOR PATIENT USE?

The essential parameters of dialyzer preparation are as follows:
- All air in the dialyzer must be removed. Any air left in the dialyzer could be dialyzed across the membrane and into the patient's vascular system. Air trapped in the walls of the hollow fibers will reduce dialyzer clearance by preventing diffusion between the blood and dialysate compartments. Also, air will promote clotting in the hollow fibers of a dialyzer.
- Any particulate matter left in the dialyzer from the manufacturing process must be flushed out with saline prime.
- All disinfectant used in the reprocessing procedures must be removed, and the dialyzer must be free of residual disinfectant.
- Dialyzers must always be flushed and primed with a physiological saline solution (0.9 g of sodium chloride in 100 mL of water) compatible with patient blood.

HOW IS AIR REMOVED FROM A DIALYZER?

To remove air from a dialyzer, prime normal saline into the dialyzer from the bottom. This is accomplished by attaching the bloodlines to the dialyzer and turning the dialyzer so that the venous end is up. Then run the saline through the arterial bloodline, through the dialyzer into the venous bloodline, and into a basin. As the dialyzer is filled, air is forced out of the top of the dialyzer. Tap the dialyzer lightly and turn it from side to side to ensure that all of the air is removed from the header.

HOW MUCH SALINE SHOULD BE USED TO PRIME THE DIALYZER?

Priming the dialyzer will require 500 to 1000 mL of saline. The amount depends on the type of dialyzer and whether it has been reprocessed. A new dialyzer should use 1000 mL of prime to remove glycerin and particulate matter remaining from the manufacturing process. A reprocessed dialyzer requires approximately 500 mL of saline because the prime will be recirculated with the dialysate, flowing counterclockwise to remove any residual disinfectant. It is always prudent to follow the manufacturer's IFU or your facility's written policy.

SHOULD ANYTHING BE DIFFERENT WHEN PRIMING A REPROCESSED DIALYZER?

Reprocessed dialyzers are filled with a disinfectant, and it is important to ensure that all disinfectant is removed and no air is introduced into the dialyzer. When air is introduced, it is very difficult to remove. All air must be removed from the arterial bloodline before attaching it to the dialyzer. This is accomplished by priming the arterial bloodline with saline, making sure that all air is removed before attaching the line to the dialyzer. After this is done, the dialyzer is turned venous end up and the priming procedure is continued.

DO MANUFACTURERS MAKE ANY RECOMMENDATIONS REGARDING THE PRIMING OF THEIR DIALYZERS?

Yes, all manufacturers make recommendations for priming their dialyzers. In some dialyzers, the blood compartment should be filled first; in others, the dialysate compartment should be filled first. Most hollow-fiber dialyzers require that you "wet" the membranes first before attaching the dialysate lines. This ensures that the dialyzer fibers will not collapse when exposed to the dialysate. Dialysis personnel should read and follow the instructions that come with the dialyzers used in the particular facility.

DIALYZER REPROCESSING

Cleaning and disinfecting a dialyzer to be used again for the same patient's treatment is considered dialyzer reprocessing or dialyzer reuse. Dialyzer reuse is safe and cost effective and has been used since the early 1960s but is no longer widely used in the United States. The guidelines in the Association for the Advancement of Medical Instrumentation (AAMI) Recommended Practice for Reuse of Hemodialyzers (RD47) must be followed because the Centers for Medicare & Medicaid Services (CMS) have adopted them as standards governing the practice. The US Food and Drug Administration (FDA) now requires dialyzer manufacturers to label their dialyzers so that users know that they are appropriate for reprocessing. The manufacturer must also recommend appropriate reprocessing techniques and the type of germicide to be used.

Dialyzer reprocessing may be performed manually or with an automated system, with the automated systems more commonly in use today. The FDA recently approved a new dialyzer reprocessing system (ClearFlux) that has the potential to significantly reduce dialyzer consumption. The "two-phase" system uses a gas and liquid flow mixture that can better penetrate and clean the hollow-fiber tubes of the dialyzer, as opposed to the standard reuse process that relies on a one-phase or liquid-only flow. This device creates a high-velocity turbulent flow in the dialyzer to more thoroughly cleanse the device and thus minimizes the loss of fiber bundle volume even after as many as 40 uses.

Reprocessing may be performed on site at the provider facility, or the dialyzers may be transported to an off-site location. Bloodlines and other disposable items have been reused, but these are regulated and restricted by the FDA and are rarely reused in the United States. The CMS has taken an official end-stage renal disease (ESRD) program position on reuse and has published specific written requirements. Some chemicals used to reprocess dialyzers are considered hazardous and are regulated by the Occupational Safety and Health Administration (OSHA).

WHAT ARE SOME ADVANTAGES OF DIALYZER REUSE?

There are purported clinical advantages of dialyzer reuse. With each dialysis treatment, the patient's blood leaves proteins on the wall of the membrane. These protein deposits create a secondary membrane that reduces the amount of exposure of the patient's blood to the artificial membrane during subsequent treatments. Bleach, however, when used in the disinfection process, will decrease this protection because it strips the protein layers from the dialyzer.

On rare occasions, a patient may react to a new dialyzer. These reactions are believed to be caused by either bioincompatible membranes or ethylene oxide residue left in the sterilized dialyzer. A reaction may occur shortly after the initiation of dialysis and be less severe, precipitating symptoms such as itching, hives, dyspnea, or back pain. Reactions can also be life threatening, causing anaphylaxis and cardiac or respiratory arrest. When the dialyzer has been reprocessed for reuse, such reactions are not observed during subsequent treatments. Other sterilization methods, however, are replacing the use of ethylene oxide in dialyzers.

Reused dialyzers also help to contain the cost of each patient treatment, and with reuse, there is a significant reduction in the amount of nonbiodegradable medical waste products and biohazardous trash.

HOW MANY TIMES CAN A DIALYZER BE REUSED?

Some centers arbitrarily settle on three or five reuses per dialyzer, whereas other centers use a dialyzer until it has been determined that its effectiveness is no longer adequate to deliver the recommended dose of dialysis for the patient. Even these small numbers represent significant savings. To determine the cost effectiveness of reuse, divide the original cost of the dialyzer by the total cost of reprocessing. To qualify for reuse, a dialyzer must meet the defined criteria: the residual volume or total cell volume (TCV) must be 80% or greater of the original TCV, it must hold at least 90% of the original clearance volume specified by the manufacturer, it must pass a pressure-holding test, and the appearance evaluation should show no more than a few clotted fibers. After each clinical use, the dialyzer is evaluated using these criteria and must meet them to be used again.

WHAT ARE THE BASIC STEPS FOR REUSE?

The basic steps in most reprocessing programs are as follows: (1) flushing the dialyzer to remove most of the blood residuals; (2) cleaning, which is usually done with chemicals (bleach or hydrogen peroxide, and reverse ultrafiltration; (3) testing to verify that the membrane is intact and that the dialyzer will remove waste products as expected; and (4) disinfection with either a chemical such as formaldehyde or Renalin (a mixture of peracetic acid, acetic acid, and hydrogen peroxide) or heat.

WHAT SPECIFIC CRITERIA ARE USED TO DETERMINE IF A DIALYZER MAY BE REUSED?

The four main criteria for reuse are as follows:

Total cell volume measurement is the most widely used method to determine whether a reused dialyzer has maintained adequate solute removal capability. In this test, the dialyzer is filled with water and pumped dry, and the contained volume is measured in a graduated cylinder. This volume is the standard for that dialyzer and the value against which it will be compared after each use. If less than 80% of the initial volume remains, the dialyzer is rejected for further patient use. A dialyzer with 80% of its initial volume still has 90% of its initial solute removal capability.

1. Pressure testing of the dialyzer is performed to determine whether there are broken fibers that would lead to a blood leak during dialysis. Pressure is applied to the dialyzer and then held. If the pressure drop is too great, the dialyzer is discarded. This is sometimes referred to as leak testing.

2. Some reuse machines test the dialyzer's k_{UF} (ultrafiltration coefficient). Although this is not a test to predict dialyzer clearance, it is an indicator of how "open" the dialyzer membrane may be to large molecules.

3. Finally, appearance or visual inspection is an important criterion. A dialyzer with larger streaks of residual blood, indicating a large number of clotted fibers, should be considered for immediate rejection. Dialyzers after use should be reprocessed within 2 hours of treatment or refrigerated to minimize clotting of the fibers and prevent bacterial growth.

Dialyzer reprocessing may be completed by dialyzer reuse technicians, or facilities may cross-train staff from other positions, such as hemodialysis technicians or clerical staff, to perform reprocessing. Each person who is assigned dialyzer reprocessing must complete all components of the training and demonstrate competency (CMS, 2008).

Is Large Solute Clearance Affected by Reprocessing?

Yes. The extent of this effect depends on the dialyzer membrane and reprocessing technique; some membranes tend to become more open when exposed to bleach cleaning. In most cases, membrane clearance of large solutes, such as β_2-microglobulin, is decreased when Renalin is used. It is very important to understand how particular dialyzers are affected by the reprocessing technique used. Dialyzers reprocessed with bleach have increased membrane permeability, which may increase the risk of bacteria and endotoxins moving from the dialysate into the blood (Nissenson & Fine, 2017). Some manufactures of dialyzers produce one type of dialyzer for use with bleach disinfection and another for use with other types of germicides to minimize membrane permeability.

How Are Reprocessed Dialyzers Disinfected?

Peracetic acid (3%–4%), formaldehyde or formalin (1%–4%), glutaraldehyde (0.8%), and heated water with citric acid (1.5%) are the most commonly used chemical disinfectants for reprocessing. High-level disinfection must be used for the blood and dialysate compartments and low-level disinfection is used for the outer casing and port caps (CMS ESRD Conditions for Coverage [CfCs], 2008).

What Types of Labeling Are Required for Reprocessed Dialyzers?

The CMS CfCs require that each dialyzer must be tested for TCV clearance before the first use and must then be labeled with the patient's name, number of previous uses, and the date and time when the dialyzer was last processed.

Meticulous care must be taken to ensure that each dialyzer is used for only one patient. Careful attention must be given to patients with same or similar names. Additional means of identification, such as a Social Security number or birth date, are recommended as an additional check to verify that the correct dialyzer is being used for the patient. Some facilities place a warning on the dialyzer to alert the staff member to exercise extra caution when placing the patient on that dialyzer. After the patient is at the treatment station, two people must verify that the first and last names on the dialyzer belong to that patient. Records that track the history of the dialyzer from its first use to when it is discarded should be maintained in the facility.

What Exposure Time Is Required for Renalin and Formaldehyde?

Renalin, a mixture of hydrogen peroxide, peracetic acid, and acetic acid, is a sterilant and requires a 0.5% solution with an 11-hour contact time. In contrast, aqueous formaldehyde, a high-level disinfectant, kills all microorganisms, including spores and viruses, with a minimum exposure time of 24 hours and a 4% concentration of formalin at room temperature. A lower concentration, 1.5% formalin, is effective at 38°C (100°F) for a 24-hour exposure.

What Happens If a Dialyzer Is Not Adequately Disinfected?

If there is not sufficient exposure (concentration and time), bacteria in the dialyzer will not be killed and may even multiply. This could result in the patient becoming bacteremic when the blood is exposed to the dialyzer during subsequent treatment.

What Information Should Be Verified Before Using a Reprocessed Dialyzer for a Patient?

Several checks must be completed before using a reprocessed dialyzer. The most important check is to verify that the dialyzer is being used for the correct patient. It is important to determine that the dialyzer had adequate contact time with the given sterilant. Other requirements include ensuring that the dialyzer contained an adequate level of disinfectant before it was rinsed and that all of the disinfectant was removed during the rinsing process. Finally, the dialyzer must pass all reuse tests, such as TCV and pressure tests.

What Precautions Are Necessary When Using Chemical Disinfectants?

The use of protective gear, including an eye shield, gloves, and a waterproof gown, is necessary when using chemical disinfectants. Adequate ventilation (in adherence with the OSHA guidelines) is also required. Any splashes on the skin or eyes should be flushed with copious amounts of water, and appropriate medical care should be sought.

Note that the OSHA requires that personnel be well informed about these hazardous chemicals and their potential toxicity. Every dialysis facility must have printed the OSHA requirements and regulations related to the use of disinfectants. Training records of staff education and health monitoring records must be maintained. Material safety data sheets (MSDSs) must be available for each chemical housed in the facility and for each chemical to which the employee may be exposed. The MSDSs must be accessible to the staff at all times.

What Precautions Should Be Taken When Working with Formaldehyde?

The OSHA standard, Title 29 of the Code of Federal Regulations, section 1910.1048, protects workers who have the potential to be exposed to formaldehyde. Formaldehyde is a suspected carcinogen associated with nasal and lung cancer.

Airborne concentrations as little as 0.1 ppm may cause irritation to the nose, eyes, and throat. Allergic reactions may occur with exposure, causing wheezing, coughing, or asthma-like symptoms.

Air quality monitoring is used to protect the staff from potentially dangerous exposure. The OSHA has set permissible exposure limits at 0.75 ppm, measured as an 8-hour time-weighted average (TWA). The OSHA standard for short-term exposure limit is 2 ppm during a 15-minute period. The action level is 0.5 ppm for an 8-hour TWA. The OSHA mandates that all staff be educated annually about the hazards of and how to work safely with formaldehyde. An emergency shower and eyewash station must also be available to the staff in the event of an exposure. Mandatory respiratory training and respirator fit testing must also be conducted for reuse personnel.

ARE CHEMICAL DISINFECTANTS STABLE OVER TIME?

Renalin is broken down fairly rapidly by temperatures greater than 27°C (80°F), exposure to light, and exposure to organic matter (e.g., blood). Time is another factor: after it has been diluted, Renalin has a relatively short shelf life. It is very important to test each dialyzer for Renalin potency just before preparing it for patient use. Formaldehyde is quite stable for long periods.

HOW SHOULD THE DIALYZER BE PREPARED BEFORE THE NEXT RUN?

After the dialyzer is filled with a disinfectant at the end of the reprocessing procedure, it is necessary to document the presence of the disinfectant using an appropriate chemical test. This helps to confirm that the dialyzer is stored with the disinfecting chemical. Before the next clinical use, the disinfectant must be removed. The bloodlines are connected to the dialyzer, and sterile saline is rinsed through the blood side of the dialyzer. Usually up to 1000 mL of saline is run through the dialyzer and discarded. The arterial and venous bloodlines are then connected to establish a closed loop. The blood pump is started, and the recirculation of saline with ultrafiltration should remove any residual chemical left in the system. Essentially, the disinfectant is simply dialyzed out of the system.

Just before use, the recirculating saline in the dialyzer is sampled using a test appropriate for the disinfectant used. After the test is performed, the absence of the disinfectant must be documented. Only after a negative test result has been confirmed is the dialyzer considered safe for patient use. Most dialysis units and state agencies require two people to verify that the dialyzer is correct for a specific patient and has a negative disinfectant test before using the reprocessed dialyzer.

WHEN THE DISINFECTANT USED IS RENALIN, IS THERE A SPECIFIC ORDER IN WHICH THE COMPARTMENTS ARE PRIMED?

Renalin is a strong acid, so it is important to prime the blood compartment with normal saline before attaching the dialysate lines. If the dialysate compartment is primed first, reaction between the dialysate and Renalin will cause some of the carbon dioxide to come out of solution as a gas. These bubbles can be trapped in the fibers, creating an air gap between the blood and dialysate, resulting in poor diffusion.

ARE THERE CIRCUMSTANCES IN WHICH REUSE IS INAPPROPRIATE FOR A PARTICULAR PATIENT?

Patients with systemic infections or sepsis are generally excluded from reprocessing programs. Patients with hepatitis B are excluded from participating in reuse programs as determined by the CMS CfCs for ESRD.

ARE PATIENTS REQUIRED TO GIVE THEIR CONSENT FOR THE REUSE OF DIALYZERS?

The CMS requires that patients give consent in writing. The consent must be made part of the patient's clinical record. If the patient does not give this written consent, reuse is not permitted.

CHAPTER 10

INFECTION CONTROL

Infection control is used in the dialysis setting to prevent patients and staff from acquiring infections specific to the dialysis unit. Infection control incorporates policies and procedures that include surveillance and monitoring activities for water treatment, dialyzer reuse, bacterial contamination, and transmission of blood-borne and other infectious diseases.

The Centers for Disease Control and Prevention (CDC) has issued and updated blood-borne infection control strategies and precautions (including standard precautions) for dialysis centers as well as other health care agencies over the years. The new Centers for Medicare & Medicaid Services (CMS) rules, which went into effect in October 2008, require dialysis providers to follow the CDC documents "Recommendations for Prevention and Transmission of Infections among Chronic Hemodialysis Patients" (*MMWR*, 50[RR-5], 2001) and "Prevention of Intravascular Catheter-Related Infections" (*MMWR*, 51[RR-10], 2002). The CDC has provided additional and updated infection control recommendations in 2016, which are outlined throughout this chapter.

The Occupational Safety and Health Administration (OSHA) has issued regulations that enforce the use of standard precautions and other infection control strategies for all health care agencies. The OSHA blood-borne pathogen regulations provide specific measures that health care workers and their employers can take together to substantially reduce the risk of health care workers contracting a blood-borne disease while on the job. The CDC has also issued recommendations for preventing the spread of drug-resistant organisms and other potentially infectious diseases such as tuberculosis (TB).

This chapter reviews information that personnel are required to know to help prevent the spread of infectious diseases in dialysis facilities. It also includes a review of blood-borne diseases and standard precautions published by the CDC, as well as strategies to prevent the spread of methicillin-resistant *Staphylococcus aureus* (MRSA), vancomycin-resistant enterococci (VRE), and TB. Questions commonly asked by dialysis personnel regarding water treatment, bacterial contamination, dialyzer reuse, and infection control issues are addressed in the specific chapters dealing with those subjects. The updated guidelines consistent with the October 14, 2008 CMS Conditions for Coverage (CfCs) are addressed to reflect the regulations applicable to both chronic in-center dialysis and home dialysis programs.

The CDC has issued specific recommendations for the prevention of blood-borne pathogens in dialysis facilities. Box 10.1 outlines these guidelines.

WHAT ARE THE STANDARD PRECAUTIONS?

The recommendation that blood and body fluid precautions be used consistently for all patients, regardless of their blood-borne infection status, is the basic tenet of Standard Precautions. Blood-borne pathogens, such as human immunodeficiency virus (HIV) and hepatitis B virus (HBV), infect people of all ages, of all socioeconomic classes, and from all geographic areas. Health care workers may not be able to identify patients who harbor a virus or who may transmit infection. The CDC defines "Standard Precautions" as the minimum infection prevention practices that apply to all patient care, regardless of suspected or confirmed infection status of the patient, in any setting where health care is delivered (2018).

Reducing exposure to and transmission of blood-borne pathogens through the use of Standard Precautions involves appropriate work practices, such as the use of barrier precautions. Appropriate barrier precautions are to be used to prevent exposure of the skin and mucous membranes to blood or any other body fluid of any patient. Health care workers should wear personal protective equipment (PPE) that is most appropriate to the anticipated potential exposure. Barrier precautions, also known as PPE, include the use of the following:

- Gloves
- Face shields, eye wear, or masks
- Gowns

Gloves are to be worn when performing procedures that have the potential for exposure to blood, dialysate, and other potentially infectious substances. This includes when touching blood and body fluids, mucous membranes, or nonintact skin of any patient; when handling items or surfaces soiled with blood or body fluids; when performing vascular access procedures such as placing or removing access needles or catheter lines where blood spillage is likely; when handling blood lines, dialyzers, and dialyzer tubing after dialysis treatment; and when cleaning and disinfecting the dialysis machine and chair after dialysis treatment (CMS, 2014). Gloves should be provided to patients and visitors if they participate in activities such as self-cannulating or holding access sites after dialysis treatment. Disposable gloves are for single use only and come in a variety of materials such as vinyl, latex, and nitrile. Gloves must be changed and hands washed after contact with each patient or station; whenever the gloves are contaminated with blood, dialysate, or other body fluids; when going from a "dirty" area to a "clean" area; when moving from a contaminated body site to a clean body site on the same patient; after touching a patient; and after handling infectious waste containers. Hand hygiene should be performed using antiseptic soap and water or a waterless alcohol-based antiseptic hand rub with a 60% to 90% alcohol content. Masks and goggles or full face shields should be worn during all procedures likely to generate droplets, blood splashes, or body fluids near the face. Masks should fully cover the nose and mouth. Goggles should fit

> **Box 10.1** Components of a Comprehensive Infection Control Program to Prevent the Transmission of Infections Among Patients Undergoing Chronic Hemodialysis
>
> Infection control practices for hemodialysis units:
> 1. Infection control precautions specifically designed to prevent the transmission of blood-borne viruses and pathogenic bacteria among patients
> 2. Routine serological testing for HBV and HBC infections
> 3. Vaccination of susceptible patients against hepatitis B
> 4. Isolation of patients who test positive for HBsAg
> 5. Dedication of all single-use injectable medications and solutions for use on a single patient, with puncture only once
> 6. Surveillance for infections and other adverse events
> 7. Infection control training and education

HBV, Hepatitis B virus; *HBC,* hepatitis C virus; *HBsAg,* hepatitis B surface antigen.

snugly over and around the eyes. Personal eyewear, such as prescription glasses, is not a substitute for protective eyewear. Face shields should cover the forehead, extend below the chin, and wrap around the side of the face when worn properly. Initiating and terminating dialysis and troubleshooting the vascular access are examples of procedures that may increase a health care worker's risk of exposure to blood-borne pathogens if barrier precautions, such as gloves, a face shield, and impervious gowns or lab coats, are not used.

Cover garments, such as impervious isolation gowns or fluid resistant lab coats, are to be worn during procedures likely to generate droplets, blood splashes, body fluids, potentially contaminated substances, or chemicals near the body. The protective garment should provide full protection to the arms and torso from the area of the neck to the thigh or knee. Before leaving the work area, all PPE should be removed and placed in a designated area or container for washing, decontamination, or disposal. Hands should be thoroughly washed after the removal of PPE and before leaving the work area. In addition to barrier precautions, employee work practices, such as diligent handwashing, are essential to reduce the risk of exposure to and transmission of blood-borne pathogens.

Employee work practices include precautions that health care workers should take to prevent injuries caused by needles, scalpels, and other sharp instruments that may be responsible for the transmission of blood-borne diseases.

Precautions should be taken when cleaning used instruments, during disposal of used needles, and when handling sharp instruments after procedures. Needles should never be recapped, purposely bent, or broken by hand. Needles should never be removed from disposable syringes or otherwise manipulated by hand. After use, disposable syringes and needles, fistula needles, scalpel blades, and other sharp items must be placed in puncture-resistant containers located as close as practical to the area of use. The safety guard or device on a fistula needle must always be activated and engaged when the needle is removed and before disposal in the sharps container. Sharps containers should not be mounted too high but should be easily accessible. They should not be allowed to overfill.

To minimize the need for emergency mouth-to-mouth resuscitation, mouthpieces, pocket masks, resuscitation bags, or other ventilation devices should be available for use in areas where the need for resuscitation is predictable.

Health care workers with exudative lesions or weeping dermatitis should refrain from direct patient care and from handling patient equipment until the condition resolves. All skin defects (cuts, abrasions, ulcers, and so on) must be covered with an occlusive bandage.

Pregnant health care workers are not known to be at a greater risk of contracting HBV or HIV infection than nonpregnant health care workers; however, if a health care worker develops HBV or HIV infection during pregnancy, the infant is at risk of infection resulting from perinatal transmission. Therefore, pregnant health care workers should be especially familiar with and strictly adhere to precautions to minimize the risk of HBV or HIV transmission.

WHY IS HANDWASHING SO IMPORTANT?

The most common method of pathogen transfer from patient to patient or staff to patient is by hands. Handwashing reduces the risk of transferring contaminants from hands to other individuals, to other areas of the body, or to other surfaces that the health care worker may later contact. Hands should be washed when entering or leaving patient care areas, before gloving and immediately after removing gloves or other PPE, in between patient contacts, and after touching an environmental surface, such as the dialysis machine, without having gloved first. Hands should also be washed upon arrival to work and just before leaving from work, before and after eating, and before and after going to the restroom. Dialysis facilities must identify and dedicate "clean" sinks used for hand washing purposes only. Care must be taken not to use the "clean" sink for draining fluids or for placing items that have been used in the course of patient treatment. Sinks must also be made available to patients to wash their access sites and hands before treatment.

It is important to remember that gloves should never be used as a replacement for handwashing.

Adherence to handwashing guidelines is essential for providing safe patient care. Handwashing should always be performed after removing gloves. The CDC has issued guidelines on the use of alcohol-based hand rubs as an alternative to using traditional soap and water when providing patient care: before patient contact; after contact with a patient's intact skin, body fluids or excretions, nonintact skin, or wound dressings; and after removing gloves. The traditional method of handwashing with soap and water is indicated when hands are visibly dirty, contaminated, or soiled.

Table 10.1 Guide to Hand Hygiene Opportunities in Hemodialysis	
HAND HYGIENE OPPORTUNITY CATEGORY	**SPECIFIC EXAMPLES**
Before aseptic procedures	• Before cannulation or accessing catheter • Before performing catheter site care • Before parenteral medication preparation • Before administering IV medications or infusions
Before touching a patient	• Before entering station to provide care to patient • Before contact with vascular access site • Before adjusting or removing cannulation needles
After body fluid exposure risk	• After exposure to blood or any body fluids • After contact with other contaminated fluids (e.g., spent dialysate) • After handling used dialyzers, blood tubing, or prime buckets • After performing wound care or dressing changes
After touching a patient	• When leaving station after performing patient care • After removing gloves
After touching patient surroundings	• After touching dialysis machine • After touching other items within dialysis station • After using chairside computers for charting • When leaving station • After removing gloves

From CDC Dialysis Collaborative: Version 11/30/2010. Retrieved from https://www.cdc.gov/dialysis/PDFs/collaborative/Hemodialysis-Hand-Hygiene-Observations.pdf.

When handwashing with soap and water, the hands should be rubbed together for at least 15 seconds followed by a rinse. When decontaminating with an alcohol-based hand rub, the product should be applied to the palm of the hand and the hands rubbed together until dry. Some dispensers can be set to deliver the exact amount of soap or hand rub recommended by the manufacturer.

The CDC has established guidelines for hand hygiene opportunities in the hemodialysis setting. Table 10.1 outlines these guidelines.

The length of fingernails should be considered because studies have documented that long fingernails (more than ¼ inch) can harbor high concentrations of bacteria. Even after careful washing, long fingernails may harbor significant numbers of pathogens, such as gram-negative rods, corynebacteria, and yeasts, in the subungual space. Artificial fingernails also contribute to the spread of certain gram-negative pathogens and should not be worn when providing care to patients with compromised immune systems. This is extremely important to keep in mind when caring for patients at a high risk of developing infections.

WHAT ARE SPECIFIC EXAMPLES OF STANDARD PRECAUTIONS IN A DIALYSIS UNIT?

Standard Precautions in a dialysis unit can be summarized into four main categories:
1. Barrier precautions, or PPE, such as gloves, face shields, masks, protective eyewear, impervious or fluid resistant gowns, and lab coats
2. Protection against penetration caused by sharps
3. Good personal hygiene, including no perfumes or colognes because of the possibility of allergies in some patients
4. Good environmental control and avoidance of environmental contamination

During the initiation and termination of dialysis or at any time when there is a risk of exposure to blood-borne pathogens, a mask, protective eyewear (goggles or face shield), and gloves must be worn. An impervious gown or lab coat should be worn if blood is likely to splash. A sharps container should be positioned within reach of the patient caregiver so that the needle or syringe can be disposed of immediately without its having to be placed down and picked up a second time. Hands must be washed after removing gloves and before touching any environmental surface, such as machine knobs, charts, phones, or other equipment. Eating, smoking, applying cosmetics, and handling contact lenses in the treatment area must be prohibited. Good environmental controls include maintaining separate clean and soiled areas as well as adequately cleaning and disinfecting the treatment area and equipment in contact with the patient, such as the chair and blood pressure cuff.

WHAT ARE THE MOST SIGNIFICANT BLOOD-BORNE PATHOGENS?

A blood-borne pathogen simply means a microorganism (usually a virus) that is transmitted in the blood or body fluids and can cause disease in humans. The most significant blood-borne pathogens are HBV, hepatitis C virus (HCV), and

HIV. The efficiency of transmission varies among the viruses because of the number of viruses present in blood. The risk of infection varies and is dependent on the pathogen involved, type of exposure, amount of blood involved, and amount of virus in a patient's blood at the time of exposure.

WHAT IS HEPATITIS?

Hepatitis is an inflammation of the liver caused by infectious agents, medications, or toxins. There are several types of infectious hepatitis, but the most common types are hepatitis A, hepatitis B, and hepatitis C. The three hepatitis viruses are transmitted through different routes. Vaccines are available for both hepatitis B and hepatitis A. A vaccine does not exist at this time for hepatitis C. The CDC reports the rate of new HBV infections declined from 1990 to 2014. The decline has been greatest among children born since 1991, when routine vaccination of children was first recommended. Since 2017, there has been an increase in the rate of new HBV infections, which is likely because of increasing injection drug use (CDC, 2017). The current prevalence of HBV in health care workers is not known but most likely mirrors that of the general population (Lewis, Enfield, & Sifri, 2015).

HOW INFECTIOUS IS THE HEPATITIS B VIRUS?

Hepatitis B virus is highly transmissible because of the high concentration of the virus in the blood of infected people (1 mL of hepatitis B surface antigen [HBsAg]–positive blood may contain 100 million infectious doses of the virus) and the ability of the virus to survive for several days on environmental surfaces at room temperature.

HOW IS THE HEPATITIS B VIRUS TRANSMITTED?

In the dialysis unit, exposure to blood with the possibility of HBV transmission can be either direct or indirect. Direct exposure consists primarily of skin penetration (percutaneous) by sharp objects, such as needles, scalpels, and broken capillary tubes, or contact of blood with broken skin and mucous membranes of the eyes, mouth, or nose.

Indirect exposure involves transmission from environmental surfaces, such as hemostats, clamps, control knobs on dialysis machines, doorknobs, or equipment not disinfected after each use.

The most common ways by which HBV is spread in dialysis units are skin penetration by contaminated sharps and contact of contaminated blood with broken skin or mucous membranes.

ARE ADDITIONAL PRECAUTIONS NECESSARY TO SAFELY DIALYZE AN HBsAg-POSITIVE PATIENT IN THE DIALYSIS UNIT?

Following the CDC guidelines, the CMS recommends routine testing of all patients for HBV before admission to the dialysis unit. All susceptible patients and staff should be offered hepatitis B vaccination. Along with standard precautions, a separate or "isolation" room should be available for dialyzing HBV-positive patients as a standard of practice. Patients with HBV infection are to use a dedicated machine and their dialyzers may not be reprocessed. Gloves and gowns are required to be worn upon entering the isolation room. The same hemodialysis equipment should not be used for both HBsAg-positive and HBsAg-seronegative patients. HBV-positive patients should also have dedicated supplies and medications. HBsAg-positive patients should not participate in a dialyzer reuse program. Ideally, dialysis staff members should not care for both HBsAg-positive and HBsAg-seronegative (susceptible) patients during the same shift but can care for HBsAg-positive and hepatitis B surface antibody (anti-HBs)–positive (immune) patients during the same shift. Staff members who are HBsAg positive may be assigned preferentially to care for HBsAg-positive patients. If for some reason staff members must care for both HBsAg-positive and HBsAg-seronegative patients during the same shift, they must change gowns between patients, wash hands, and change gloves to prevent cross-contamination.

WHAT ARE THE CDC RECOMMENDATIONS FOR HEPATITIS B SEROLOGICAL SCREENING?

Patients should be screened for HBsAg, total hepatitis B core antibody (anti-HBc), anti-HBs, and alanine aminotransferase (ALT) to determine their serological status before they first enter a dialysis unit (Table 10.2). Patients may be identified as HBsAg positive (indicating that the patient has tested positive for the presence of HBsAg), HBsAg negative (indicating that the patient does not have HBsAg), or HBsAg susceptible (indicating that the patient does not have sufficient anti-HBs levels to achieve immunity to HBV). The results of the anti-HBs assay should be quantified numerically; a simple "positive" or "negative" result is not acceptable. The CDC recommends periodic screening for each of the serological status categories. Refer to Box 10.2 for the hepatitis B screening panel information.

WHAT ARE THE CDC RECOMMENDATIONS FOR HEPATITIS B VACCINE?

The CDC strongly recommends the administration of hepatitis B vaccine to susceptible patients and staff as an additional means of preventing HBV in the hemodialysis unit. In addition, if a health care worker has the potential to be exposed to HBV on the job, the employer is required by law to make hepatitis B vaccination available at no cost. The CDC recommends a higher vaccine dosage or increased number of doses for patients undergoing hemodialysis (CDC, 2012).

Today's vaccines are safe and effective. Hepatitis B vaccines now used in the United States are made using yeast and therefore cannot be infected with HIV or blood-borne pathogens. More than 2 million US health care workers have already been vaccinated. The complete series of hepatitis B vaccinations is 85% to 97% effective at protecting a person from contracting the disease or becoming a carrier.

Table 10.2 How do I Interpret Some of the Common Hepatitis B Panel Results?

TESTS	RESULTS	INTERPRETATION	VACCINATE?
HBsAg Anti-HBc Anti-HBs	Negative Negative Negative	Susceptible	Vaccinate if indicated
HBsAg Anti-HBc Anti-HBs	Negative Negative Positive with $\geq$10mIU/mL*	Immune due to vaccination (or may represent passive transfer of antibodies from receipt of HBIG)	No vaccination necessary
HBsAg Anti-HBc IgM anti-HBc Anti-HBs	Negative Positive Negative Positive	Immune due to natural infection	No vaccination necessary
HBsAg Anti-HBc IgM anti-HBc Anti-HBs	Negative Positive Positive Positive	Acute resolving infection	No vaccination necessary
HBsAg Anti-HBc IgM anti-HBc Anti-HBs	Positive Positive Positive Negative	Acutely infected	No vaccination necessary
HBsAg Anti-HBc IgM anti-HBc Anti-HBs	Positive Positive Negative Negative	Chronically infected	No vaccination necessary (may need treatment)
HBsAg Anti-HBc Anti-HBs	Negative Positive Negative	Four interpretations possible[†]	Use clinical judgment

*Postvaccination testing, when it is recommended, should be performed 1-2 months after the last dose of vaccine. Infants born to HBsAg-positive mothers should be tested for HBsAg and anti-HBs after completion of at least 3 doses of a licensed hepatitis B vaccination series, at age 9-18 months (generally at the next well child visit).

[†]1. May be distantly immune, but the test may not be sensitive enough to detect a very low level of anti-HBs in serum
2. May be susceptible with a false positive anti-HBc
3. May be chronically infected and have an undetectable level of HBsAg present in the serum
4. Passive transfer of antibody following HBIG administration or from an HBsAg-positive mother to her newborn

Modified from Immunization Action Coalition: Ask the Experts: Hepatitis B. Retrieved from http://www.immunize.org/askexperts/experts_hepb.asp.

Box 10.2 Hepatitis B Screening Panel

- **Hepatitis B surface antigen (HBsAg)** is a protein on the surface of the hepatitis B virus (HBV); its presence indicates that the person is infectious. It persists indefinitely in chronic carriers.
- **Hepatitis B surface antibody (anti-HBs)** is a marker of immunity. Its presence indicates recovery and immunity from HBV infection, either from past infection or through vaccination.
- **Total hepatitis B core antibody (anti-HBc)** appears at the onset of symptoms in acute hepatitis B and indicates previous or ongoing infection with HBV.
- **IgM antibody to hepatitis B core antigen (IgM anti-HBc)**, if positive, indicates recent infection with the HBV (<6 months) and acute infection.
- **Hepatitis B early antigen (HBeAg)** is a protein produced and found in the serum during acute and chronic HBV infection. Its presence indicates that the virus is replicating and the infected person has high levels of HBV and increased infectivity. It is positive during both acute infection or through vaccination.
- **Hepatitis B early antibody (HBeAb or anti-HBe):** A serum marker for hepatitis B appearing 8 to 16 weeks after infection. It is produced by the immune system temporarily during acute HBV infection or consistently during or after a burst in viral replication. Spontaneous conversion from e antigen to e antibody (a change known as seroconversion) is a predictor of long-term clearance of HBV and indicates resolution of acute infection.

IgM, Immunoglobulin M.

Modified from Mast EE, Margolis HS, Fiore AE, et al: A comprehensive immunization strategy to eliminate transmission of hepatitis B virus infection in the United States: recommendations of the Advisory Committee on Immunization Practices, part 1: Immunization of infants, children, and adolescents. *MMWR Recommendations and Reports* 54(RR-16):1–31, 2005.

What If I Lose Antibody Protection After a Couple of Years?

The Public Health Service Advisory Committee on Immunization Practices states: "Individuals who have initially responded to the hepatitis B vaccine with protective levels of anti-HBs, and then lose detectable antibodies, do not need to receive booster shots. They are protected and will not develop clinical hepatitis." However, dialysis patients may have less complete vaccine-induced protection that may persist only as long as the antibodies remain at a certain level. Dialysis patients may need a booster dose and should undergo antibody testing annually.

What Steps Should Be Taken After Occupational Exposure to Blood?

Institutions have in place a plan for occupational exposure that includes reporting, evaluating the risk of infection, available treatments, and postexposure monitoring. When exposed to blood, administration of first aid to the exposed individual is the first step. Needlestick injuries and cuts should be washed with soap and water, and splashes to the mouth, nose, or skin should be flushed with water. Eyes that have been exposed to blood should be irrigated with clean water, saline, or sterile saline solution. The exposure should then be reported to the immediate supervisor so that appropriate evaluation and counseling can take place. Postexposure blood testing of the exposed and source patient should be completed as soon as possible. PEP will be offered if indicated to reduce the chance of becoming infected with HIV or hepatitis. It is important to be prompt when seeking PEP because the prophylaxis for HIV should be instituted within hours after exposure. The medications used for PEP have numerous side effects, which is why they are recommended only when the exposure is a risk of transmission. PEP for hepatitis B should begin within 24 hours after exposure, which can significantly reduce the risk of acquiring the virus. PEP is not recommended for health care personnel who have experienced exposure to HCV. The risk of positive conversion after exposure to HCV is approximately 1.8%. Baseline testing for anti-HCV and ALT is recommended within 48 hours of exposure and again in 3 weeks (CDC, 2018). Health care workers should always protect themselves and their coworkers by using Safe Needle Devices (SNDs) when indicated, using SNDs as the manufacturer suggests, disposing of needles and sharps immediately into an appropriate container, and reporting all sharps and needlestick exposures.

What Is HIV?

HIV attacks the body's immune system, causing the disease known as acquired immunodeficiency syndrome (AIDS). HIV weakens the immune system by destroying cells that fight disease and infection. Currently, there is no vaccine to prevent HIV infection.

How Infectious Is HIV?

The efficiency of HIV transmission in the dialysis setting is much less than that of HBV because of the lower concentration of HIV in blood compared with the concentration of HBV. The concentration of HIV in blood is approximately 10 to 10,000 infectious viruses per milliliter. As of December 2013, the CDC had received voluntary reports of 58 documented and 150 possible episodes of HIV transmission to health care personnel in the United States. Of the 57 documented episodes, 48 transmissions were from percutaneous exposure. Health care workers exposed to needle stick involving HIV-infected blood have a 0.23% risk of becoming infected if untreated. The risk of transmission from body fluids and fluid splashes to intact skin or mucous membranes is considered low risk of HIV transmission, whether blood is or not involved (CDC, 2016).

How Is HIV Transmitted?

Like other blood-borne pathogens, HIV is present in the blood of infected individuals. HIV is transmitted primarily through sexual contact but may also be transmitted through contact with blood and body fluids. The virus can also be passed to a newborn infant from an infected mother. Transmission through contact with contaminated environmental surfaces has not been documented. The virus is very sensitive to chemical disinfection and is completely inactivated by a 10% solution of 0.5% sodium hypochlorite (bleach) within 1 minute of exposure.

No airborne transmission of HBV or HIV has been documented. However, splashing, splattering, centrifuge accidents, or removal of stoppers from tubes can produce droplet transfer into the mouth or eyes or onto defects in the skin surface. HIV cannot reproduce, and it cannot survive on inanimate objects.

What HIV-Related Precautions Are Necessary in a Dialysis Unit?

Standard Precautions are the only thing necessary to protect patients and staff from HIV infection in a dialysis setting. Patient isolation is not necessary because of the lack of an environmental route for transmission of the virus and the low number of viruses in blood. It is not necessary to cohort or group together HIV-positive patients. HIV testing is not recommended as a part of infection control in a dialysis unit. Also, it should not be used as a prerequisite for admission to a dialysis unit but may be helpful for optimal medical management and counseling. HIV testing should be part of a transplant workup because a transplant could be contraindicated in some patients who are already immunosuppressed because of HIV. If HIV antibody testing is performed, informed consent, appropriate confirmation testing, appropriate professional counseling, and confidentiality of test results must be ensured.

Can Dialyzers Be Reused for Known HIV-Positive Patients?

Although the CDC believes that dialyzer reuse poses no specific threat if performed correctly, there are dialysis units that do not reuse dialyzers of known HIV-positive patients.

What If I Am Exposed to Blood From Someone Known to Be Positive for or Who Tests Positive for HIV?

As with any blood exposure, you should immediately notify your supervisor because this is an urgent medical concern. The source patient should be tested for evidence of HIV infection after consent is obtained. The CDC recommends that workers with occupational exposure to HIV should receive follow-up counseling and medical evaluation, including HIV antibody tests at baseline and periodically for at least 6 months after exposure (e.g., 6 weeks, 12 weeks, and 6 months), and should observe precautions to prevent possible secondary transmission.

In 1996, the Public Health Service published source materials and provisional recommendations for chemoprophylaxis (preventive drug therapy) after occupational exposure to HIV by the type of exposure. Although these recommendations are provisional because they are based on limited data, chemoprophylaxis should be recommended to exposed workers after occupational exposure associated with the highest risk for HIV transmission. A 4-week, two-drug PEP regimen is recommended to begin within 72 hours for a warranted exposure. For exposure with a lower but nonnegligible risk, PEP should be offered, balancing the lower risk against the use of drugs with uncertain efficacies and toxicities. If exposed, a physician should be consulted to determine whether antiretroviral medication is warranted (CDC, 2016).

What Is Hepatitis C?

Hepatitis C is a serious liver disease that results from infection with HCV. It is the most common form of hepatitis in the United States, and the CDC estimates 2.7 to 3.9 million persons are chronically infected nationwide (CDC, 2018). A vaccine for HCV prevention does not exist.

How Infectious Is the Hepatitis C Virus?

Hepatitis C virus is less concentrated in blood than HBV and does not survive long on environmental surfaces. The concentration of infectious viruses is thought to be less than 1000 viral organisms per milliliter. However, outbreaks have occurred in dialysis units and are thought to be caused by poor infection control practices. People at an increased risk of acquiring HCV include intravenous drug users, health care workers with occupational exposure to blood, hemodialysis patients, and transfusion recipients. Long-term dialysis patients are at an increased risk of contracting HCV. The number of years on dialysis, history of blood transfusion, and volume of blood transfused are all risk factors associated with HCV infection.

Hepatitis C virus transmission may also occur because of inadequate infection control practices. Cross-contamination between patients can be a problem when machine and other environmental surfaces are not disinfected between patient use, when supplies are shared between patients, and when blood spills are not cleaned up promptly. The estimated number of new HCV infections in the United States in 2016 was 41,200 (CDC, 2018).

How Is the Hepatitis C Virus Transmitted?

Like HBV and other blood-borne pathogens, HCV is transmitted through percutaneous exposure to infected blood. HCV transmission within the dialysis environment can be prevented by strict adherence to the infection control precautions recommended for all hemodialysis patients.

Are Additional Precautions Necessary to Safely Dialyze a Patient in the Dialysis Unit Who Is Hepatitis C Positive?

Patients who are positive for the HCV antibody do not need to be isolated or dialyzed separately on dedicated machines. They may participate in dialyzer reuse programs if their liver enzyme values are acceptable.

What Are the CDC Recommendations for Hepatitis C Serological Screening?

Routine screening of patients or staff for the HCV antibody is not necessary for purposes of infection control. However, dialysis centers may wish to conduct serological surveys of their patient populations to determine the prevalence of the virus in the center and to determine medical management for patients or staff with a diagnosis of HCV. Diagnostic blood tests for HCV infection include the HCV antibody and HCV ribonucleic acid (RNA) tests (Table 10.3).

Although the HCV antibody test has a sensitivity of about 90%, it does not distinguish between acute and chronic infection. In addition, the test does not distinguish between people who are infectious and those who have completely recovered and cannot transmit the disease to someone else. Although the CDC does not recommend routine screening for HCV, regular monitoring of liver enzymes is recommended for the detection of all types of hepatitis, including hepatitis C.

All patients should be monitored monthly for liver enzymes, ALT, and aspartate aminotransferase (AST) to detect HCV. Elevations in liver enzymes are currently more sensitive indicators of acute HCV infection than is the detection of the HCV antibody.

In the absence of unexplained ALT elevations, testing for anti-HCV every 6 months should be sufficient to monitor the occurrence of new HCV infections. If unexplained ALT elevations are observed in patients who are anti-HCV negative, repeat anti-HCV testing is warranted. If unexplained ALT elevations persist in patients who repeatedly test anti-HCV negative, testing for HCV RNA should be considered (CDC, 2001). See recommended testing sequence for identifying current HCV infection in Fig. 10.1 (CDC, 2013).

Table 10.3 Interpretation of Results of Tests for Hepatitis C Virus Infection and Further Actions

TEST OUTCOME	INTERPRETATION	FURTHER ACTIONS
HCV antibody nonreactive	(i) No HCV antibody detected	Sample can be reported as nonreactive for HCV antibody. No further action required. If recent exposure in a person tested is suspected, test for HCV RNA.[a]
HCV antibody reactive	(ii) Presumptive HCV infection	A repeatedly reactive result is consistent with current HCV infection, past HCV infection that has resolved, or biologic false positivity for HCV antibody. Test for HCV RNA to identify current infection.
HCV antibody reactive, HCV RNA detected	(iii) Current HCV infection	Provide the person tested with appropriate counseling and link the person tested to care and treatment.[b]
HCV antibody reactive, HCV RNA not detected	(iv) No current HCV infection	No further action is required in most cases. If distinction between true positivity and false biological positivity for HCV antibody is desired and if the sample is repeatedly reactive in the initial test, test with another HCV antibody assay. In certain situations,[c] follow up with HCV RNA testing and appropriate counseling.

[a]If hepatitis C virus (HCV) RNA testing is not feasible and the person tested is not immunocompromised, perform follow-up testing for HCV antibodies to demonstrate seroconversion. If the person tested is immunocompromised, consider testing for HCV RNA.
[b]It is recommended before initiating antiviral therapy to retest for HCV RNA in a subsequent blood sample to confirm HCV RNA positivity.
[c]If the person tested is suspected of having HCV exposure within the past 6 months or has clinical evidence of HCV disease or if there is concern regarding the handling or storage of the test specimen.
From CDC: Testing for HCV infection: an update of guidance for clinicians and laboratories. *MMWR Morbidity and Mortality Weekly Report* 62(18):362–365, 2013.

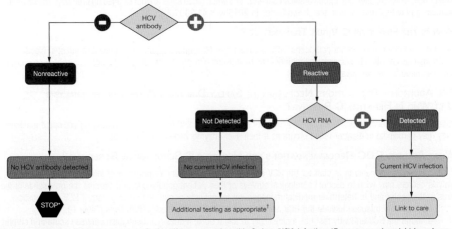

Fig. 10.1 Recommended testing sequence for identifying current hepatitis C virus (HCV) infection. *For persons who might have been exposed to HCV within the past 6 months, testing for HCV RNA or follow-up testing for HCV antibody is recommended. For persons who are immunocompromised, testing for HCV RNA can be considered. †To differentiate past, resolved HCV infection from biologic false positivity for HCV antibody, testing with another HCV antibody assay can be considered. Repeat HCV RNA testing if the person tested is suspected to have had HCV exposure within the past 6 months or has clinical evidence of HCV disease or if there is concern regarding the handling or storage of the test specimen. (From Centers for Disease Control and Prevention (CDC): Testing for HCV infection: an update of guidance for clinicians and laboratorians. *MMWR Morbidity and Mortality Weekly Report* 62(18):362–325, 2013.)

What Should Be Done If I Am Exposed to the Hepatitis C Virus?

Postexposure prophylaxis for HCV is not recommended for health care personnel after blood or other body fluid exposure. Testing for the HCV antibody should be done within 48 hours of exposure and repeated at 6 months. The CDC reports that after a needlestick or sharps exposure to HCV positive blood, the risk of HCV infection is approximately 1.8% (CDC, 2018).

What Is Tuberculosis?

Tuberculosis is an infectious disease caused by the bacterium *Mycobacterium tuberculosis* and usually attacks the lungs but can attack any part of the body.

How Is Tuberculosis Transmitted?

The bacteria are carried in airborne particles (droplet nuclei) that are generated when people with pulmonary or laryngeal TB who are not receiving effective antituberculosis medication cough or sneeze. The small droplets can remain suspended in air for prolonged periods. While airborne on normal room currents, these droplet nuclei can infect individuals as soon as the inhaled droplets containing the bacilli become established in the alveoli of the lungs.

A healthy immune system usually limits further multiplication 2 to 10 weeks after initial infection, and the person does not become ill. A positive TB skin test result is usually the only evidence of infection.

Approximately 10% of these healthy individuals with latent TB develop active TB months or years later. However, for people infected with HIV, the risk of progression to active infectious disease is markedly increased. The CDC estimates that approximately one fourth of the world's population is infected with TB, with 1.3 million TB-related deaths annually. The rate of TB in the United States is declining, with a 1.6% decrease from 2016. Approximately 9105 TB cases were reported in the United States in 2017, representing the lowest number of reported cases since recording began in 1953 (CDC, 2017).

What Is the Difference Between Tuberculosis Infection and Active Tuberculosis?

Patients who progress to active contagious TB are capable of transmitting the disease. Those who are infected but who have not progressed to active TB will have no symptoms, will not be contagious, and will not know they are infected unless they have a positive Mantoux skin test result. It may take months or years before the person progresses to active TB, or the person may never develop active TB. Symptoms of active TB include prolonged coughing for 3 weeks or more, fatigue, fever, weight loss, and night sweats. Medication and therapy are available.

Is Tuberculosis a Problem in Dialysis Units?

Tuberculosis rates have decreased in US citizens, both born in and out of the United States. Outbreaks have been reported in correctional facilities, hospitals, and some dialysis units. The level of transmission risk varies by the type of health care facility. For example, the risk of acquiring TB may be greater in emergency departments where patients are provided care before screening and diagnosis take place.

Can a Patient with Active, Contagious Tuberculosis Be Safely Dialyzed in an Outpatient Facility?

Patients with active TB disease should not be dialyzed in ambulatory settings while infectious. These patients must be referred to hospitals with appropriate isolation accommodations (separate room, negative pressure, and so on) as prescribed by the CDC guidelines. The CMS end-stage renal disease (ESRD) program regulations require freestanding dialysis units to have backup agreements with a hospital. This may provide a mechanism for referring active TB patients for dialysis treatment until they are no longer infectious.

What Are the CDC Recommendations for Tuberculosis Screening?

Two types of tests are available to detect TB bacteria: the tuberculin skin test (TST) and TB blood tests. A positive skin or blood test result reveals that a person has been exposed to TB and whether he or she is currently infected with the TB bacteria. Chest radiography and sputum analysis are required to confirm TB active infection. Health care workers should be screened at the onset of employment. TB screening is often done at least annually or as determined by state regulations (CDC, 2017). The frequency of TB screening is often based on an institution's risk assessment, including the community TB profile. If you live and work in an area with a high incidence of TB, screening may be more frequent.

Patients should be screened on or before their first dialysis treatment. The CDC recommends that all dialysis patients be tested at least once for baseline TST results and be rescreened if TB exposure is detected.

New dialysis patients may arrive after hospitalization or an extensive workup. If a recent (within the past year) chest radiography or TST was included, initial screening may not be necessary unless risk factors are present.

The CDC recommends that the two-step Mantoux skin test be used for baseline screening. The Mantoux technique involves intradermal injection of 0.1 mL of purified protein derivative (PPD) tuberculin containing 5 tuberculin units. The two-step procedure (if the initial PPD result is negative, the test is repeated 1–3 weeks later) is used for baseline testing in people who periodically receive TB skin tests to reduce the likelihood of mistaking a booster reaction for a new infection.

Nonroutine screening of patients and staff should be conducted as needed in response to clinical symptoms or documented exposure, such as an active case identified among patients or staff.

A new method of TB surveillance is the interferon-gamma release assay (IGRA), which is a whole blood test that can help diagnose *M. tuberculosis*. There are currently two IGRAs approved by the Food and Drug Administration (FDA). IGRA does not differentiate between latent and active TB but measures a person's immune reactivity to *M. tuberculosis*. The advantages of IGRA include the availability of results within 24 hours and elimination of the probability of a boosted response on subsequent testing. This test is not yet widely used but can be an alternate testing method, with each institution evaluating the benefits and indications for its use (CDC, 2012).

WHAT ARE DRUG-RESISTANT ORGANISMS?

Drug-resistant organisms are bacteria that have mutated to defend themselves against commonly used antibiotics. Resistant strains develop quickly and crossbreed, transferring their resistance to other bacteria. VRE and MRSA are two bacteria known to be resistant to antibiotic therapy. Both have become important nosocomial pathogens in US hospitals and health care facilities. MRSA and VRE may cause infections in patients who are immunosuppressed, including dialysis patients, cancer and HIV patients, older adults, newborns, and those being treated with multiple antibiotics. Those at an increased risk of acquiring infections from drug-resistant organisms include nursing home patients, patients with frequent hospital admissions or prolonged hospital stays, patients with chronic illnesses requiring steroid therapy, patients with catheters (e.g., subclavian catheters), and patients with incisions and other openings into the body. TB can also become drug resistant and occurs when the drugs used to treat TB are not taken correctly, such as not completing the full course of treatment or when prescribed the wrong medications.

HOW ARE MRSA AND VRE TRANSMITTED?

MRSA

The main route of transmission of MRSA is by health care workers' hands that have become contaminated by contact with a patient who either is infected with or carries the organism. People may carry the organism in their noses or on their skin. Some people are carriers; others can become infected through boils, wound infections, or pressure ulcers. MRSA commonly infects wounds, exit sites, and access sites. Environmental surfaces may also be contaminated with MRSA and act as a reservoir for the bacteria.

VRE

Enterococci are normal flora of the gastrointestinal and female genital tracts. Because of this, most infections with these microorganisms have been attributed to sources within the patient. However, recent reports indicate that enterococci, including VRE, can spread by direct person-to-person contact or indirectly via transient carriage on the hands of personnel or contaminated environmental surfaces and patient care equipment.

CAN A PATIENT WITH MRSA OR VRE BE SAFELY DIALYZED IN AN OUTPATIENT FACILITY?

Standard infection control or standard precautions recommended by the CDC should provide sufficient protection against the transmission of MRSA in the dialysis unit.

The CDC Standard Precautions include the following:

- Wash hands after touching blood, body fluids, excretions, and contaminated items, even when wearing gloves. Also, wash hands after gloves are removed, between tasks, and between procedures on the same patient to prevent cross-contamination of different body sites.
- Wear gloves when touching blood, body fluids, excretions, and contaminated items. Gloves should be put on before touching mucous membranes and nonintact skin, and they should be removed promptly after use.
- Wear a mask and eye protection or face shield. These will protect the mucous membranes of the eyes, nose, and mouth during procedures that are likely to cause splashing or spraying of body fluids.
- Wear a gown for protection from skin contamination and soiling of clothing during procedures and patient care activities.
- Handle patient care equipment that is soiled with body fluids and excretions in a manner that prevents skin exposures and contamination of clothing. Make sure reusable equipment is not used for the care of other patients until it has been sanitized.

In addition to these standard precautions, patients with VRE who have draining wounds not contained by dressings, who have diarrhea or are incontinent, who have poor hygiene, or who are confused and are handling their dressings should be dialyzed in a separate room or area. It is important to dedicate the use of noncritical items, such as stethoscopes or sphygmomanometers, to a single patient or group of patients who are infected with or are carriers of VRE. If such devices are to be used on other patients, adequate cleaning and disinfecting must first take place.

WHAT ARE CARBAPENEM-RESISTANT ENTEROBACTERIACEAE?

Carbapenem-resistant Enterobacteriaceae (CRE) are a family of bacteria that are highly resistant to common antibiotics and therefore very difficult to treat. *Klebsiella* spp. and *Escherichia coli* are examples of Enterobacteriaceae, which form normal part of the human intestines (gut). These bacteria sometimes spread outside the gut and cause serious infections such as pneumonia; bloodstream, urinary, and wound infections; and meningitis. Carbapenem is an antibiotic frequently used to treat infections caused by bacteria such as *E. coli* and *Klebsiella pneumoniae*. Because antibiotics have been overused, many Enterobacteriaceae have become resistant to the antibiotics used to treat these organisms. CRE most often occur in individuals who are ill or those in acute or long-term health care settings. Other individuals at risk are those who are immune compromised, have diabetes, on mechanical ventilation, or have an invasive device such as an indwelling catheter.

Carbapenem-resistant Enterobacteriaceae are of concern because they are associated with a high mortality rate of up to 50% (CDC, 2015). Contact precautions should be taken when a patient is colonized or infected with CRE. Strict adherence to hand hygiene recommendations should always be followed when caring for all patients to avoid transmission via health care workers' hands. Minimizing devices such as central venous and urinary catheters should be encouraged to help reduce the risk of infection.

ARE DIALYSIS PATIENTS SUSCEPTIBLE TO *CLOSTRIDIUM DIFFICILE* COLITIS?

Clostridium difficile is a bacteria that causes inflammation of the colon, or colitis. It is often seen in individuals who require prolonged use of antibiotics. Those taking antibiotics are 7 to 10 times more likely to get *C. difficile* while taking antibiotics or 30 days after the treatment has ended. It is experienced more frequently in those greater than 65 years of age and in those who reside in nursing homes or are hospitalized. Because dialysis patients are frequently exposed to antibiotics, they are susceptible to *C. difficile* infection, and the infection is higher than in the general population. Symptoms include watery diarrhea, fever, diminished appetite, nausea, and abdominal pain and tenderness. The CDC (2015) recommends wearing gloves and gowns when treating patients with *C. difficile* and handwashing with soap and water because hand sanitizer does not kill the bacteria.

WHAT ARE THE STERILIZATION AND DISINFECTION PROCEDURES IN A DIALYSIS UNIT?

All dialysis units must have written policies and procedures that deal with disinfection of the dialysis fluid pathway of the hemodialysis machine. These procedures are targeted to control bacterial contamination and do not involve preventing blood-borne infections. The procedures generally consist of using sodium hypochlorite (bleach) on a regular basis (according to the manufacturer's instructions) and a sterilant overnight at certain intervals (e.g., every 100 hours of use). Studies have shown that HIV is inactivated rapidly after being exposed to commonly used chemical germicides at concentrations much lower than those used in practice. The more resistant HBV is also known to be inactivated by common household bleach. Suggested concentrations of sodium hypochlorite for daily preparation range from 500 ppm (1:100 dilution of household bleach) to 5000 ppm (1:10 dilution). It is important to follow the manufacturer's label instructions for correct dilution of disinfectant. Environmental Protection Agency–registered disinfectants such as sodium hypochlorite are preferred over household bleach products for surface disinfection. Routine disinfection can be done using a low-level disinfectant, but intermediate-level disinfectants should be used when surfaces are visibly contaminated with blood or body fluids. Intermediate-level disinfectants are potent enough to inactivate mycobacteria and are tuberculocidal. It is advisable to use intermediate level disinfectant for routine and intermediate disinfection to minimize confusion when selecting products to disinfect (CDC, 2016).

HOW SHOULD OTHER SURFACES BE CLEANED?

Machine surfaces, patient chairs, and other surrounding furniture and equipment, such as infusion pumps, should be routinely wiped with a 1:100 to 1:10 bleach solution after every patient treatment. Environmental surfaces such as walls, floors, and other surfaces should be routinely cleaned, consistent with good housekeeping practices. Disinfection must adhere to the minimum wet contact duration as specified by the product label. Patients should not be present at the station during disinfection. The CDC specifies that routine disinfection after treatment should not take place until it is patient-free or when the patient who just received treatment at that station has physically left that station. A patient-free interval is necessary to ensure thorough disinfection to minimize the risk of cross contamination as well as prevent the patient from being exposed to disinfection fumes (CDC, 2016). Special attempts to disinfect or sterilize these surfaces are not necessary. Blood spills should be cleaned immediately. Linen soiled with blood or body fluids should be transported in leak-proof bags. A facility-wide procedure for cleaning and disinfection of priming buckets should be established to include cleaning, disinfecting, and air drying. Prime buckets should be dry before being attached to the machine after disinfection. All disposable supplies brought to the patient station but not used should be discarded posttreatment. Chairside computer stations, keyboards, and touchscreens on dialysis machines should be disinfected after patient treatment with the manufacturer's recommended disinfecting agent.

WHAT ARE SOME KEY AREAS OF OBSERVATION MADE DURING A BASIC ESRD CMS SURVEY FOR INFECTION CONTROL?

Guidelines from the CDC as well as some specific CMS developed guidelines are applied to both chronic dialysis in-center facility and home dialysis programs. CMS has developed a core survey process to ensure a culture of safety for patients undergoing dialysis therapies. The survey is completed by direct observation of patient care practices and seeks to identify that patient care is provided by qualified staff who are knowledgeable and have the resources to deliver care in meeting with the ESRD CfCs (CMS, 2014). The survey process includes observation of the delivery of patient care, staff and patient interviews, and review of medical records and facility logs. Staff performing direct patient care are observed and interviewed with regard to infection control practices and techniques. Staff are monitored for appropriate use of standard precautions and application of PPE. Also monitored are disinfection processes, hand hygiene techniques, and disinfection and handling of medical supplies, including disposables, linens, and medications. The facility's infection control program is reviewed for policies for the prevention of transmission of blood-borne viruses and bacteria among patients, routine serology testing and vaccination for HBV, isolation policies, infection surveillance, and infection control training and education.

What About Waste Disposal?

Two kinds of wastes are seen in dialysis units: regular trash and infectious waste. Regular trash, which is mostly paper and plastic, can be disposed of by the usual practice. Infectious waste, which is usually defined in a dialysis unit as "bloody," must be disposed of in specially labeled red bags. Various states have laws regarding the definition of infectious waste and its disposal.

Has Peritoneal Dialysis Waste Tested Positive for HIV?

HIV antibody has been detected in the dialysate waste of patients infected with HIV. To date, there are no national guidelines for the disposal of the dialysate waste of patients infected with HIV.

Should Additional Precautions Be Taken When Caring for Patients on Home Peritoneal Dialysis?

Standard Precautions must be observed with all patients when there is a possibility of contact with blood or body fluids. In addition, each renal unit devises its own criteria for the safe disposal of waste fluids for patients both at home and in a unit setting. Patients at home should be instructed to drain their bags into the toilet and then seal the empty bag in a plastic bag before disposal with household garbage. In the continuous ambulatory peritoneal dialysis unit, a toilet or sluice should be used whenever possible. Many units use a 1:10 bleach solution following the dialysate. Some units suggest adding 10 mL of bleach to the bag before disposal. If a sink is used for waste disposal, a bleach solution should follow the waste and should be preferably maintained for 30 minutes.

CHAPTER 11

ANTICOAGULATION AND HEPARIN ADMINISTRATION

Blood tends to clot when it encounters any surface other than the lining of a normal blood vessel. This mechanism is vital for preserving the life of an individual. Blood will therefore clot soon after entering the extracorporeal circuit of the hemodialysis system, rendering treatment impossible unless the ability to clot is interrupted. There are several methods to prevent blood coagulation in the extracorporeal circuit, each with advantages and drawbacks for the patient or the practitioner. It is essential that the dialysis practitioner be familiar with more than one method to safely and effectively meet the needs of each hemodialysis patient.

WHAT IS ANTICOAGULATION?

Anticoagulation is the blocking, suppression, or delaying of blood clotting. Clot formation occurs when blood contacts "foreign" surfaces, such as when it enters the bloodlines and dialyzer. Normally, blood does not clot within the vascular system. However, clots can form under certain conditions, most commonly after an injury, when the clot serves to seal the damaged vessel and prevent further blood loss. Anticoagulation therapy in hemodialysis is intended to reduce clotting within the extracorporeal circuit and to optimize dialyzer efficiency leading to a more efficacious dialysis treatment.

WHAT CAUSES BLOOD TO CLOT?

Clotting is part of a complex body process called *hemostasis.* This process involves (1) retraction and contraction of the injured vessel, (2) sticking of blood platelets to the injured area, and (3) a complex interaction of coagulation factors, resulting in a clot. These coagulation factors are present in normal blood and are identified by roman numerals I through V and VII through XIII. Platelets are damaged by contact with a foreign surface. Platelet factor III is released, causing platelets to stick or adhere to the wall of the vessel and start the clotting process. Plasma factors XI and XII are also activated by contact with a foreign surface and contribute to clotting.

WHY DOES BLOOD NOT CLOT WITHIN THE NORMAL VASCULAR SYSTEM?

The lining of the blood vessels, the endothelium, is smooth, allowing the blood to flow freely through the vessels. The surfaces of other cells—vascular endothelial cells, platelets, and red blood cells—are gelatinous and hydrophilic, with a high water content. They have low interfacial tensions and little tendency to adhere when intact.

WHY IS ANTICOAGULATION NEEDED DURING DIALYSIS?

Blood coagulates when it comes in contact with foreign surfaces, such as dialyzers and bloodlines. To avoid this, anticoagulants are used. The first anticoagulant was hirudin, obtained from the heads of medicinal leeches. In 1916, Jay McLean found an anticoagulant in the livers of animals. He called this extract heparin; however, it was not purified for human use until 1936. Its potency was finally standardized in the United States in 1966.

WHAT IS THE NATURE OF HEPARIN?

Heparin is an acid mucopolysaccharide and is neutralized by strong basic compounds such as protamine sulfate, toluidine blue, and quinidine, causing it to lose its anticoagulant properties. Heparin for clinical use includes a number of fractions, with molecular weights (MWs) ranging from 8000 to 14,000 Da. Heparin composed of only low MW (4000–6000 Da) fractions is available in the United States, and although more expensive, it has the benefits of single-dose administration, reduced bleeding risk, and reduced effect on circulating lipases, potentially resulting in lower triglyceride and cholesterol levels in long-term hemodialysis patients. This latter factor may be significant because high triglyceride and cholesterol levels are associated with cardiovascular disease.

HOW DOES HEPARIN PREVENT COAGULATION?

Heparin combines with a blood protein fraction called the heparin cofactor (antithrombin III). The complex of heparin–antithrombin III combines with and inactivates thrombin, activated factor X, and activated factor XI, thus preventing clotting at all three stages of coagulation (Fig. 11.1). The conversion of prothrombin to thrombin is inhibited, as is the conversion of fibrinogen to fibrin. Peak anticoagulant activity is reached 5 to 10 minutes after injection. The half-life of heparin is about 90 minutes for doses usually used in dialysis. The mechanism of heparin inactivation is not completely clear; it is metabolized by the liver and is taken up by the reticuloendothelial system.

ARE THERE DIFFERENT KINDS OF HEPARIN?

Most heparin is derived from pork intestinal mucosa or beef lung. Pork mucosal heparin is more abundant, less expensive, and most commonly used. The US Pharmacopeia (USP) unitage (units of activity per milliliter) for both forms of heparin is the

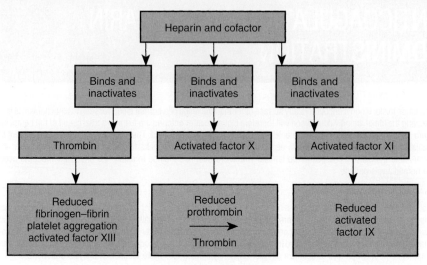

Fig. 11.1 Diagram of the effect of heparin.

same, but there is a difference in their anticoagulant actions on a weight basis; that is, 1 mg of porcine heparin has more anticoagulant activity than 1 mg of beef lung heparin. Beef heparin is no longer commercially available. The reasons for this include the greater expense of beef heparin as well as concerns of beef heparin being associated with a higher incidence of thrombocytopenia. Beef heparin is also less potent than porcine heparin.

What Drugs Interact with Heparin?

Some medications such as aspirin, nonsteroidal antiinflammatory agents, and dextran may enhance the effectiveness of heparin and cause bleeding. Cardiac glycosides, nicotine, quinine, and tetracycline interfere with or decrease the effectiveness of heparin.

How Is the Heparin Dosage Determined?

A patient's heparin dosage is prescribed by the physician and is generally based on the patient's dry weight. Dosage adjustments need to be made if the patient has a change in weight, if the duration of treatment changes, or if the dialyzer membrane changes. Erythropoietin may increase heparin requirement, necessitating an increase in the prescribed amount. The heparin dosage must be low enough to reduce the risk of bleeding yet high enough to prevent clotting in the extracorporeal circuit. With adequate heparinization, the patient will have better clearance of solutes through the dialyzer membrane. Adequate heparinization will also help the dialyzer to clear more thoroughly, allowing the patient to receive as many of the red blood cells as possible when the blood is returned to him or her at the end of the treatment. Because chronic outpatient dialysis units are not able to monitor clotting times on account of Clinical Laboratory Improvement Act (CLIA) mandates, dialysis personnel must be attentive to indications suggesting that the patient may require more or less heparin. Clotting in the dialysis system, poor clearance of the dialyzer after treatment, and inadequate urea clearance may indicate a need to increase heparin dosing. Excessive bleeding or bruising after treatment may indicate a need to decrease heparin dosing.

What Techniques Are Used in Heparin Administration?

Different protocols are available for the administration of heparin for hemodialysis. Systemic heparinization is the most commonly used method. Standard or systemic heparinization is when an initial loading dose of heparin is given before the dialysis treatment. This is typically a dose ordered by the physician and is based on the patient's body weight. An initial bolus of heparin is administered into the venous access needle and no further heparin is administered. Dialysis personnel may administer an additional or a maintenance dose of heparin in the form of repeated separate boluses, or as a continuous infusion based on physician order.

What Is the Continuous Intravenous Heparin Infusion Technique?

A priming or "loading" dose of heparin is administered, as described previously. Heparin is then slowly injected into the extracorporeal system at a constant rate by an infusion pump. This is continued throughout the dialysis treatment, usually at a rate of 1000 to 2000 units/hr. Clotting is evaluated at intervals, usually by saline flushes and visual inspection of the drip chambers or dialyzer fibers (or both), and the heparin infusion rate is adjusted accordingly. Infusion is normally stopped 30 minutes to 1 hour before the end of the treatment to allow the clotting time to begin its return to normal, especially for patients from whom needles must be removed after dialysis.

WHAT IS THE RISK OF BLEEDING WHEN HEPARIN IS USED FOR HEMODIALYSIS?

There is always a risk of bleeding when heparin is used. End-stage renal disease patients tend to bleed more easily because of a platelet dysfunction associated with uremia. One must be particularly concerned about patients who have had surgery within the preceding 24 to 48 hours or are scheduled for surgery immediately after dialysis, those who have recently been injured, those with pericarditis, or those who might have a hemorrhagic lesion of the gastrointestinal tract or uterus. Patients with any coagulopathies should undergo normal saline solution flushes as part of their treatment to prevent clotting in the extracorporeal circuit.

ARE THERE SPECIAL TECHNIQUES FOR USING HEPARIN IN HEMODIALYSIS WHEN THERE IS A RISK OF BLEEDING?

Three approaches have been used in this situation: regional heparinization; low-dose or "tight" systemic heparinization; and no heparin-saline flush techniques.

WHAT IS REGIONAL HEPARINIZATION?

In regional heparinization, an anticoagulant is infused continuously into the inlet (arterial) line of the dialyzer while simultaneously being neutralized by infusing an antidote into the outlet (venous) line before the blood returns to the patient.

In the past, heparin was used as the anticoagulant and protamine sulfate, a low-MW protein derived from salmon sperm, was infused into the venous line. Protamine, a strongly basic protein, bound the acidic heparin and thus neutralized its effect on the coagulation system. However, because of a number of difficulties, such as the precise balancing of the dosage of each infusion, a tendency toward rebound anticoagulation several hours after dialysis, and protamine-induced anaphylaxis, this method is rarely used today.

An alternative method of regional anticoagulation involves the use of sodium citrate. Regional citrate anticoagulation works by binding the ionized calcium present in the extracorporeal circuit. Calcium ions are a required component for the clotting pathway and essential for clot formation. This technique involves infusing trisodium citrate into the arterial line of the dialyzer. A calcium-free dialysate must be used. Because returning blood with decreased ionized calcium to the patient would be dangerous, the process is reversed by the infusion of calcium chloride into the venous line as close as possible to the vascular access connection.

The major disadvantages of this technique are that frequent laboratory tests must be performed to check the patient's total calcium level as well as clotting times. Citrate metabolism produces bicarbonate. The plasma level of bicarbonate thus increases, occasionally to significantly alkalotic levels. (An alternative version uses a large volume of dilute sodium citrate, normal dialysate, and no calcium infusion. The disadvantages are minimized, but the ultrafiltration goals must be adjusted to remove the extra fluid.)

Both types of regional anticoagulation methods require a high level of experience, skill, and attention to detail. With the low-dose or "tight" systemic and heparin-free techniques available today, regional methods are generally reserved for the most critically ill acute dialysis patients.

WHAT IS CITRASATE DIALYSATE, AND HOW IS IT USED AS AN ANTICOAGULANT?

An alternate to regional citrate anticoagulation is Citrasate dialysate, which is an acid concentrate containing a small amount of citric acid that provides mild anticoagulation in the extracorporeal circuit. The concentration of citrate in Citrasate is only 2.4 milliequivalents per liter (mEq/L) or only about one fifth of the concentration used to achieve anticoagulation via traditional regional citrate infusions. Citrasate is particularly useful for challenging patients, including those with heparin-induced thrombocytopenia (HIT), heparin antibodies, severe clotting problems, or bleeding risk factors such as active bleeding, trauma, and prior or subsequent surgery. Citrasate also works well with sustained low-efficiency daily dialysis (SLEDD).

Citrasate contains citric acid, which is an anticoagulant. Citric acid provides an anticoagulative effect in the dialyzer and bloodlines and is quickly neutralized after it enters the systemic circulation. Performing dialysis using a citrate dialysate is no different than dialyzing a patient with a regular bicarbonate dialysate. There is no need to perform additional patient monitoring beyond ordinary measures. Additional blood tests or monitoring are not needed because there are no concerns regarding hypocalcemia, risk of bleeding, or low blood mineral levels from citrate use.

Major benefits of using a citrate dialysate are improved anticoagulation, which leads to a higher dose of dialysis and prevents clotting of fibers in the dialyzer, resulting in better clearances, and the lack of concern regarding hypocalcemia (Advanced Renal Technologies, 2015).

WHAT IS LOW-DOSE OR "TIGHT" HEPARINIZATION?

Low-dose or "tight" heparinization consists of monitoring the patient with frequent clotting times and administering only enough heparin to keep the clotting time at 90 to 120 seconds by activated clotting time (ACT) testing. Low-dose or "tight" heparinization is usually the most practical technique for managing patients who are at risk of bleeding. These include patients who have recently had surgery, those who are menstruating, and those who will undergo central venous catheter removal after treatment. The baseline clotting time is drawn through the first dialysis needle inserted and acts as a guide to the size of the priming dose and maintenance heparin requirements. After administration of the minimal priming dose, usually 10 units/kg of body weight, the heparin dosage is adjusted to provide an ACT of 110 $\pm$ 10 seconds.

In some centers, low-dose or "tight" heparinization is used for patients' first dialysis treatment. A consistent heparin dosage can be established after several treatments. However, because of CLIA restrictions, anticoagulation methods that require the use of clotting time determinations present a problem.

CAN PATIENTS BE HEMODIALYZED WITHOUT HEPARIN?

Heparin-free dialysis has become the method of choice when treating patients with active bleeding and those with an increased risk of bleeding, pericarditis, coagulopathy, or thrombocytopenia. Several techniques are available, including priming the bloodlines and dialyzer with heparinized saline, setting the blood flow rate as high as possible, or rinsing the dialyzer and bloodlines with 100 to 200 mL of normal saline every 15 to 30 minutes.

Most facilities do not prime the system with heparin when the patient is being dialyzed heparin free and use only half-hourly or hourly saline rinses to monitor clotting in the dialyzer or venous drip chamber.

CAN BLOOD BE TRANSFUSED INTO AT-RISK PATIENTS DURING HEPARIN-FREE DIALYSIS?

Blood transfusions can complicate heparin-free dialysis, especially because they commonly involve packed red blood cells. The transfused blood increases the viscosity of the blood in the dialyzer and may infuse clinically significant amounts of normal (i.e., nonuremic) clotting factors. Saline rinses help to keep the system patent and allow for observation of the fibers for any dark streaks that may indicate clotting. The other parameters (saline flushes, blood flow rate, and so on) remain the same as those used in heparin-free dialysis.

WHAT ARE THE CONTRIBUTING FACTORS THAT PREVENT HEMORRHAGE DURING HEMODIALYSIS?

Success in preventing hemorrhage during the dialysis procedure rests on the general management of the patient and the care with which dialysis is performed. The bleeding tendency of uremic patients is correctable with adequate dialysis. The technique used for anticoagulation during dialysis is an important part of the process because any coagulation in the extracorporeal circuit will impair treatment outcome. Thus timely institution of an adequate dialysis program is an important initial factor in the prevention of hemorrhage, but subsequent success depends on careful and continuous attention to all of the factors related to optimal treatment adequacy.

CHAPTER 12

ACCESS TO THE BLOODSTREAM

HISTORICAL BACKGROUND

Effective hemodialysis became a reality in the 1940s. Each treatment required a surgical cutdown. Hollow tubes (cannulas) of glass or metal were inserted into an artery and a vein. The glass and metal tubes were later replaced with cannulas made of polyvinyl chloride or other plastic materials. During the 1950s, attempts were made to leave the cannulas in place for more than one treatment. Different methods of maintaining patency were attempted. At best, these attempts lasted only a few treatments.

In 1960, Scribner, Quinton, and Dillard at the University of Washington devised a cannula that could be left in place much longer. It consisted of Teflon tubes, one placed in an artery and the other in a vein. These tubes were connected externally, allowing for continuous rapid flow of blood through the device. This technique was improved in 1962 with the use of Silastic (silicone rubber) for the external shunt loop and Teflon for the vessel tips. This allowed greater flexibility of the tubing and increased comfort for the patient. This innovation not only was effective for a single hemodialysis but also offered a method for repeat treatments.

Another major development came in 1966 when Cimino, Brescia, and colleagues developed the forearm internal arteriovenous (AV) fistula. It was created by performing a surgical anastomosis between a forearm artery and vein. The subsequent flow of arterial blood into the vein permitted percutaneous puncture of this vessel and offered adequate flow for hemodialysis.

Use of internal synthetic graft materials began in 1974. Today the most common type of synthetic graft is polytetrafluoroethylene (PTFE). A "button" needle-free form of vascular access was developed in 1980. The button needle-free form worked but not as well as the other internal synthetic graft materials. These new synthetic grafts and devices offered new possibilities for patients who did not have adequate vessels for a Cimino fistula.

In 1961, Shaldon described temporary access for hemodialysis via cannulation of the femoral vein. In 1979, Uldall devised a special catheter for temporary access in the subclavian or internal jugular vein. Introduction of double-lumen catheters further enhanced the means of temporary access by allowing one catheter to function as both the inlet and the outlet ports.

Vascular access, as used for hemodialysis in the early 1960s, has evolved considerably during the past 30 years or more. However, maintaining patent access with adequate blood flow remains one of the major problems in chronically hemodialyzed patients (Fig. 12.1).

INTERNAL ACCESSES

The percentage of prevalent hemodialysis patients in the United States with an AV fistula as their primary vascular access was 52.6% at the beginning of 2009. By May 2017, this percentage had increased to 62.8% (United States Renal Data System [USRDS], 2016).

The goal of the Centers for Medicare & Medicaid Services (CMS), which is based on achievable practice, is a prevalent AV fistula use rate of 66%. The National Kidney Foundation (NKF) Kidney Disease Outcomes Quality Initiative (KDOQI) has established guidelines for the selection of a permanent vascular access for chronic hemodialysis. Current guidelines recommend fistula rates of 50% or greater for incident and at least 40% for prevalent hemodialysis patients. (NKF, 2006).

The Fistula First Breakthrough Initiative (FFBI) was established in 2005 by the CMS to increase AV fistula use in all appropriate hemodialysis patients and to decrease the placement of central venous catheters. A group consisting of the CMS and End-Stage Renal Disease (ESRD) Networks has created a coalition that supports and promotes 13 "Change Concepts" that can provide all hemodialysis patients the opportunity to receive an AV fistula. These Change Concepts are strategies for providing the patient and staff with the resources, tools, and best-demonstrated practices to implement the KDOQI guidelines for vascular access placement.

The order of preference for a vascular access in patients undergoing chronic hemodialysis is as follows: (1) a wrist (radial-cephalic) primary AV fistula (Fig. 12.2A), (2) an elbow (brachiocephalic) primary AV fistula, (3) an AV graft of synthetic material (Fig. 12.2B), or (4) a transposed brachiobasilic vein fistula. If an AV fistula cannot be placed, an AV graft is acceptable. A long-term catheter, such as a cuffed tunneled central venous catheter, should be discouraged as a permanent vascular access. Short-term catheters may be used for acute dialysis but only for a limited duration of time (NKF KDOQI Vascular Access Clinical Practice Guidelines Update, 2006).

Vascular access placement should occur well before the need for dialysis treatment. The 2006 NKF KDOQI Clinical Practice Guidelines for chronic kidney disease (CKD) recommend initiation of a vascular access when the glomerular filtration rate (GFR) is less than $30 \, mL/min/1.73 \, m^2$ (stage 4 CKD). KDOQI guidelines recommend a fistula should be placed

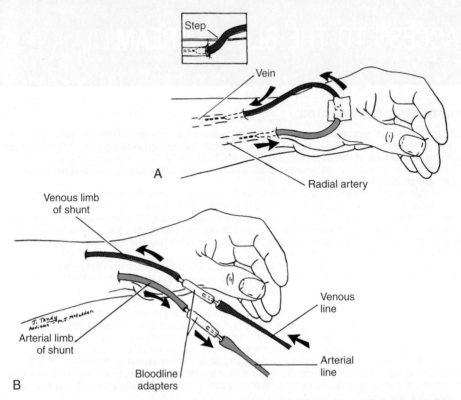

Fig. 12.1 A, Quinton-Scribner shunt with a connector in place between dialysis runs. **B,** Shunt arms separated and connected to dialyzer bloodlines. (From Larson E, Lindbloom I, Davis KB: *Development of the clinical nephrology practitioner,* St. Louis, 1982, Mosby.)

at least 6 months before the anticipated start of hemodialysis treatments, and a graft should be placed at least 3 to 6 weeks before the initiation of maintenance dialysis.

The goal is for the patient to have permanent and functioning access at the time when hemodialysis therapy is initiated. Early referral and placement provide the time needed for the fistula to properly mature and develop. Duplex ultrasound is the preferred method for preoperative vascular mapping and should be performed on all patients before placement of the vascular access. In patients with stage 4 or 5 CKD, veins that could be used for placement of a vascular access, such as those in the forearm and upper arm, should not be used for venipuncture. All patients and staff should be educated on the need to protect potential access vessels. Patients should be encouraged to wear a Medic Alert bracelet that would signal others to avoid using those vessels for venipuncture unless it is an emergency. The timing of access placement is critical so that the patient has a fully functioning access when maintenance dialysis is required. A fistula should be placed at least 6 months before and a graft should be placed at least 3 to 6 weeks before the anticipated start of hemodialysis therapy (NKF Clinical Practice Guidelines and Recommendations, 2006).

ARTERIOVENOUS FISTULAS

WHAT IS AN ARTERIOVENOUS FISTULA?

An AV fistula is an internal access surgically created by a vascular surgeon using the patient's own blood vessels. In an internal AV fistula, a small (5-mm) opening is created surgically in an adjoining artery and vein, and the two vessels are joined at this opening, creating an AV fistula. The two blood vessels used are anastomosed in a side-to-side, end-to-side, or end-to-end connection (Fig. 12.3). The diversion of arterial blood into the vein causes the vein to become enlarged, distended, and prominent, allowing the placement of large-gauge needles for dialysis treatment. The blood flow rate (Qb) and diameter of the access will increase in response to the high pressure of the arterial blood entering the venous system. The KDOQI has issued the "rule of 6s" as an objective measure used to assess maturation of the access. At 6 weeks after creation, the fistula should have a diameter of at least 6 mm with discernible margins while a tourniquet is in place, and the depth should be no more than 0.6 mm below the skin surface. The FFBI defines a fully matured AV fistula as one that can sustain three consecutive two-needle cannulations with no infiltrations at the prescribed needle gauge and support a blood flow rate of 600 mL/min (NKF, 2006; FFBI Coalition, Clinical Practice Workgroup, 2010).

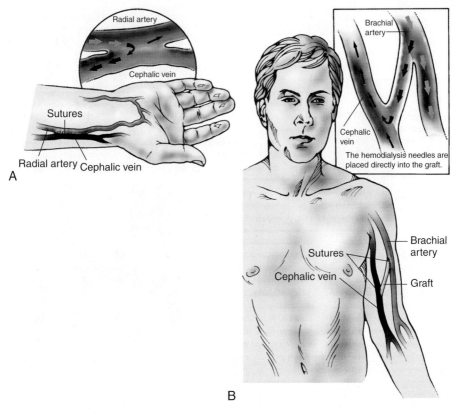

Fig. 12.2 Options for long-term vascular access for hemodialysis. **A,** A surgically created venous fistula. The increased pressure from the artery forces blood into the vein. This process causes the vein to dilate enough for fistula needles to be placed for hemodialysis. When the vein dilates in this manner, the fistula is said to be "developed." **B,** A surgically placed straight vascular graft in the upper arm. The graft creates a shunt between arterial and venous blood. (From Ignatavicius DD, Workman ML: *Medical-surgical nursing: critical thinking for collaborative care*, ed. 6, St. Louis, 2010, Saunders.)

Maturation occurs when there is dilation and thickening of the venous segment of the fistula. This is caused by the increase in the flow and pressure of arterial blood. The vein used to create the AV access will sometimes develop additional branches, which will also enlarge and mature enough to be cannulated for dialysis. This is called *collateral circulation,* and it increases the available surface area for cannulation. However, if collateral circulation prevents development of the main vein, ligation is necessary.

The AV fistula can be placed in the upper or lower arm. The radial artery and cephalic vein (lower arm) (Fig. 12.4) and brachial artery and cephalic vein (upper arm) are commonly used. Proper evaluation of the vasculature and physical assessment play a role in determining the access of choice for each patient. A major cause of early AV fistula failure is the selection of suboptimal vessels. Venography allows identification of appropriate veins and helps to rule out sites that are not suitable for use. Doppler flow studies may also be used if venography is not available.

Every attempt is made to use a patient's nondominant arm to help the patient maintain the present standard of living and to facilitate self-cannulation if the patient performs his or her own dialysis care. The patient must have sufficient arterial blood flow to maintain the access and to provide adequate dialysis treatment. The AV fistula may take up to 4 months or longer to mature enough to allow cannulation.

What Is Basilic Vein Transposition?

Basilic vein transposition is a technique used to create a vascular access in patients with inadequate vessels in the wrist. Vein transposing can be accomplished by either elevating the vessel to bring it closer to the skin or moving it laterally to permit easier cannulation. This transposed vessel technique involves dissecting the basilic vein and transposing it anteriorly and subcutaneously while anastomosing it to the brachial artery (Fig. 12.5). This transposed vessel provides a large surface area for cannulation and requires only one anastomosis. The incision for this access is rather large, with the start of the incision being at the mid-antecubital fossa and extending to the medial aspect of the arm to the axilla. The main

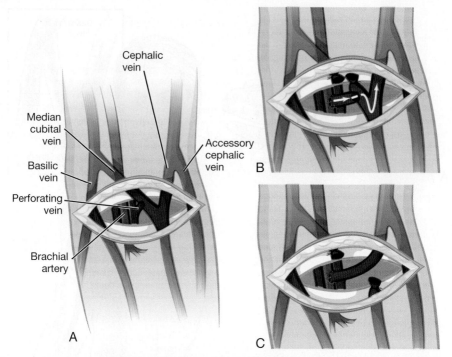

Fig. 12.3 A, Vessels for the creation of an elbow arteriovenous (AV) fistula. **B,** Brachiocubital AV fistula. **C,** Brachiocephalic AV fistula. (From Floege J, Johnson RJ, Feehally J: *Comprehensive clinical nephrology,* ed. 4, St. Louis, 2011, Mosby.)

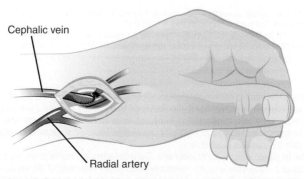

Fig. 12.4 Midforearm radiocephalic fistula is used if the distal radial artery is not suitable. (From Tordoir JH: Vascular access for dialytic therapies. In Feehally J, Floege J, Tonelli M, Johnson RJ, eds: *Comprehensive clinical nephrology,* ed. 6, Philadelphia, 2019, Elsevier, pp. 1050–1061.)

advantage of this type of access placement is the avoidance of using a synthetic graft. As with other autologous grafts, you will see a longer patency rate and fewer risks of infection.

WHAT IS A PROXIMAL RADIAL ARTERY ARTERIOVENOUS FISTULA?

The proximal radial artery arteriovenous fistula (PRA-AVF), also known as a "reverse flow" fistula, is a newer advanced surgical procedure for native AV fistula placement. In this type of access, the proximal radial artery is used for the arterial inflow. The arterial anastomosis is made higher in the arm, and the vein develops both above and below the anastomosis. With this configuration, blood will tend to flow in two directions at the same time, allowing cannulation in both the forearm and the upper arm. When cannulating, if both needles are to be placed in the forearm, the venous needle should be placed downstream (retrograde), with the needle top pointing toward the hand, which is the direction of

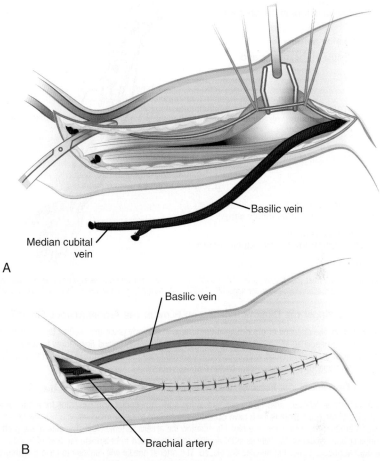

Fig. 12.5 Transposed brachiobasilic arteriovenous fistula. **A,** Dissection of the basilic vein. **B,** Anterolateral transposition and brachial artery anastomosis. (From Floege J, Johnson RJ, Feehally J: *Comprehensive clinical nephrology,* ed. 4, St. Louis, 2011, Mosby.)

blood flow. If the upper arm is used for the venous return, the flow goes toward the heart, so that the needle would be placed upstream (antegrade), with the needle top pointing toward the shoulder (Jennings, Ball, & Duval, 2006) (Fig. 12.6). A PRA-AVF is useful when a patient's forearm veins are damaged or when the patient has advanced arteriosclerotic and calcified radial arteries. This approach has an acceptable survival rate and does not produce circulatory complications such as steal syndrome.

WHAT IS AN ARTERIOVENOUS GRAFT?

When a patient is not a candidate for a native AV fistula, a vascular graft is substituted. An AV graft can be of biological or synthetic material; however, synthetic grafts are used most frequently. The graft material is implanted subcutaneously into either the forearm or the upper arm. In some circumstances when the arm cannot be used, the chest or leg area may be used. The graft bridges an artery on one end and a vein on the other end. The tissue surrounding the graft will grow into and around the graft, helping to stabilize the vessel. The blood flow direction is from the artery to the vein. With the AV graft, the needles for cannulation are placed directly into the graft material.

The graft may be placed in several configurations: straight, looped, or curved. The NKF KDOQI guidelines recommend the use of synthetic over biological materials. Synthetic grafts are made of plastic polymers, such as PTFE or polyurethane (PU). The AV graft may be used as early as 2 to 6 weeks after placement, with the surgeon's approval. The NKF KDOQI guidelines recommend the AVG not be cannulated for at least 2 weeks after placement and after all swelling has subsided (NKF, 2006).

The synthetic graft is used most often in patients who do not have adequate vessels to create an internal AV fistula. With the prolonged time necessary for AV fistula maturation and concomitant catheter exposure, certain patient populations may benefit from AV graft placement versus the preferred AV fistula (USRDS, 2018).

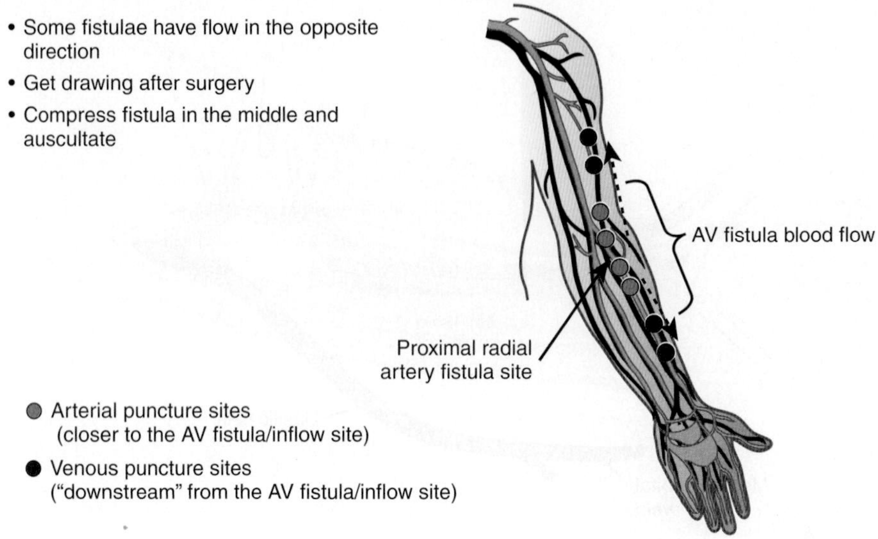

- Some fistulae have flow in the opposite direction
- Get drawing after surgery
- Compress fistula in the middle and auscultate

AV fistula blood flow

Proximal radial artery fistula site

● Arterial puncture sites
  (closer to the AV fistula/inflow site)
● Venous puncture sites
  ("downstream" from the AV fistula/inflow site)

Fig. 12.6 Direction of flow. What you "KNOW" about the "FLOW" is really important with reverse flow arteriovenous fistulas, such as a proximal radial artery fistula. (Courtesy William Jennings, MD, FACS; Lynda Ball, BS, BSN, RN, CNN; and Linda Duval, RN, BSN.)

DO YOU NEED TO KNOW THE DIRECTION OF BLOOD FLOW IN THE ARTERIOVENOUS GRAFT?

It is necessary to know the direction of blood flow in the access to properly place the needles for the hemodialysis treatment. The venous needle should always be placed in the direction of the blood flow (artery to vein). Placing the venous needle against the flow of blood will cause increased resistance to the blood returning to the patient. This will be signified by a high venous pressure reading on the dialysis machine.

HOW DO YOU DETERMINE THE FLOW OF BLOOD IN A LOOPED ARTERIOVENOUS GRAFT?

In a looped or horseshoe AV graft, after gently depressing the graft at midpoint, you can listen for a bruit or feel for a thrill on each side of the graft. Because you have occluded the flow of blood at midpoint, you will still be able to feel a thrill or hear a bruit on the side where the blood is entering the access (arterial side). The side of the graft with little or no thrill or bruit would be the venous side. Another technique used to determine the flow of blood is to palpate the graft at midpoint after the needles are placed. The arterial needle will continue to have a flashback of blood when the graft is compressed at midpoint.

WHAT TYPES OF ARTERIOVENOUS GRAFTS ARE AVAILABLE?

Synthetic grafts are the most common AV grafts currently in use. Many synthetic materials (e.g., Dacron, PTFE) are available in various diameters and lengths. A newer form of PTFE allows for needle insertion immediately after placement, although the manufacturer recommends waiting 5 to 7 days. Fig. 12.7 shows several types of placement for synthetic grafts.

WHAT ARE THE ADVANTAGES OF AN ARTERIOVENOUS GRAFT?

Arteriovenous grafts can be used sooner than AV fistulas, usually after 2 weeks. Maturation time for the vessel to enlarge is not required. The larger vessel size allows for easier cannulation. Table 12.1 lists the advantages and disadvantages of internal accesses.

WHAT ARE THE SPECIAL CARE NEEDS AND POTENTIAL PROBLEMS WITH THE USE OF AN ARTERIOVENOUS FISTULA FOR ACCESS TO THE BLOODSTREAM?

Needle insertions are necessary for each hemodialysis. With repetitive venipuncture, scar tissue forms over the fistula, making the insertion of needles more difficult and painful. Furthermore, if a needle becomes accidentally dislodged and passes through a vessel wall (infiltration), bleeding into the tissues may result in the formation of a painful hematoma. If this occurs, use of the fistula may be difficult or impossible until swelling decreases. At the end of each hemodialysis treatment, after the needles are withdrawn, firm pressure must be applied over the puncture area for 12 to 20 minutes to prevent persistent bleeding.

ARE THERE SPECIAL PROBLEMS WITH AN INTERNAL ARTERIOVENOUS FISTULA?

The size and location of arterialized veins are important. It is often a matter of weeks, and sometimes months, before the veins enlarge sufficiently for large-gauge needles to be inserted without difficulty. This process takes longer in

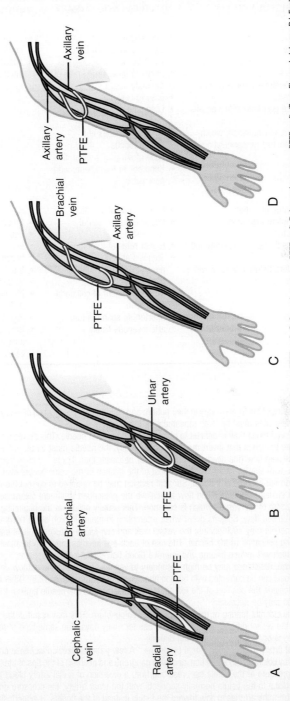

Fig. 12.7 Polytetrafluoroethylene (PTFE) grafts in the arm. **A,** Straight forearm PTFE graft. **B,** Loop forearm PTFE graft. **C,** Curved upper arm PTFE graft. **D,** Looped upper arm PTFE graft. (From Floege J, Johnson RJ, Feehally J: *Comprehensive clinical nephrology*, ed. 4, St. Louis, 2011, Mosby.)

Table 12.1 Advantages and Disadvantages of Internal Accesses

ARTERIOVENOUS FISTULA	ARTERIOVENOUS GRAFT	VENOUS CATHETER
Advantages		
• Permanent • Excellent patency rate • Can last for decades • Highest blood flow rates • Lowest rate of complications (infection, steal syndrome, and stenosis) • Improved performance over time as the access develops • Development of collateral circulation, which creates additional branches for cannulation	• Permanent • Large surface area for cannulation • Ability to span large areas of the body • Easy to cannulate • Less time required for maturation (2 wk) • Variety of shapes and configurations • Ease of surgical implantation • Good option for patients with poor veins	• Can be used immediately • Allows time for the internal access to mature
Disadvantages		
• Failure of vein to enlarge or mature • More difficult to cannulate than graft • Cosmetically unattractive • Must find healthy veins that are in proximity and not too tortuous • Requires time to mature before use (6–8 wk)	• Higher rates of infection • Possible graft material rejection • Higher rates of thrombosis • Stenosis at venous anastomosis from intimal hyperplasia • No development of collateral circulation • Shorter life span than an arteriovenous fistula	• High rates of infection • Greater risk of sepsis • Usually temporary • Increased hospitalizations • Short life span • Inadequate blood flow • Provides inadequate dialysis • High thrombosis rates • Risk of damaging subclavian or other veins

women than in men. The veins of the forearm vary in their pattern and distribution. The location of easily accessible vessels may be limited so that a few sites must be used repeatedly for insertion.

Occasionally, the desired blood flow is difficult to obtain through the inlet needle. This problem may result from the size of the vein or from the branches that divert the flow. Occasionally, the needle must be placed very near the anastomosis to obtain sufficient flow (the needle tip should never be closer than 1½ to 2 inches from the anastomosis). Sometimes, with side-to-side AV fistulas, most of the dilation of the veins occurs over the back of the hand, and the arm veins do not become prominent. Surgical revision may be required to correct the flow of blood when the AV fistula is unable to sustain adequate blood flow to achieve the prescribed treatment clearance.

A third problem is spasm of the vessel, which is common. This usually occurs at the beginning of hemodialysis, causing decreased arterial blood flow. Spasms occur when attempting to maintain high blood flows in an immature fistula. The lumen of the needle may suck against the vessel wall and can cause spasms. This is painful and is accompanied by a fluttering sensation at the needle. The use of back-eye needles may help to minimize the need to flip the dialysis needle, which will reduce trauma and improve blood flow while avoiding spasms.

On the return flow side, resistance may be high secondary to venous stenosis in the outflow vessel above the anastomosis. Venous stenosis can be corrected with balloon angioplasty or dilatation (Fig. 12.8). Other mechanical causes of return flow resistance include the position of the extremity and placement of the needle against the vessel wall. Repositioning of the needle may be necessary.

A fourth problem is accidental tearing of the vessel during venipuncture. This may result in the formation of a large hematoma, making the vessel difficult or impossible to use for many days. The same type of accident may occur if the patient suddenly moves or thrashes about during dialysis.

In addition, the radial artery may develop "steal syndrome." A few patients develop ischemic changes in their fingers. This is manifested by coldness, poor function, and even gangrene and necrosis of the tips of the fingers. The "steal" is caused by low arterial pressure at the fistula site, resulting from a diversion of radial artery blood to the vein. Because the radial artery distal to the fistula normally connects with the ulnar artery, the pressure gradient causes ulnar blood to be diverted from the arteries to flow toward the fistula instead of the fingers. Hypoperfusion of the palm and fingers results, causing pain and coldness that worsens during dialysis treatment. If recognized early, the syndrome may be corrected by surgically tying off the radial artery distal to the fistula. Older adult patients, patients with hypertension,

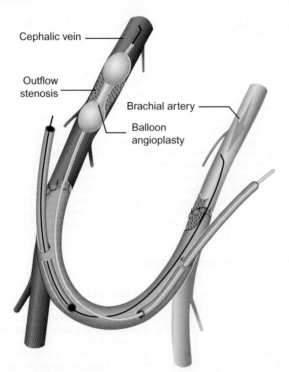

Fig. 12.8 Hemodialysis access intervention. Balloon dilation of outflow stenosis. The outflow stenosis is commonly found at or near the venous outflow anastomosis but can be encountered anywhere in the peripheral vein. (From Bittl JA: Catheter interventions for hemodialysis fistulas and grafts. *JACC Cardiovascular Interventions* 3(1):1–11, 2010.)

patients with diabetes, and patients with a history of peripheral arterial occlusive diseases are particularly prone to developing ischemic steal syndrome.

Infections, thromboses, and aneurysms are three additional potential AV fistula problems. Infection of the fistula can occur secondary to poor personal hygiene or poor aseptic technique during cannulation. Whereas fistula infection is rare, local infection can lead to thrombosis or sepsis if not treated. Signs and symptoms include redness and swelling of the access or pain and fever. Diagnosis is confirmed by culturing the drainage or by blood cultures. Antibiotic therapy is then used. Any infection at the AV anastomotic site requires immediate surgery.

Thrombosis is the most common complication of AV fistulas. In addition to infection, it can be caused by hypotension or stenosis of the fistula. Thrombosis can also be secondary to compression of blood flow caused by the use of tight bandages or a fistula-needle–holding device, the patient sleeping on the fistula arm, or hematoma formation. The use of fistula-needle–holding devices is discouraged, and these should never be used on new and developing AV fistulas. The bruit should always be auscultated after placing a fistula-needle–holding device on a patient's access. A thrombosed fistula can be declotted mechanically or by pharmacomechanical thrombolysis that involves installation of a thrombolytic agent such as tissue plasminogen activator in small doses. The clot may be mechanically fragmented with a device and then removed with suction.

Finally, aneurysms (outpouchings of the vessel wall) can occur from repeated cannulations of the same site and from infection. Large aneurysms limit the available cannulation sites. Care must be taken to assess skin integrity that could become compromised over time. Aneurysms should never be cannulated because of the risk of rupture along with hemorrhage or exsanguination.

How Does One Assess the Internal Access Before Needle Insertion?

Assessment cannot be overemphasized and is the key to skillful cannulation. A thorough access assessment will help to increase the longevity of the access, as well as minimize other complications. A complete assessment of the access must be performed before cleaning the site or actual cannulation. Hands should be thoroughly washed and gloves should be worn before assessment of the internal access. Assessment of the internal access involves several steps:

- Visibly observe the access, noting any signs of infection. Look for signs of redness or inflammation. The access extremity should have a normal skin temperature and be neither too hot nor too cold. The skin should be of a normal temperature for the patient. A hot feeling may indicate an infection, and an access that is noticeably cool might be thrombosed. Observe previous needle insertion sites for proper healing and scab formation. Make note of any open areas or drainage. A registered nurse should be informed of any unusual findings. A culture of drainage may be indicated, and the nurse in consultation with the nephrologist must determine whether the access may be cannulated.

- The skin should not be discolored or bruised, and the patient should not complain of any pain or numbness in the access or extremity. Swelling may be seen in an access that has recently been placed. Some patients have poor venous drainage in the access limb, causing swelling. Finally, swelling may be present because of a previous needle infiltration. Elevation of the affected limb is helpful to increase the venous return and decrease the swelling. Swelling should be monitored from treatment to treatment for improvements or worsening conditions. The circumference of the arm may be measured with a tape measure and compared for any increases or improvements. A registered nurse should be informed of any unusual findings before cannulation of the patient is attempted.
- Check for circulation or patency. Palpate the internal access for a "thrill," which should be felt over the entire length and resembles a gentle vibration. The thrill will diminish in strength the further away you move from the anastomosis. A thrill is indicative of adequate blood flow (450 mL or greater) throughout the vessel. A pulse will indicate less than adequate blood flow through the access. Listen with the bell of the stethoscope for a continuous low-pitched bruit or a swooshing sound. This should be clearly audible over the entire length of the access. The bruit should be heard with greater intensity over the anastomosis. Intensification of the normal sound of the bruit may indicate a stenotic area in the access. The absence of a bruit or thrill indicates that the access is clotted or no longer patent. A clotted access should never be cannulated. The patient or caregiver should be taught to assess the access daily by palpating for a thrill.

WHAT IS THE PROPER ASEPTIC PREPARATION FOR CANNULATION OF AN INTERNAL VASCULAR ACCESS?

Always assess, inspect, palpate, and identify cannulation sites before cleansing and preparing the skin for cannulation. An antiseptic solution, such as 10% povidone–iodine, 70% alcohol, or 2% chlorhexidine, should be used to cleanse the skin over and around the fistula. Apply the antiseptic in a circular motion away from the puncture site until a circle 2 inches in diameter has been covered. Be sure to follow the directions provided by the antiseptic manufacturer for effective disinfection. Povidone–iodine must be allowed to dry on the epidermis before needle insertion. If the patient is allergic to povidone–iodine, isopropyl alcohol may be used. Alcohol has a short bacteriostatic action time, so it is important to complete needle insertion just before the alcohol dries. The access should be reprepped should the site be touched by the patient or cannulator after the initial skin prep if cannulation has not yet taken place.

WHAT TYPES OF NEEDLES ARE USED FOR PUNCTURING AN INTERNAL VASCULAR ACCESS?

Large-gauge, thin-wall, and back-eye needles are preferred for maximum blood flow. A larger gauge needle is used for the high blood flow rates necessary for high-flux or high-efficiency dialysis. Blood flow rates of 400 to 500 mL/min may be attained with 14-gauge needles. The smallest needle available such as a 17-gauge needle is typically used for initial cannulation attempts (NKF, 2006). Smaller 17-gauge needles are used in children or infants to accommodate their small vessel size and decreased blood flow rate requirements. It is generally recommended to use at least a 15-gauge needle with blood flow rates of 350 mL/min or greater. Dialyzing a patient at a high blood flow rate with a small-gauge needle may cause hemolysis of the red blood cells as they pass through the small needle opening with such shear force.

Fistula needles may have fixed or rotating wings. Rotating wings allow the needle to be rotated or "flipped" after being inserted into the vascular access. Care must be taken not to damage the wall of the access when rotating the needle. Additionally, the needle should be rotated back to its original placement before removal to avoid coring the vessel. If you flip the needle and do not rotate it before removal, the hole may enlarge and cause trauma to the vessel wall. For this reason, flipping needles is strongly discouraged and the reason why a needle with a back eye is always used for the arterial needle. The back eye maximizes blood flow from the access and minimizes the need to "flip" the needle.

ARE THERE PARTICULAR POINTS TO BE OBSERVED WHEN PLACING THE NEEDLES?

The flow of blood through the access determines needle placement because the venous needle must always be placed in the direction of blood flow. Blood flow is sometimes identified as antegrade and retrograde, with the former meaning in the direction of blood flow and the latter meaning against blood flow. The arterial needle should be placed nearest the anastomosis but at least 1½ to 2 inches away from the site. A thorough assessment must be performed to ensure that the needle is placed far enough away from the anastomotic connection to avoid cannulating this site. The arterial needle may point toward the hand or the heart or either antegrade or retrograde. The venous needle should be placed so that it is at least 1½ to 2 inches proximal to the arterial needle. It should always be directed toward the heart or in the direction of blood flow (antegrade).

The AV fistula and AV graft are cannulated at different angles. The angle of entry depends on the depth of the access: the deeper the access, the steeper the angle required. The angle of insertion ranges from 20 to 45 degrees.

Cannulation of a new AV fistula must be approached with extreme care. The vessel is very fragile in its early stages and prone to infiltration. Preferably, only the most seasoned cannulators will initially access the fistula. Many facilities have adopted cannulation protocols in which the AV fistula is initially cannulated using only one needle (arterial outflow), and the venous return is through the central venous catheter for the first few treatments. Smaller gauge needles as well as lower blood flow rates are also used for the first few treatments. The temporary catheter is usually removed when cannulation with two needles has been successfully performed over consecutive treatments. It is important to remember that hands must be thoroughly washed and gloves worn before cannulating a patient's vascular access.

WHY IS POSITIONING THE NEEDLES IMPORTANT?

The manner in which needles are placed will affect the long-term patency rate of the access. Care must be taken to avoid placing the needles in the same general area during each treatment. Over time, this would cause the vessel walls to thin and aneurysms to develop. Aneurysms are weakened areas of the vessel that actually dilate, enlarge, and balloon out. These areas are generally avoided as sites for cannulation. Needle sites should be rotated at each treatment, and it is best to use the entire length of the access to achieve maximum surface area and development.

Placing the arterial needle near the anastomosis will achieve the best blood flow. The tip should not be closer than 1½ to 2 inches from the anastomosis. Placement of the needle toward or away from the anastomosis depends on the optimal blood flow. The usual practice is to place the arterial needle point in the direction of the flow. Finally, spacing the needles at least 1 inch apart minimizes the recirculation of blood that may result in inadequate dialysis.

WHAT CONDITIONS FAVOR RECIRCULATION?

A fistula with a low blood flow rate leads to recirculation. The low flow can be caused by stenosis at the arterial end or more commonly by stenosis at the venous end. It is usually associated with an increase in venous pressure and, if the recirculation is sufficiently great, may result in the "black blood" syndrome. This may also be caused if the dialysis needles are placed too close to one another. The result is a decrease in dialysis efficiency because the patient's blood is not being cleaned sufficiently.

WHAT IS "BLACK BLOOD" SYNDROME?

When recirculation is severe, the blood becomes acidotic, and the red blood cells cannot carry oxygen. The pH of this blood is usually below 7, and the blood appears very dark.

HOW IS THE OCCURRENCE OF RECIRCULATION DETERMINED?

The concentration of any substance (urea or creatinine) in the arterial bloodline going into the dialyzer should be the same as in the patient's systemic circulation. If the arterial concentration is less, the substance may have been diluted by venous blood returning from the dialyzer, indicating that some blood is passing through the dialyzer more than once without returning to systemic circulation. To calculate the percentage recirculation, three blood samples are obtained simultaneously. One represents the systemic circulation *(S)* or peripheral. The others are specimens from the inflow line just before it enters the dialyzer (arterial blood or *A*) and from the outflow line just after it leaves the dialyzer (venous blood or *V*). The estimated recirculation is calculated as follows:

$$\text{Percent recirculation} = 100\left[(S - A)/(S - V)\right]$$

Example: Where $S = 100$, $A = 90$, and $V = 20$

$$\text{Percent recirculation} = 100\left[(100 - 90)/(100 - 20)\right]$$
$$= 100[10/80]$$
$$= 100[0.125]$$
$$= 12.5\%$$

Given a good fistula and the use of two well-placed needles, the percentage of recirculation should be less than 10%. With double-lumen catheters, recirculation may often be as high as 15%. Recirculation greater than 15% is excessive and should be investigated and corrected.

HOW IS THE PERIPHERAL BLOOD SAMPLE OBTAINED?

Peripheral veins are no longer used. The peripheral sample is obtained from the arterial line before the dialyzer using the slow-stop flow technique for measuring access recirculation (Box 12.1).

DOES THE PATIENT REQUIRE AN ANESTHETIC BEFORE NEEDLE PLACEMENT?

Some patients, particularly those with newer or never-used accesses, experience discomfort with needle insertion. An anesthetic, such as lidocaine 1% (Xylocaine), may be used intradermally. Lidocaine is administered at an angle of 15 degrees just under the top tissue of the skin. You must always aspirate before giving lidocaine to make sure that you are not in a blood vessel. If you do withdraw blood with aspiration, you must discard that syringe and begin again. With repeated cannulations, scar tissue develops and the patient experiences less pain with cannulation. Another topical anesthetic is available in the form of a cream. The patient applies this cream before arriving for treatment. The cream must be removed before the patient is cannulated.

Box 12.1 Protocol for Urea-Based Measurement of Recirculation

Perform the test after approximately 30 minutes of treatment and after turning off ultrafiltration.
1. Set the pump speed to 500 mL/min (or maximum achievable rate).
2. Draw the arterial (A) and venous (V) line samples.
3. Immediately reduce the blood flow rate to 120 mL/min.
4. Turn the blood pump off exactly 10 seconds after reducing the blood flow rate.
5. Clamp the arterial line immediately above the sampling port.
6. Draw a systemic (S) arterial sample from the arterial line port.
7. Unclamp the line and resume ultrafiltration and dialysis.
8. Measure BUN in A, V, and S samples, and calculate the percent recirculation (R) using the formula

$$R = [(S - A)/(S - V)] \times 100.$$

BUN, Blood urea nitrogen.
From Nissenson AR, Fine RN: *Handbook of dialysis therapy*, ed. 4, Philadelphia, 2008, Saunders.

Can Anything Be Done To Cause the Veins of an Arm with an Arteriovenous Fistula To Enlarge More Quickly?

Nothing should be attempted for 4 to 5 days after the fistula is created. Thereafter the physician will recommend a variety of isometric exercises to help the AV fistula mature after placement. Hand exercises, such as squeezing a rubber ball, fingertip touches, and hammer and bicep curls, may help to increase blood flow and enhance vein maturation. The physician may or may not recommend the use of a light tourniquet with any of these exercises. Warm compresses or soaks several times a day may speed up venous distention. Correction of anemia along with increasing cardiac output may also potentially increase the blood flow through the fistula to enhance maturation.

What Care Is Required for the Fistula Arm Between Dialyses?

An arm with a new fistula should be elevated on a pillow between treatments to decrease swelling in the extremity. It is important to maintain adequate pressure, either by hand or with a light pressure dressing over the puncture sites, for 10 to 20 minutes after the needles are removed. Most patients still experience some heparin effects at the end of dialysis, and bleeding can be a serious problem. Even oozing under the skin can cause hematoma and scar formation, which eventually make the vessel difficult to use. After the bleeding has stopped, bandages are sufficient to protect the puncture sites. If bleeding continues from the puncture site more than 20 minutes after removal of the needles, the heparin dose should be evaluated and readjusted. Daily cleaning of the fistula arm with soap is advised. Some people like to use an ointment to keep the skin soft.

What Is the Buttonhole Technique of Cannulation?

The buttonhole technique, or constant site technique, has been used to cannulate AV fistulas on a limited basis for approximately 25 years but has now grown in popularity, particularly for self-care patients. In the buttonhole technique of cannulation, the access is cannulated in exactly the same spot and angle of insertion from treatment to treatment. A tunnel tract of scar tissue eventually develops, which then allows the needle to be easily inserted into the same channel with each cannulation. Because the same sites are cannulated during each treatment, the scab formed from the previous treatment must be removed before cannulation. Care must be taken to remove the scabs aseptically to prevent infection. The access should be disinfected after scab removal as per the facility protocol. The track or tunnel usually becomes well established after approximately 8 to 10 cannulations. This type of cannulation is associated with less pain and fewer incidents of infiltration. Other benefits include fewer infections, fewer missed needle sticks, and less time spent in cannulating the access. This method is a useful alternative for patients who self-cannulate or those dialyzing at home. Medisystems offers a buttonhole needle set with antistick dull bevels. This blunt needle (Fig. 12.9) can be used after the buttonhole develops. The antistick dull bevel prevents cutting of the tissue surrounding the scar tissue tunnel track. The 2006 KDOQI Clinical Practice Guidelines and Recommendations suggest that patients who are capable and who have a well-positioned access be encouraged to self-cannulate with the preferred buttonhole technique method. Box 12.2 provides details regarding cannulating an access using the buttonhole technique.

What Is the HeRO Vascular Access Device?

The HeRO vascular access device is a vascular access option for patients who have limited peripheral access sites for fistulas or grafts because of central venous stenosis or superior vena cava occlusion and who have become catheter dependent. The HeRO access is a subcutaneous graft with a central outflow that requires no venous anastomosis and is thus able to bypass any stenosis of the central veins. The device is implanted surgically and can be used as a long-term vascular access. The HeRO device consists of two components: a venous outflow component and an arterial graft component. The venous outflow component is inserted directly into the internal jugular vein, with the tip positioned in the right atrium. The arterial graft component consists of a 6-mm PTFE upper arm graft that has a titanium connector on its end. The arm graft is then joined to the outflow component with the titanium connector. Blood will begin flowing from the artery through the graft and outflow component to the heart (Fig. 12.10).

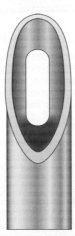

Fig. 12.9 Cannulating mature constant sites in native fistulas using an antistick dull bevel. (From National Kidney Foundation [NKF]: KDOQI clinical practice guidelines and clinical practice recommendations for 2006 updates: hemodialysis adequacy, peritoneal dialysis adequacy and vascular access. *American Journal of Kidney Disease* 48(suppl 1):S1-S322, 2006.)

Box 12.2 Buttonhole Cannulation Guidelines

- Use the same angle of insertion with every cannulation.
- Use the same cannulator until a tunnel has formed.
- Use a tourniquet on all arteriovenous fistulas during every cannulation.
- Anchor the fistula by pulling the skin taut.
- Switch to blunt needles to prevent damaging the vessel.

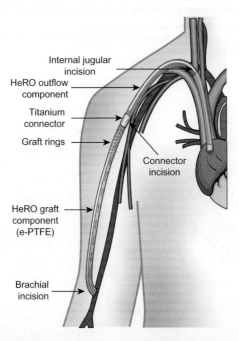

Fig. 12.10 HeRO vascular access device. A diagram of the Hemoaccess Reliable Outflow (HeRO) device is shown with the arterial anastomosis at the brachial artery near the antecubital fossa and the tip of the venous catheter position in the right atrium. The titanium connector links the graft and venous components. The device was inserted using a brachial incision in the proximal upper arm for the arterial anastomosis, an incision at the base of the neck for the initial venous cannulation, and an incision near the deltopectoral group to facilitate passage of the two components. *e-PTFE,* Expanded polytetrafluoroethylene; *PTFE,* polytetrafluoroethylene. (From Glickmann MH: HeRO vascular access device. *Seminars in Vascular Surgery* 24(2):108–112, 2011.)

ARE THERE SPECIAL TECHNIQUES TO CANNULATE THE HeRO DEVICE?

The HeRO device has been approved by the Food and Drug Administration as a graft and can be treated as such. The KDOQI guidelines for cannulation should be followed. The HeRO device is cannulated like a conventional upper arm graft. Cannulation should be deferred until any swelling has subsided. Standard fistula needles should be used, and the facility algorithm protocol may be followed. Cannulation should take place at an angle of 45 degrees and the cannulation sites should be rotated. The thrill may be less prominent than with a conventional graft due to the absence of a venous anastomosis.

ARE VENOUS CATHETERS USED IN DIALYSIS?

Dialysis catheters are used in the management of hemodialysis patients in certain situations: (1) as an access for acute dialysis, (2) for patients who are imminently awaiting a kidney transplant, (3) when allowing maturation of the AV access, (4) as a permanent access when the availability of vessels for a permanent internal access is limited, (5) for patients undergoing plasmapheresis, (6) for patients receiving continuous venovenous renal replacement therapy, and (7) for patients undergoing peritoneal dialysis requiring temporary hemodialysis because of peritonitis. It should be noted that prolonged use of subclavian vein catheters would result in subclavian vein stenosis.

The NKF KDOQI guidelines suggest that only 10% of chronic maintenance hemodialysis patients should have catheters as their permanent vascular access. The rate of AV fistula utilization for prevalent hemodialysis pattens has improved while the rate of central venous catheter utilization at the initiation of dialysis (80%) has remained relatively stagnant (USRDS, 2016).

The use of central venous catheters as a permanent access for hemodialysis is not the best choice but is an alternative in access selection. Patients with stage 4 CKD should be informed of the risks and benefits associated with catheters and should be strongly encouraged to opt for the placement of a permanent vascular access, such as a fistula, well before the need to initiate dialysis. Although it is not the access of choice, in patients with stage 4 or 5 CKD, catheterization of the subclavian vein and use of peripherally inserted central catheter lines should be avoided to prevent the risk of venous stenosis and thrombosis, thus preserving the vessel for use. Table 12.1 lists the advantages and disadvantages of venous catheters.

WHICH VEINS ARE USED FOR A VENOUS CATHETER?

The subclavian, internal jugular, and femoral veins are used for temporary access (Fig. 12.11A). The vessels are accessed using double-lumen catheters (Fig. 12.11B).

WHAT ARE THE CONTRAINDICATIONS FOR USING SUBCLAVIAN OR JUGULAR CATHETERS?

Subclavian or jugular catheters should not be used in the following patients:
- Patients with acute respiratory distress who cannot be positioned in the supine or Trendelenburg position
- Patients with known subclavian vein stenosis

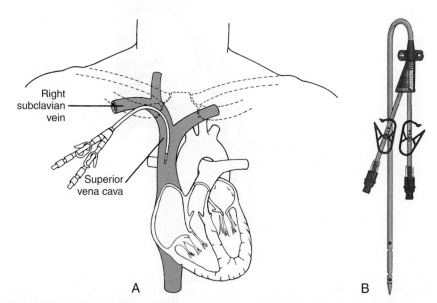

Right subclavian vein

Superior vena cava

A

B

Fig. 12.11 A, Temporary vascular access using subclavian double-lumen venous catheter. **B,** Double-lumen temporary catheter. (Courtesy MEDCOMP Corp., Harleysville, PA.)

How Is the Subclavian or Jugular Catheter Placed?

The physician uses a strict aseptic technique. The patient lies supine in the Trendelenburg position with the head turned to the opposite side. The skin around the area is cleaned and covered with sterile drapes. With local anesthesia, the catheter is inserted and sutured into place. Verification of correct placement by chest x-ray examination is required before the catheter may be used.

What Complications Can Occur with Subclavian or Jugular Catheters?

Immediately after insertion of the catheter, pneumothorax, hemothorax, or air embolism may occur. Bleeding is another complication if the artery is inadvertently punctured during insertion.

What Are the Indications for Using a Femoral Catheter?

A femoral catheter is used in the following types of cases:
- Acutely ill patients confined to bed
- CKD patients with clotted accesses but who require urgent dialysis
- Patients receiving continuous renal replacement therapy
- Patients who may have subclavian vein stenosis

What Complications Can Occur with Femoral Catheters?

Although femoral catheters are not widely used, some complications that might occur as a result of their placement are retroperitoneal hemorrhage from venipuncture during insertion, bleeding at the insertion site, hematoma, and infection.

Are Double-Lumen Catheters Available for Permanent Use?

Permanent catheters are becoming more widely used. A silicone rubber catheter is inserted intraoperatively. The catheter has a subcutaneous Dacron graft that impedes infection. These catheters are usually placed in the internal jugular vein, and a subcutaneous tunnel is created that allows the catheter to exit through the chest wall (Fig. 12.12A). Permanent catheters are also placed in the subclavian, mammary, and femoral veins. Another type of permanent catheter is a Tesio catheter (Fig. 12.12B), which uses two single-lumen catheters placed side-by-side in the same vein. This allows for customized catheter placement with an increased blood flow rate. Permanent catheters are useful in pediatric patients whose small arteries and veins prohibit placement of an AV graft.

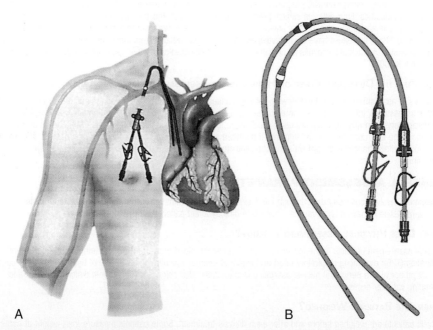

A

B

Fig. 12.12 A, Internal jugular permanent vascular access using the Tesio catheter. **B,** Permanent catheter modified by Tesio. (Courtesy MEDCOMP Corp., Harleysville, PA.)

CHAPTER 13

PATIENT AND MACHINE MONITORING AND ASSESSMENT

Initial and ongoing assessment of the patient and continuous monitoring of the dialysis equipment are among the most vital functions of dialysis personnel. Both registered nurses and patient care technicians (PCTs) have defined roles and responsibilities. State boards of nursing regulate the practice of nursing, including the direct supervision of nonprofessionals to whom specific tasks may be delegated. Readers are advised to review the regulations guiding practice in the states in which they practice.

In some states, only registered nurses are allowed to perform assessments as described by the Nurse Practice Acts or a licensed practical nurse (LPN) or licensed vocational nurse (LVN) as permitted by some state laws. Some states, however, have special laws that allow unlicensed dialysis PCTs to perform certain tasks. In many states, PCTs are permitted by the state to infuse normal saline intravenously for priming and hypotension, to inject intradermal lidocaine (Xylocaine) before inserting dialysis needles into the vascular access, and to administer intravenous heparin for anticoagulation as per the protocol or the physicians' orders. These tasks are allowed under the direct supervision of a registered nurse.

In this chapter, assessment refers to the role of the nurse. Monitoring or collection of data is the role of the PCT. After data are collected, the nurse and PCT work together to initiate changes in the dialysis treatment as per the physicians' orders or the protocols.

WHAT IS PATIENT MONITORING?

Patient monitoring is a series of repeated or continuous observations and documentation of the patient's physiological state and response to dialysis. Machine monitoring is continuous and includes the following: arterial and venous pressures, blood flow rate, transmembrane pressure (TMP), ultrafiltrate removal, dialysate temperature, dialysate flow and conductivity, and remaining treatment time. Dialysis personnel are responsible for reading, documenting, and evaluating these parameters. Vital signs are measured at least every hour or more frequently in unstable patients or where the facility policy dictates. Assessments determine the appropriate dialysis intervention to attain the goals of treatment.

WHAT ARE THE DIALYSIS TREATMENT OUTCOME STANDARDS?

The National Kidney Foundation (NKF) Kidney Disease Outcomes Quality Initiative (KDOQI) provides guidelines with indicators of outcomes. Four different clinical practice guidelines, that is, those related to hemodialysis adequacy, peritoneal dialysis adequacy, treatment of anemia, and vascular access, are used to assess and improve the outcome of each dialysis. Other guidelines have been developed, including those related to nutrition, dyslipidemia, bone disease, and hypertension. Additional guidelines for pediatrics have also been developed. (See Appendix A for additional information on the NKF KDOQI.)

WHAT ARE THE DIFFERENT TYPES OF HEMODIALYSIS ASSESSMENT?

The types of assessment include the following: physical assessments, laboratory data analysis and interpretation, first dialysis assessment, intradialytic assessment (predialysis, postdialysis, and monitoring of hemodialysis procedure), and interdisciplinary team (IDT) assessment using the Centers for Medicare & Medicaid Services (CMS) clinical practice guidelines. The IDT must develop and implement a written and individualized comprehensive plan of care. The plan of care should reflect changes in the patient's condition and must include measurable and expected outcomes within a defined time frame.

GENERAL ASSESSMENT PARAMETERS

Assessment involves collecting data through interviews, physical examination, performance of laboratory tests, and interpretation of patient observations. These data directly affect patients' care.

WHAT DOES PHYSICAL ASSESSMENT INCLUDE?

Physical assessment consists of the following: assessing weight, blood pressure (BP), and temperature, pulse, and respiration (TPR); evaluating respiratory effort and extent of edema; auscultating for quality of heart and breath sounds; comparing apical and peripheral pulses; assessing skin integrity, skin color, and jugular vein distension (JVD); and evaluating vascular access.

WHEN ARE PATIENTS WEIGHED?

Dialysis patients are weighed before and after each dialysis treatment. Some patients measure their weight at home to guide the adjustment of their fluid intake between dialyses.

WHY IS MEASUREMENT OF WEIGHT IMPORTANT?

Weight is a good indicator of how well the patient is controlling fluid balance between dialyses. Predialysis weight indicates how much ultrafiltration (UF) is required during treatment. Postdialysis weight is the best indicator of how much UF occurred during the hemodialysis procedure.

WHAT IS MEANT BY THE PATIENT'S DRY WEIGHT?

Dry weight is the ideal postdialysis weight after the removal of all or most excess body fluid. Patients who are at dry weight are usually normotensive. If the postdialysis weight suggests that the volume status is too high, the patient may be on the borderline for fluid overload and may be hypertensive. If the postdialysis weight is too low, the patient may be hypovolemic and at risk of hypotension and clotting of the vascular access.

HOW MUCH WEIGHT GAIN IS PERMISSIBLE BETWEEN DIALYSIS TREATMENTS?

Weight gain between dialysis procedures is due to fluid retention. Most dialysis units encourage patients to limit their weight gain to 0.5 kg (or 1 lb) per day. (Refer to Chapter 14 for further discussion and calculation of fluid restrictions.)

WHY IS BLOOD PRESSURE MEASUREMENT IMPORTANT?

Blood pressure is often related to volume. Hypertension may indicate volume overload. Hypotension may indicate dehydration. BP is measured while the patient is sitting and standing to evaluate orthostatic changes requiring intervention. It is important to monitor and treat hypertension in chronic kidney disease (CKD) patients to reduce the risk of cardiovascular disease and other complications. Hypertension occurs in more than 80% of patients with stage 5 CKD.

WHAT IS NORMAL BLOOD PRESSURE?

Hypertension is very common in CKD patients, and as many as 75% of patients with a glomerular filtration rate (GFR) of less than 60 mL/min have a BP of greater than 140/90 mm Hg. Normal BP is an individual matter. In CKD patients, BP is analyzed for trends rather than absolute values. The KDOQI 2003 Guidelines on Goals of Antihypertensive Therapy for CKD patients on dialysis recommend predialysis and postdialysis BP goals should be less than 140/90 mm Hg and less than 130/80 mm Hg, respectively.

WHERE CAN THE CUFF BE PLACED FOR BLOOD PRESSURE MEASUREMENT?

The upper arm is the most common cuff placement site, but there are two alternative placements. A large thigh cuff can be applied around the mid-thigh area. The pulse is audible via a stethoscope at the popliteal space. In addition, a regular cuff may be applied above the ankle, with auscultation over the posterior tibial or dorsalis pedis artery. This usually yields an audible BP, but the readings obtained will be 20 to 40 mm Hg higher than the arm pressure. A notation should be made in the patient's chart whenever leg pressure readings are taken. BP cuffs should never be placed on an extremity with a deep vein thrombosis, grafts, ischemic changes, or an arteriovenous (AV) fistula or graft. Inaccurate BP readings will occur if using a cuff that does not fit properly. For example, if the cuff is too wide for the patient, the BP reading will be artificially low, and if the cuff is too narrow, the reading will be artificially high. Cuffs are available in different sizes to best match the patient's limb being measured. Ideally, the width of the cuff should be 40% of the circumference (or 20% wider than the diameter) of the midpoint of the limb on which the cuff is used to measure BP. If taking a measurement on an obese patient and a large cuff is not available, wrap a standard size cuff around the patient's forearm and palpate over the radial artery. If taking a measurement of a very thin patient, consider using a pediatric sized cuff (Ball et al, 2019). The bladder, which is enclosed by the cuff, should encircle at least 80% of the upper arm of an adult (Potter & Perry, 2013) (Fig. 13.1).

WHY ARE TEMPERATURE, PULSE, AND RESPIRATION MONITORED?

Temperature, pulse, and respiration observations serve as a baseline at the start of dialysis. Temperature elevation suggests infection or complicating illness. An elevated temperature is often a sign of vascular access infection. Fever during dialysis may be caused by a high dialysate temperature or a pyrogen reaction. A rapid pulse may result from anemia or fluid overload. Irregular heart rate (dysrhythmia) may indicate cardiac complications, including those associated with serum potassium levels. An increase in the pulse rate during dialysis may be associated with a falling blood volume (from UF) and may occur just before a drop in BP. Increased respiratory rate may indicate excessive fluid gain. Any unexpected finding should be reported to the physician.

WHAT IS EDEMA?

Edema is the excessive accumulation of fluid in tissue spaces. Excessive weight gain between dialyses results in edema. Edema appears in different areas of the body in different patients. It may present at the ankle or sacrum, facial or periorbital areas, or peripherally. The jugular veins are often distended when the patient is fluid overloaded. Fluid status assessment determines the amount of UF required during dialysis.

ARE THERE OTHER PHYSICAL ASSESSMENTS?

Predialysis assessment includes subjective analysis of the patient's health since the previous dialysis treatment. Ask whether the patient has experienced symptoms such as headaches, fever, cramping, dizziness, hypotension, bleeding,

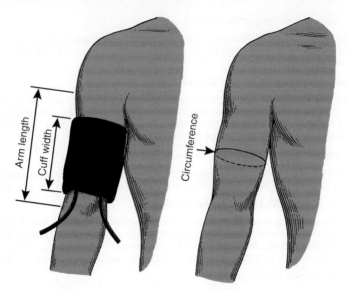

Fig. 13.1 Guidelines for proper blood pressure cuff size. Cuff width should be 20% greater than the upper-arm diameter or 40% of the circumference and two thirds of the arm length. (From Potter P, Perry A, Stockert P, Hall A: *Fundamentals of nursing,* ed. 8, St. Louis, 2013, Mosby.)

angina, nausea, vomiting, or diarrhea. Dialysis personnel can assess changes in mentation, speech, mobility, or thought processes while patients describe their health and any problems between dialysis sessions.

FIRST HEMODIALYSIS ASSESSMENT

WHY IS THE FIRST HEMODIALYSIS PROCEDURE SO IMPORTANT?

The CMS conditions for coverage require that the registered nurse complete the first nursing assessment prior to the initiation of the dialysis treatment (Department of Health and Human Services, 2008). The first hemodialysis is critical because it sets the atmosphere for all future treatment procedures. The first hemodialysis is sometimes performed in the hospital. The patient may be unstable and feel sick. Information that the nurse gives the patient during this first dialysis is often forgotten or misunderstood. Therefore, the nurse and dialysis personnel must often reiterate teaching instructions regarding medications or access care. Written manuals and instructions are helpful so that patients have a reference as needed. Sometimes the first dialysis is performed in an outpatient dialysis facility. When this is the case, it is imperative that the dialysis personnel be cognizant of the emotional status of the new patient. The patient may be fearful because of the myths about dialysis he or she has heard or because of the appearance of the equipment. These fears, combined with the fact that the patient is chronically ill, are strong reasons for the patient to be in emotional shock and to not recall the instructions given during the first dialysis. See Chapter 25 for information on how to assess a patient's readiness to learn. The dialysis nurse and personnel must make the first dialysis as smooth and uneventful as possible.

WHAT PROCEDURES TAKE PLACE BEFORE THE FIRST HEMODIALYSIS?

The physician evaluates and prescribes the dialysis orders for the new patient. The nurse reviews the orders and starts predialysis assessment after the fluid composition and machine settings are programmed. Before the first meeting with the patient, medical records should be reviewed. This information will be helpful during physical assessment. After introductions, a brief tour around the facility should be conducted. The first visit should be as simple and as pleasant as possible. Remember that instructions will have to be repeated many times.

Make certain that signed consent for dialysis treatment has been completed and retained in the patient's medical records. Physical assessment begins with the patient's weight, BP, and TPR observations. A general assessment of the patient's fluid status and overall well-being follows. Some questions that should be asked include the following: Is edema present? Is the patient in any respiratory distress or experiencing any pain? Is there any bleeding or bruising? Is there residual kidney function? Are bowel movements regular? Are there sleep problems? Are there any allergies to food or medication? Many units have assessment forms that offer guidelines for the caregiver.

During this first procedure, some of the dialysis parameters will be set, such as heparin requirements, tolerance of fluid removal, arterial and venous pressure readings, saline requirements, tolerance to the dialyzer, and dialysate composition. Because the first dialysis is so critical, the physician usually prescribes a slow blood flow and only 2 hours of dialysis in some instances.

PREDIALYSIS ASSESSMENT

WHAT IS PREDIALYSIS ASSESSMENT?

Before the initiation of hemodialysis, the patient and machine are both evaluated. The patient's physiological status is assessed to ascertain the need to adjust the dialysis orders or prescribed medications. The machine parameters are assessed to ensure that the prescribed procedure is implemented correctly.

WHAT IS INCLUDED IN THE PATIENT'S PREDIALYSIS ASSESSMENT?

Predialysis assessment includes the following:
- Fluid status (respiratory rate and effort, JVD, heart sounds, breath sounds, and presence of edema)
- Interdialytic weight gain
- Sitting and standing BP
- TPR, including apical and peripheral pulse evaluation
- Skin color, temperature, turgor, and integrity
- Vascular access patency and freedom from bleeding and infection
- Interpretation of physical assessment and laboratory data for appropriate intervention and medication administration

WHAT OTHER CHECKS SHOULD BE DONE ON THE DIALYSIS MACHINE BEFORE PATIENT USE?

It is necessary to ensure that the machine functions have been checked and are working correctly. All extracorporeal alarms should be tested to ensure that they respond appropriately. Arterial pressure, venous pressure, and air detector alarms should all cause the blood pump to stop and the venous line clamp to close. In addition, the conductivity and temperature of the dialysate should be tested to ensure that they are within the proper range. These alarms must be working at all times so that if any problem arises, the dialysate will be diverted from the dialyzer, and a major complication will be avoided. Finally, the dialysate concentrate should be adequate to meet the patient's treatment.

WHY IS IT NECESSARY TO PERFORM SUCH A THOROUGH ASSESSMENT OF THE PATIENT AND THE MACHINE BEFORE INITIATION OF DIALYSIS TREATMENT?

The accuracy of assessment and appropriateness of the interventions directly affect the patient's outcome and will ensure that the goal of adequate dialysis is achieved.

WHAT IS ULTRAFILTRATION?

Ultrafiltration is the process of removing fluid from the blood during a dialysis treatment. It is the result of hydrostatic forces across the dialysis membrane. The difference in the hydrostatic pressure between the blood and fluid is the TMP. When the pressure on the dialysate side is lower than the pressure on the blood side, water then moves from the blood side to the dialysate side. The rate of UF is the sum total of the positive and negative pressures plus the filtration factor, known as the UF coefficient (k_{UF}), of each individual dialyzer. The k_{UF} ranges from 0.5 to 80.0 mL/hr/mm Hg, depending on the specific dialyzer characteristics (see Chapter 6).

WHAT INFORMATION IS NEEDED TO CALCULATE THE RATE OF ULTRAFILTRATION?

All of the following questions must be answered to calculate the rate of UF:
- What is the patient's dry weight?
- What weight loss is needed (in kilograms)?
- What is the target postdialysis weight?
- How much fluid will the patient receive orally and/or intravenously during treatment?
- What is the k_{UF} of the dialyzer?
- How much saline will be infused to rinse the blood circuit?
- What is the length of time that the patient will be dialyzed?

HOW IS FLUID REMOVAL CALCULATED?

The following steps are performed for calculating fluid removal:

1. *Add*   Amount of weight in mm to be removed
     Amount of fluid intake in mm
  $+$ $\dfrac{\text{Amount of intravenous fluid in mm to be removed}}{\text{Total amount of fluid to be removed in mm}}$

2. *Divide* $\dfrac{\text{Number of hours of dialysis}}{\text{Total amount of fluid in mm to be removed}}$

3. *Divide* $\dfrac{\text{Total from step 2}}{k_{UF}\text{ of dialyzer}} = \text{TMP}$

An example of how to calculate fluid removal follows. Dialyze for 3 hours and remove 2.3 kg; the conventional dialyzer k_{UF} equals 4.

1. *Add*   Weight in mm to be removed   2300 mL
                Oral intake   600 mL
                Saline rinsed back   100 mL
                Total amount of fluid to be removed   3000 mL

2. *Divide* $\dfrac{\text{Fluid to be removed } (3000 \text{ mL})}{\text{Number of hours of dialysis } (3 \text{ hr})} = 1000 \text{ mL/hr}$

3. *Divide* $\dfrac{\text{Total from step 2 } (1000 \text{ mL})}{k_{UF} = 4} = 250 \text{ TMP}$

In a conventional dialysis delivery machine, the TMP must be set manually. Most systems now provide a programmable function for controlled UF. Controlled UF allows the machine to adjust and control fluid removal.

ARE THERE LIMITATIONS TO HOW MUCH FLUID CAN BE REMOVED DURING A STANDARD HEMODIALYSIS TREATMENT?

When it is necessary to remove large amounts of fluid during the dialysis treatment, a high ultrafiltration rate (UFR) is required. High UFRs are associated with intradialytic hypotension. Intradialytic hypotension occurs in 20% to 30% of dialysis treatments and can potentially damage the brain, gut, heart, and kidneys and is known as "organ stunning" as the organs become hypoperfused (Feehally et al, 2019). CMS has set guidelines for the recommended maximum UFR for patients at 13/mL/kg/hr or less. This UF maximum helps to avoid extreme hypotensive episodes with the potential for organ stunning and increased mortality risk.

To calculate the UFR in mL/kg/hr:

$$\text{Fluid weight to remove} = 1800 \text{ mL}$$
$$\text{Prime and rinseback} = 300 \text{ mL}$$

$$\text{Total } = 2100 \text{ mL}$$
$$\text{UFR as mL/hr}$$
$$\text{UF goal} \div \text{treatment time} = \text{UFR in mL/hr}$$

$$2100 \text{ mL} \div 4 \text{ hours} = 525 \text{ mL/hr}$$
$$\text{UFR in mL/kg/hr (goal is} \leq 13 \text{ mL/kg/hr)}$$
$$\text{UFR in mL/hr} \div \text{target weight} = \text{mL/hr}$$
$$525 \div 51 \text{ kg} = 10.29 \text{ mL/kg/hr}$$

WHAT IS SEQUENTIAL ULTRAFILTRATION AND DIALYSIS?

In 1947, Alwall instituted the application of UF as a means of fluid removal during dialysis. The concept of convective transport rather than diffusion (see Chapter 7) is currently used in the hemofiltration approach. Several dialyzers have membranes or fibers of sufficient permeability and strength to yield UF of several liters per hour at safe TMPs.

Application of UF alone before conventional dialysis with minimal UF is known as sequential or isolated UF and dialysis. During the UF phase, blood circulates normally through the dialyzer, but the dialysis fluid does not. UF resulting from the negative pressure gradient across the membrane is collected at the outflow side and measured. Patients tolerate fluid removal by this method at a rate and quantity greater than those with conventional dialysis without hypotension or symptoms. Severely hypertensive patients are able to achieve better BP control than would otherwise be obtainable. This therapy is particularly useful for maintenance dialysis patients with chronic large fluid gains (see Chapter 18 for more information).

INTRADIALYTIC ASSESSMENT AND MONITORING

WHAT IS INTRADIALYTIC MONITORING?

Intradialytic monitoring is the ongoing assessment of the patient and equipment during hemodialysis treatment. The patient and machine are monitored at least every half hour by the caregivers. Monitoring is done more frequently in unstable patients. The vital signs and machine monitors are assessed.

The patient must also be monitored for consciousness, and the caregiver must always perform a visual check to ensure that the patient's access is visible and the needles and lines are secure. If the patient is on a heparin pump, the volume administered must be documented. Arterial and venous drip chambers should be observed and adjusted to appropriate levels as necessary. External transducer protectors should be observed for the presence of saline or blood and changed if found to be contaminated.

These parameters are adjusted as needed in accordance with the treatment goals. All assessments are logged in the dialysis flow records. In computerized fluid delivery systems, the machine parameters are automatically monitored and recorded in the dialysis flow sheets.

Are Any Other Patient Assessments Performed During Dialysis?

An important assessment, not subject to numerical recording, is the general condition and response of the patient during the procedure. Nausea, apprehension, shortness of breath, restlessness or agitation, irritability, itching, flushing, twitching, irrational behavior, sensation of faintness, and complaints of pain are some of the many signs or symptoms that can occur. A person undergoing regular dialysis has an individual response pattern, and any change in this pattern is significant. Acute dialysis patients must be evaluated more often because of their less stable condition and unknown response to therapy. All observed clinical conditions are documented in the chart and reported to the physician. Sometimes reactions or complications are reported to the continuous quality improvement committee for the purpose of ongoing monitoring or corrective action.

Is There Any Way to Know How Well a Patient's Blood Is Being Cleaned During Treatment?

Noninvasive assessment tools can monitor the amount of clearance the patient is receiving during the actual dialysis treatment. One such tool is the OnLine Clearance Adequacy Monitoring Program, which is available in several types of machines. For example, the Fresenius 2008 K and 2008 T machines use a monitoring system called OnLine Clearance. This monitoring tool uses sodium chloride, which has a molecular weight (MW) of 58 g/mol, as a surrogate marker for urea, which has an MW of 60 g/mol. Sodium can move across the dialyzer membrane similarly to urea. The OnLine Clearance test occurs in two phases. The first phase or half of the test involves elevating the dialysate sodium concentration above the normal sodium concentration in the blood. The dialysate sodium concentration is elevated to achieve conductivity as high as 15.5 millisiemens/cm. Because of the concentration gradient now created, sodium will cross the dialyzer membrane into the blood. The second half of the OnLine Clearance test involves lowering the dialysate sodium concentration to achieve a conductivity of 13.5 millisiemens/cm, allowing diffusion to take place again, with sodium moving from the blood compartment into the dialysate compartment. Conductivity monitors are located at both the dialyzer inlet and the dialyzer outlet flow paths. The difference between the two conductivity readings generates the clearance value. Because of the similarities in urea and sodium chloride, the degree of urea removal can be predicted. The machine performs up to six OnLine Clearance tests during a 4-hour treatment. This allows the dialysis nurse or technician to see how well the treatment prescription is working for the patient. The patient's volume of urea distribution is entered into the OnLine Clearance program before treatment is initiated because this is used to determine the effective clearance. Certain variables contribute to nonoptimal patient dialysis, including poor needle positioning, dialyzer clotting, access recirculation, or incorrectly set blood or dialysate flow rates. The OnLine Clearance program is a tool that can greatly improve the adequacy of treatment, which will in turn help to improve the quality of life of the patients. One advantage of using these types of tools is that the dialysis caregiver will know during treatment whether optimal adequacy is being provided and also be able to troubleshoot early in the treatment to correct any problems.

What Are Potential Hemodialysis Complications?

During the hemodialysis procedure, many potential complications can occur in both the patient and the equipment. These complications may result from the process itself or from complex interactions between the patient and the dialysis procedure.

What Is the Most Common Complication During Hemodialysis Treatment?

The most common complication during hemodialysis treatment is hypotension related to a rapid decrease in the circulating blood volume caused by UF. Lack of vasoconstriction caused by antihypertensive medications or other cardiac factors is another cause of hypotension. During UF, fluid is removed from the vascular space. For continued UF, the vascular space must be refilled. When fluid is being removed faster than the vascular space can be refilled, hypotension will occur.

Ingestion of food during dialysis treatment may contribute to hypotension because of vasodilation. This is commonly referred to as postprandial hypotension and usually occurs about 2 hours after eating as blood pools in the intestines to aid digestion. Thus, it is prudent for the patient to avoid eating during treatment; in addition, loss of consciousness may occur with untreated hypotension, placing the patient at risk of obstruction of the airway if he or she is eating.

What Causes Hypotension as Dialysis Begins?

Hypotension at the beginning of dialysis occurs in some patients with a relatively small blood volume (children and small women). This is the result of volume shifts as the dialyzer fills with the patient's blood. It is much less frequent with small-volume dialyzers than with larger ones. This type of reaction is rarely serious and usually does not last long. It will respond to an infusion of small amounts of saline or albumin. A careful technique when starting dialysis will minimize the occurrence of these episodes.

What About Hypotension Occurring Later During Dialysis?

Hypotension later during dialysis is usually attributable to the removal of fluid from the vascular space (UF) in excess of the patient's ability to compensate. Hypotension may be asymptomatic until there is a decrease of 40 to 55 mm Hg in systolic pressure. It usually responds to fluid replacement. Most modern dialysis machines remove fluid at a steady rate set by the practitioner. Removing more than 1% of a patient's dry body weight as fluid per hour often results in hypotension.

Why Do Some Patients with Gross Edema Become Hypotensive Early During Dialysis?

Patients with gross fluid overload may have heart failure or low serum albumin. Dialysis removes fluid from the vascular compartment, but the low serum protein does not exert sufficient oncotic pressure to mobilize fluid from the interstitial space. There is another group of patients in whom cardiac failure or hypoproteinemia are not obvious causes but who have problems with overhydration and vascular instability during dialysis. During conventional dialysis with UF, these people become symptomatically hypotensive with tachycardia, nausea, and vomiting. Other symptoms of hypotension are shortness of breath, cool and clammy skin, paleness, restlessness, excessive yawning, diaphoresis, and decreased mental status. The causes are likely multifactorial. Changes in serum osmolality, effects of acetate if used as the buffer, and norepinephrine depletion have been suggested or demonstrated. Infusion of hypertonic saline or mannitol or use of higher than usual sodium concentrations in the dialysis fluid may be beneficial. Sequential UF followed by dialysis may also give good results.

How Is Hypotension Prevented and Treated Intradialytically?

Sodium modeling and UF profiling, discussed earlier, are excellent methods of preventing severe hypotension. BP monitoring, with careful observation or use of an in-line hematocrit monitor, is also helpful in reducing hypotensive episodes. If hypotension is treated early by placing the patient in the Trendelenburg position, by decreasing the UF pressures, or by giving replacement fluid, more serious complications may be avoided. It is helpful to be aware of the signs of hypotension, such as the patient complaining of feeling hot or lightheaded. Some patients will complain of blurred vision or nausea. It is prudent to check a patient's BP whenever he or she complains of these symptoms. The treatment for hypotension is administering a normal saline bolus, placing the patient in the Trendelenburg position, decreasing the UFR, and using a volume expander if ordered.

What Is the Crit-Line Instrument?

The Crit-Line monitor (CLM) is an arterial in-line medical instrument that provides noninvasive continuous measurement of the absolute hematocrit, percent blood volume change, and oxygen saturation in real time. The CLM assesses how well the patient is tolerating fluid removal, assists in identifying fluid overload, and allows visualization of plasma refilling or the amount of fluid that the body is able to shift or refill into the bloodstream from the tissues during any given treatment session. It measures blood volume changes on the basis of hematocrit because these two values have an inverse relationship. As fluid is removed from the intravascular space, the density of blood increases. This is displayed as the percent blood volume change on a grid-like graph on the Crit-Line screen. With this device, it is possible to maximize UF safely and prevent hypotension, cramping, and other intradialytic complications associated with volume depletion. A disposable blood chamber is attached to the arterial side of the dialyzer and photometric technology is used. This device will also measure access recirculation. The CLM is exempt from the Clinical Laboratory Improvement Act.

Does Hypertension Occur During Dialysis?

A small minority of patients develop a rise in BP during dialysis. Some experience a gradual rise in BP throughout dialysis, whereas others experience an elevation soon after starting. In some patients, the rise in BP is the result of increased cardiac output as the fluid overload is relieved. In other instances, there may be an increase in peripheral vascular resistance on a reflex or hormonal basis. Angiotensin-converting enzyme inhibitor therapy or bilateral nephrectomy may be indicated in cases where high renin levels are present, whereas hypertension in very young and old patients may respond to a lower blood flow rate and use of a smaller surface area dialyzer.

Are Arrhythmias Common During Dialysis?

As a larger number of older patients and people with complicating diseases are entering end-stage renal disease programs, arrhythmias have become more frequent during dialysis. Underlying heart diseases most often causes arrhythmias. The physician should make the presence of such problems and their significance known to the dialysis personnel. Evaluation of a new or different rhythm that develops during dialysis requires an electrocardiogram. The patient should be queried regarding medications, and a review of the recent serum potassium, calcium, and magnesium values should be made. Patients with myocardial damage may develop arrhythmias of various types in response to volume changes or shifts in electrolytes, particularly potassium. Patients receiving digitalis may pose particular problems.

What If a Patient Develops Chest Pain During Dialysis?

Some patients have chest pain that begins at the start of or during dialysis. Often these people have a history of an underlying heart disease, and the pain must be presumed to be angina. It may be alleviated if the blood flow is slowed, UF is decreased, oxygen is applied, or saline is infused. Some patients occasionally have vague chest distress or low back pain. The mechanism is obscure but often seems related to blood volume changes or decreased hematocrit. New or unexpected chest pain that occurs in a patient with no known history of cardiac disease should be reported immediately to the physician.

What Causes Muscle Cramping During Dialysis?

Muscle cramping during dialysis is probably caused by fluid shifts or osmolar changes, although pH changes may also play a role. Adjusting the dialysis prescription may sometimes relieve the cramps. Use of sodium modeling may be preventive, and infusion of hypertonic saline or a 50% dextrose solution usually brings relief when cramps occur but is generally discouraged because of the postdialysis thirst and its associated increased interdialytic weight gain. Applying heat and pressure over the painful area are temporary measures. Adjusting fluid and sodium intake between dialysis treatments may also help to prevent cramping during treatment. The best antidote is prevention by keeping interdialytic weight gains at a reasonable amount.

WHAT ARE OTHER SERIOUS COMPLICATIONS DURING DIALYSIS?

Other complications that can occur during dialysis are hemolysis and air embolism.

WHAT IS HEMOLYSIS?

Hemolysis is the lysis (breakup) of red blood cells, resulting in the release of intracellular potassium. Hemolysis may be caused by chemical, thermal, or mechanical events. The chemical causes of hemolysis include exposure of the blood to chemicals such as sodium hypochlorite, formaldehyde, copper, or nitrates. Thermal hemolysis is caused by the exposure of blood to an overheated dialysate. Dialysate temperatures greater than $42°C$ are considered dangerous. The mechanical causes of hemolysis include kinking of the bloodlines, overoccluded blood pumps, excessive negative pressure from a small-gauge needle with a high blood flow rate, or a poorly positioned needle. Other causes of hemolysis include dialyzing the patient against a hypotonic bath and blood transfusions. Hemolysis may be acute or chronic. It may be slight and require no immediate treatment or it may be a life-threatening emergency. Acute hemolysis during dialysis treatment is a medical emergency. The patient may also experience symptoms after returning home from dialysis treatment and present in the emergency department. For unknown reasons, pancreatitis will sometimes occur following an episode of acute hemolysis.

WHAT ARE THE SYMPTOMS OF HEMOLYSIS?

With hemolysis, the blood in the extracorporeal circuit may appear transparent, with a "cherry soda pop" color; however, the blood also may appear very dark and opaque. Other symptoms of hemolysis are a burning sensation in the access extremity, usually the venous needle, from the release of large amounts of potassium from the ruptured red blood cells. The patient will often complain of abdominal pain or cramping, low back pain, chest pain, nausea and vomiting, shortness of breath, or indigestion. Cardiac changes may be seen as potassium is released from the cells, causing arrhythmias and bradycardia with hypotension or hypertension. An acute drop in hematocrit will be seen as the red blood cells rupture.

WHAT STEPS SHOULD BE TAKEN IF YOU SUSPECT HEMOLYSIS IN A PATIENT?

Monitors should detect a hypotonic dialysate solution or high dialysate temperature; however, machines are not infallible. Careful monitoring by dialysis personnel is essential to avoid this potentially life-threatening complication. If hemolysis is suspected, the bloodlines should be clamped immediately, the blood pump stopped, and the patient's symptoms treated. The patient's blood should not be reinfused. The dialysate should be sampled for pH and conductivity. A blood sample from the patient should be obtained and checked for hematocrit, electrolytes, free hemoglobin, and haptoglobin. If hemolysis is suspected, a blood sample in a serum separator tube will have red serum when centrifuged. It is important to remember that hemolyzed blood cells should never be reinfused. Returning hemolyzed blood could cause hyperkalemia. The patient's symptoms should be treated and the physician should be notified immediately.

WHAT IS AN AIR EMBOLISM?

Air embolism occurs when air or a large amount of foam (microbubbles) is introduced into a patient's vascular system. Air embolism can occur when arterial or venous lines become disconnected or when blood or saline infusion bags run dry. The resultant vacuum causes microbubbles or foam. The dialysis personnel are responsible for setting and monitoring the air/foam detector throughout the entire dialysis procedure.

WHAT SYMPTOMS ARE ASSOCIATED WITH AN AIR EMBOLISM?

Symptoms will vary depending on the volume of air introduced, the site of introduction, patient's position, and the speed at which air is introduced (Feehally, 2019). The patient may complain of chest pain or tightness or shortness of breath and may cough. If the patient is sitting upright, air may be introduced into the cerebral venous system and cause neurologic symptoms, such as visual problems, loss of consciousness, and convulsions.

WHAT ACTION IS TAKEN IF A PATIENT RECEIVES AN INFUSION OF AIR?

Air embolism is a serious complication and should be treated as a medical emergency. When a patient receives air, treatment must be immediate. The bloodlines are clamped, and dialysis is stopped. The patient's blood should not be reinfused. The patient is placed on the left side in the Trendelenburg (head-down) position. This position decreases the movement of air to the brain and traps air in the right atrium above the tricuspid valve. This minimizes foaming, which occurs primarily in the right ventricle of the heart. It is important to maintain the patient's airway and to administer oxygen if needed. The patient must be moved as little as possible and must be maintained in the Trendelenburg position. It takes several hours for all of the air, particularly nitrogen, to be totally reabsorbed. A chest x-ray examination should be done to evaluate the amount of air present in the heart.

What Is Disequilibrium Syndrome?

The disequilibrium syndrome is a situation that produces neurologic and other symptoms soon after a patient begins dialysis treatments. New patients are at the highest risk of developing this complication, particularly when initiated on dialysis with high-flux dialyzers with large surface areas and shorter dialysis times. The risk factors include young age, severe uremia, low dialysate sodium concentration, and preexisting neurologic disorders (Feehally, 2019). Urea has the ability to move freely between the cells and serum. Theories suggest that when a patient who is very uremic is dialyzed for the first time, the plasma becomes more hypotonic as the urea is removed, causing water to shift from the plasma into the brain tissue, which is less hypotonic and contains higher amounts of urea. This usually occurs in patients with very high blood urea nitrogen levels or those with acute kidney injury. As water flows to the higher urea concentration, the brain cells begin to swell, causing neurologic symptoms ranging from headache, nausea, vomiting, restlessness, and twitching to the more severe tremors, disorientation, and convulsions. Symptoms usually develop toward the end of dialysis but may be delayed for up to 24 hours posttreatment. Treatment includes administration of a hypertonic solution, such as hypertonic saline, 50% dextrose, or mannitol. The patient's symptoms should be treated. Delivering a less effective treatment by using lower blood and dialysate flow rates, decreasing the treatment time, or running the patient with a concurrent flow will help to minimize these symptoms until the blood urea nitrogen levels stabilize.

Happens During a Dialyzer Reaction?

Dialyzer reactions are sometimes referred to as "first-use syndrome" because some patients develop allergic-type symptoms when exposed to the dialyzer membrane for the first time. Dialyzer reactions are now more commonly referred to as type A and type B reactions.

Type A reactions are the more severe of the two and often present with anaphylactic-type symptoms. These reactions usually occur within the first 5 minutes of treatment, with the patient experiencing the following symptoms: dyspnea, chest and back pain, feeling of warmth, sense of impending doom, and cardiac arrest. Less threatening symptoms include itching, urticaria, coughing, sneezing, watery eyes, and abdominal cramping. Type A reactions are usually caused by the factory sterilant ethylene oxide (ETO). This type of reaction is less common today because some dialyzer manufacturers are using alternative sterilization methods such as gamma irradiation, electron-beam sterilization, or steam sterilization. For those using dialyzers sterilized with ETO, proper priming of the dialyzer may help to prevent pockets of ETO remaining in the fibers that are released during dialysis treatment.

Type B reactions are less threatening but more commonly seen. The symptoms usually occur as soon as the patient's blood is exposed to the dialyzer and returned to the patient. Symptoms include chest pain, hypotension, and occasionally back pain. The treatment for both types of reactions is based on symptoms. Dialysis treatment should be discontinued until the cause of the symptoms is determined and the physician is notified. The patient's blood should not be reinfused. Oxygen is generally administered for breathing difficulties. Intravenous antihistamines or epinephrine may be ordered for anaphylaxis. BP support may also be necessary for hypotension.

What Is a Formaldehyde Reaction?

A formaldehyde reaction occurs when the patient's blood is exposed to this sterilant. This may occur when a formaldehyde-filled dialyzer is incorrectly rinsed of the sterilant or from improper testing for the presence of residual formaldehyde. Symptoms include a bitter peppery taste in the mouth, anxiety, burning in the venous needle, numbness around the mouth or lips, chest and back pain, and shortness of breath. It is important to recognize and treat formaldehyde reactions immediately because hemolysis of red blood cells may also occur. The dialysis treatment should be stopped, and the patient's symptoms should be treated. Approximately 10 mL of blood should be removed from each needle so that the patient receives no further formaldehyde. Proper rinsing of the system and attention to safety testing for residual formaldehyde will help alleviate this complication.

What Causes a Pyrogen Reaction?

A pyrogen reaction may occur from an improperly sterilized dialyzer, bacteria in the water system or dialysate, a break in the aseptic technique, or improper access preparation. A pyrogen is a fever-producing substance, usually an endotoxin, which is a byproduct of dead bacterial cell walls. Bacteria are too large to cross the dialyzer membrane, but an endotoxin is small enough to cross and cause the symptoms. A patient will experience chills after the commencement of dialysis treatment, along with a decrease in systolic BP. Headache, fever, myalgia (muscle pain), nausea, and vomiting may also be experienced. The symptoms will usually subside after the patient's treatment is discontinued. Hypotension and fever may need to be treated. Blood cultures may be ordered. It is imperative to practice scrupulous infection control techniques when accessing a patient's catheter or internal access. Dialyzers should never be used if they have been recirculating for longer than allowed by the manufacturer's directions and the facility's policy. Care must be taken to disinfect dialysate jugs, mixing tanks, and machines as per the facility's policy. It is important to rule out septicemia because the symptoms are very similar to those of a pyrogen reaction.

What Are the Potential Problems with Hemodialysis Equipment?

Hemodialysis equipment is designed to protect the patient from complications that may occur during treatment. However, machines are not infallible and will periodically malfunction. A malfunction of the temperature control device can cause hyperthermia, resulting in hemolysis. If not detected, this condition could cause death. Its opposite, hypothermia, can also occur; this condition can cause extreme chills and violent shaking.

ARE THERE OTHER EQUIPMENT COMPLICATIONS?

Other equipment complications may occur when dialyzers and bloodlines become disconnected, leak, or clot. Careful monitoring can prevent most machine complications. Machine maintenance also plays an important role in the prevention of machine-related accidents. Chapter 6 discusses the equipment and the preventive maintenance.

WHAT IS ARTERIAL PRESSURE?

Arterial pressure is a measurement of the extracorporeal blood circuit pressure between the patient's needle site and a site proximal to the blood pump. It is not the equivalent of the patient's systemic arterial pressure but rather the negative pressure created by the blood pump. Prepump arterial pressure indicates the ease with which the blood pump is able to draw blood from the fistula. Arterial monitoring guards against excessive suction in the vascular access. For example, if the patient's arterial pressure has been reading -100 mm Hg and it suddenly increases to -200 mm Hg, this could indicate a clotted or dislodged needle, a drop in the patient's systemic BP, or a kink in the arterial line. If the arterial negative pressure increases or decreases, as long as the monitor is properly set, the alarm will be activated, and the blood pump will shut off. This audible and visual alarm alerts the caregiver to a dialysis complication and always requires immediate attention. The alarm will remain activated, and the blood pump will not work until the abnormality is corrected. A high negative arterial pressure must always be assessed, and steps must be taken to correct the problem. A high negative arterial pressure may damage the vascular access and may cause hemolysis in the patient. Arterial pressure monitoring is effective for identifying flow problems and may be the earliest indication of AV fistula dysfunction.

WHAT IS VENOUS PRESSURE?

Venous pressure is a measurement of the extracorporeal blood circuit pressure at some point after the dialyzer and before the blood reenters the patient's body. The monitoring line is usually attached to the top of the venous bubble trap. Venous extracorporeal pressure measures the resistance of the blood returning to the patient via the venous needle. For example, if the patient's venous pressure reading suddenly increases from 50 to 150 mm Hg, this increase would indicate that the venous line may be kinked, the bubble trap may be clotted, the venous needle may be clotted or misaligned, or the vascular access may be in danger of failing. If, however, there is a sudden and marked decrease in venous pressure, the venous needle may have been pulled out, the transducer may be wet, or the arterial chamber may be clotted. The venous pressure alarm is similar to the arterial pressure alarm in that, when activated, the abnormal condition must be corrected before the machine will allow the blood to continue flowing through the blood circuit.

Note that all alarms must be set properly at the initiation of dialysis. This ensures that if any complication occurs, an audible and visual alarm will activate and alert caregivers to a potential problem.

WHAT EFFECT DOES THE DIALYSIS SOLUTION (DIALYSATE) FLOW RATE HAVE ON DIALYZER CLEARANCE?

The dialysis solution flow rate affects the clearance of small solutes such as urea. The usual dialysis solution flow rate is 500 mL/min, although some types of dialysis equipment (e.g., Sorb System's Redy 2000) use a rate of 250 mL/min. The slower flow rate leads to slightly lower dialyzer urea clearance. Dialysis solution flow rates up to 800 mL/min are used to increase clearance for high-efficiency dialysis. A higher dialysate flow rate can be used to enhance urea clearance when the blood flow rate is reduced for any reason. Clarkson et al (2010) state that studies have demonstrated the practical upper limit of effective dialysate flow is twice the blood flow rate, beyond which the gain in solute removal is minimal.

WHY SHOULD PATIENTS WITH CHRONIC KIDNEY DISEASE CONTROL THEIR FOOD AND ORAL FLUID INTAKE DURING DIALYSIS TREATMENT?

There are several reasons for controlling food and oral fluid intake during dialysis treatment. First, the amount of fluid removed by UF is the net change in weight from the predialysis weight to the postdialysis weight. If the patient consumes large amounts of food and fluids during dialysis, this net weight change does not reflect a realistic fluid loss. The quantity of food or fluid ingested during dialysis should always be taken into consideration when calculating the amount of fluid to ultrafiltrate during the dialysis procedure. If it is permissible for patients to eat during dialysis, it is best to limit this to very small snacks. Food in the digestive tract causes pooling of blood and may cause hypotension, vomiting, and an increased risk of aspiration. Still, with more efficient dialysis and removal of fluid, dialysis patients have fewer restrictions with respect to oral intake than previously. See Chapter 14 for more on nutrition.

POSTDIALYTIC THERAPY ASSESSMENT

WHAT IS POSTDIALYTIC ASSESSMENT?

Postdialytic assessment is the total evaluation of the patient and treatment and an interpretation of the predialytic goals. The factors to be included are listed in Box 13.1.

Box 13.1 Patient Parameters Evaluated After Dialysis

- Patient's weight and weight loss
- Vital signs (e.g., temperature, pulse, and respiration and blood pressure)
- Resolution or improvement of problematic predialysis parameters (improvement of fluid status)
- Total infusions given, both saline and blood
- Patient's subjective physical assessment (e.g., any pain or complaints)
- Access assessment
- Bleeding status

ARE THERE OTHER POSTDIALYTIC ASSESSMENTS?

The dialysis prescription plan is assessed for any changes that will be implemented in the next dialysis. Finally, the date for the next dialysis is scheduled.

CHAPTER 14

NUTRITION MANAGEMENT

Nutrition plays a critical role in the management of kidney disease. The diet will vary considerably depending on the type and stage of kidney disease as well as on patient and treatment modality–specific factors. Diet may slow the progression of kidney disease in any of the first four stages. Researchers have determined that people with normal kidney function who consume a poor-quality diet, high in red and processed meats, sugar-sweetened beverages, and sodium, were more likely to develop kidney disease. A "renal diet" that can be applied to all patients does not exist. Each situation must be evaluated individually. Certain commonalities may apply to patients with chronic and acute kidney injury (AKI); however, dietary requirements change with the progression of chronic kidney disease (CKD). Dietary restrictions are often considered the most difficult challenge that CKD patients may encounter. Fluid restrictions add an additional burden on CKD patients undergoing maintenance dialysis.

Dialysis therapy for patients with either acute kidney disease or CKD can provide optimal patient outcomes when combined with effective and appropriate nutrition management. Although diet management is ultimately the responsibility of the patient or caretaker, members of the interdisciplinary team play a vital role in educating and reinforcing diet information that is tailored to the individual and monitored for effectiveness.

WHY IS DIET IMPORTANT FOR PEOPLE WITH KIDNEY DISEASE?

Diet therapy offers the following potential benefits:
- It may be helpful in delaying the need for dialysis.
- Diet can help minimize many of the complications of kidney disease (e.g., phosphorus restriction to aid in the prevention of bone disease).
- Adequate protein and calorie nutrition can influence morbidity and mortality in patients with kidney disease.
- It can manage coexisting comorbidities such as diabetes, hypertension, and hyperlipidemia.
- The quality of life of CKD patients may be improved by individualization of the diet to suit lifestyle, ethnic, and socioeconomic variables.

WHAT IS THE ROLE OF A REGISTERED DIETITIAN?

The renal dietitian must be a registered dietitian with the Commission on Dietetic Registration and have a minimum of 1 year of professional work experience in clinical nutrition as a registered dietitian.

The registered dietitian is part of the facility's interdisciplinary team and, as such, makes recommendations for the patient's treatment plan. The dietitian will also work with the nephrologist and make recommendations for the patient's diet prescription. The patient and family are taught specifics of the diet by the dietitian who monitors nutrition-related parameters and reevaluates needs. Communication between the dietitian, nurses, technicians, physician, and social worker regarding changes in a patient's medical condition, dialysis treatment, medications, psychosocial situation, and nutritional status is critical to providing optimal patient care.

WHAT NUTRITIONAL PARAMETERS ARE ASSESSED IN THE PATIENT WITH CHRONIC KIDNEY DISEASE?

The patient's nutritional status must be monitored and evaluated by a qualified dietitian. The dietitian will monitor the patient's nutritional status, hydration status, appetite, gastrointestinal (GI) status, laboratory data, ability to chew and swallow, and use of dietary or herbal supplements. Glycemic control monitoring is important in patients with diabetes. The dietitian will also assess the patient's ability to prepare food and make recommendations to help the patient modify current dietary habits to better meet the requirements of the renal diet.

WHAT DIET CONCERNS ARE PRESENT BEFORE THE INITIATION OF DIALYSIS?

Before dialysis, the diet is constructed to achieve several goals. One goal is to delay the need for dialysis by slowing the decline of kidney function. At present, studies are inconclusive as to whether protein or phosphorus restriction can help slow the progression of kidney disease. The Kidney Disease Outcomes Quality Initiative (KDOQI) clinical practice guidelines for CKD suggest that patients with a glomerular filtration rate (GFR) of less than 60 mL/min/1.73 m^2 should undergo assessment of dietary protein, energy intake, and nutritional status.

The number one preventable risk factor for CKD is obesity because it is directly linked to both diabetes and hypertension. High caloric intake itself may increase the risk for developing CKD (Wickman & Kramer, 2013). Feehally (2019) suggests weight loss may be appropriate in early CKD because it is associated with a more rapid decline of kidney function.

In addition to possibly delaying the progression of kidney disease, protein restriction, when used with adequate caloric intake, can be helpful in minimizing nitrogenous wastes and can aid in the control of uremic symptoms. Diet management can often be effective in delaying the need for dialysis until the GFR falls below about 15 mL/min/1.73 m^2, at which time some type of renal replacement therapy is necessary. Preservation of the nutritional status by provision of adequate calories to maintain or achieve a desirable body weight and avoid endogenous protein catabolism is of prime importance during this period. Reducing protein intake may be beneficial in delaying the progression of kidney disease, and KDIGO has suggested that protein intake should be lowered to 0.8g/kg/day in adults with CKD and a GFR less than 30 mL/min/1.73 m^2 (Feehally, 2019).

Phosphorus control through limiting high-phosphorus foods or the use of phosphate-binding medications is often necessary when the GFR falls below 20 mL/min/1.73 m^2. (Phosphorus control is discussed later in this chapter.)

Another diet concern before the initiation of dialysis is sodium control for patients who are edematous or hypertensive. Sodium should be restricted to less than 5 g/day and education provided on the use of salt substitutes which contain potassium chloride. Potassium restriction is generally not necessary until urine output falls below 1000 mL/day; therefore, potassium restriction may not be necessary until after dialysis is initiated.

WHAT ARE THE DIET MODIFICATIONS FOR HEMODIALYSIS?

The need for dietary modification after initiating hemodialysis is highly individualized and is dependent on factors such as height, weight, nutritional status, residual kidney function level, laboratory data, intercurrent illnesses, and prescribed medications. Maintenance of good nutritional status, as evidenced by adequate anthropometric measurements and biochemical indices, is critically important during this period. Achieving and maintaining normal serum albumin levels is the primary goal of nutrition therapy for hemodialysis patients. Various studies have demonstrated that the primary biochemical predictor of mortality in hemodialysis patients is low serum albumin levels. In the absence of proteinuria or significant liver disease, albumin levels can be maintained with the provision of adequate protein and calories. Although the diet is highly individualized, certain diet commonalities do apply to most hemodialysis patients.

WHY DO WE MONITOR ALBUMIN IN DIALYSIS PATIENTS?

Albumin is a biomarker that is monitored to assess the nutritional status of patients with CKD. The level will be suboptimal with a poor protein dietary intake or with impaired digestion. Albumin is also decreased from non-nutritional factors such as infection, inflammation, liver disease, catabolism, surgery, and peritoneal dialysis (PD). You will see an elevated serum albumin with dehydration. Symptoms of hypoalbuminemia or a low albumin are weight loss, fatigue, low energy, delayed wound healing, hair loss, edema, and muscle wasting.

WHAT AMOUNT OF PROTEIN IS APPROPRIATE FOR HEMODIALYSIS PATIENTS?

The NKF KDOQI Clinical Practice Guidelines for Nutrition in Chronic Renal Failure suggest a predialysis or stabilized serum albumin equal to or greater than the lower limit of the normal range of 4.0 g/dL as the outcome goal and those out of range evaluated for protein energy malnutrition (2000). Protein requirements, as suggested by current research, are thought to be 1.2 ± 0.2 g/kg/day, with the upper end of the range considered appropriate for protein-malnourished patients. In general, at least 50% of this protein should be derived from high biological value protein sources, such as meat, fish, poultry, tofu, eggs, dairy, and cheese. Such protein sources contain a full complement of essential amino acids. Examples of low biological value protein sources are fruits, vegetables, legumes, and grains or starches such as bread, pasta, cereal, and rice; however, a carefully planned vegetarian diet can be used without compromising the nutritional status (Fig. 14.1). The protein needs of hemodialysis patients are higher than those of the general population, in part because of the loss of 5 to 10 g of amino acids during each hemodialysis treatment.

WHAT CALORIC LEVEL IS ADVISABLE?

Energy requirements for hemodialysis patients are not well defined, although they are generally accepted to be 35 kcal/kg/day for maintenance. With stress or malnutrition, caloric needs may be as high as 40 to 45 kcal/kg/day. For obese patients, 25 to 30 kcal/kg/day may be appropriate. Some patients may need to modify their diet to maintain an acceptable body mass index for transplant consideration.

WHAT ABOUT POTASSIUM CONTROL?

Almost all foods contain potassium, and certain fruits and vegetables are particularly rich sources. Approximately two thirds of all potassium in our diet comes from fruits and vegetables. The kidney is the main route for potassium excretion. When urine output falls below 1000 mL/day, and in some cases before this happens, potassium should be controlled in the diet. The NKF's expert panel recommended potassium restriction to 2 g/day or less for individuals with advanced CKD (e.g., stage 4 CKD and estimated GFR values <30 mL/min/1.73 m^2). For patients on maintenance dialysis, a potassium restricted diet is typically about 2 g/ day. The specific dietary potassium intake depends on the size of the patient; level of potassium in the dialysate; and other factors that may affect serum potassium levels such as residual urine output, missed treatments, or catabolism. Factors other than dietary indiscretion may contribute to hyperkalemia, including severe acidosis, constipation, catabolism, insulin deficiency, and use of certain medications such as β-adrenergic-blocking agents and angiotensin-converting enzyme inhibitors, herbal supplements, and nonsteroidal antiinflammatory drugs. The potassium content of selected foods may be found in Appendix B.

Protein Tips for Patients with Chronic Kidney Disease

Protein is found in many foods and comes from either animals or plants.

Protein helps to maintain and repair muscles, organs, and other parts of the body.

Animal proteins are high biological value proteins and include all of the building blocks your body needs.

Plant proteins are low biological value proteins and need to be combined to get all of the building blocks your body needs.

Animal Protein Foods

- Meat, such as pork, beef, chicken, turkey, duck
- Eggs
- Dairy products, such as milk, yogurt, cheese
- Fish

Plant-Protein Foods

High Protein

- Beans, peas, lentils
- Soy foods, such as soy milk, tofu
- Nuts and nut spreads such as almond butter, peanut butter, soy nut butter
- Sunflower seeds

Low Protein

- Bread, tortillas
- Oatmeal, grits, cereals
- Pasta, noodles, rice
- Rice milk (not enriched)

Protein Needs for Modality

If you are on **hemodialysis**, you should aim for 1.2 grams pf protein per kg of body weight.

If you are on **peritoneal dialysis**, you should aim for 1.3 grams of protein per kg of body weight.

How to Eat the Right Amount of Protein

Eat smaller portions of meat and dairy. This will help you to lower the amount of phosphorus in your diet because phosphorus is found in meat and dairy products.

Meat, poultry, fish: A cooked portion should be about 2 to 3 ounces or about the size of a deck of cards.

Dairy foods: A portion is 1/2 cup of milk or yogurt or one slice of cheese.

Plant-based foods: These should make up the rest of the protein that you eat. A serving is:

- 1/2 cup of cooked beans
- 1/4 cup of nuts
- A slice of bread
- 1/2 cup of cooked rice or noodles

Fig. 14.1 Renal diet teaching aids: tips on protein intake. (Data from Eating Right for Chronic Kidney Disease. Retrieved from https://www.niddk.nih.gov/health-information/kidney-disease/chronic-kidney-disease-ckd/eating-nutrition#protein. Accessed July 13, 2019.)

How Much Sodium Is Acceptable?

An intake of approximately 87 mEq or 2000 mg/day (2 g/day) of sodium is appropriate for most hemodialysis patients. Adjustments can be made depending on the blood pressure, urine output, and presence or absence of edema. Hypertension in CKD patients is largely volume related, and dry weight should be constantly reassessed in hypertensive patients. Renin-mediated hypertension is present in a small percentage of dialysis patients. Appropriate antihypertensive medications, rather than further sodium and fluid restrictions, are necessary for this subgroup. It is wise to caution your patients about the hidden potassium found in some low-sodium products and salt substitutes that contain potassium chloride. The sodium content of specific foods may be found in Appendix C.

What Level of Fluid Intake Is Acceptable?

Generally, the recommended fluid intake is 1000 mL/day or 1000 mL plus an amount equal to the urine output. Fluids contained in foods, such as fruits and vegetables, are not usually counted in this total. Foods that are liquid at room temperature, such as popsicles, soups, gelatin, and ice, are counted in the daily fluid allotment. The volume of fluid in solid foods, approximately 500 to 800 mL/day, is roughly equivalent to insensible fluid losses; therefore, the remaining "visible" fluid intake will correlate with interdialytic weight gain. An acceptable interdialytic weight gain is 1.5 kg or less than 3% of the body weight. The fluid restriction is a physician order and may be determined in consultation with the renal dietitian. Excessive fluid contributes to high blood pressure, edema, and results in left ventricular hypertrophy.

What About Phosphorus and Calcium Intake?

Phosphorus intake should be limited to 800 to 1200 mg/day in those with stage 5 CKD (KDOQI Clinical Practice Guidelines for Bone Metabolism, 2003). Because the phosphorus content of the diet correlates with protein intake, it may be necessary to include some high-phosphorus foods to achieve adequate protein intake. Phosphorus is also controlled by the intake of phosphate-binding antacids, such as calcium carbonate or calcium acetate. Aluminum-containing antacids should be avoided to minimize the risk of aluminum bone disease. Calcium-containing antacids are given with meals and snacks and are ideally titrated to the phosphorus content of the diet. The calcium content in the diet is typically low because foods high in phosphorus also tend to be rich sources of calcium. Calcium supplements, apart from the calcium in phosphate-binding antacids, may not be necessary to maintain the calcium balance when either oral or intravenous 1,25-dihydroxycholecalciferol is used. Calcium requirements vary considerably depending on the intake of phosphate, use of vitamin D, calcium content of the dialysate, and presence of hyperparathyroidism. This is discussed in greater detail in Chapter 17.

Phosphorus additives are commonly found in many best-selling processed groceries and convenience foods. Foods that contain higher levels of phosphorus additives are also less expensive, making them more attractive to purchase. This may contribute to difficulties with phosphorus control for dialysis patients while unknowingly increasing their intake of highly bioavailable phosphorus. Additives are particularly common in prepared frozen foods, dry food mixes, packaged meats, bread and baked goods, soups, and yogurt (León, Sullivan, & Sehgal, 2013). It is crucial to educate patients on how to read food labels to help avoid phosphorus additives and adequately manage serum phosphorus levels.

Are Vitamin Supplements Necessary?

Dialysis patients may be at a risk of deficiencies of certain water-soluble vitamins because of poor nutrient intake, malabsorption, drug–nutrient interactions, altered vitamin metabolism, and dialysis losses. Although evaluation of specific requirements and recommendations is ongoing, supplementation with the US Recommended Daily Allowances (US RDA) of vitamins B_1, B_2, B_{12}, biotin, pantothenic acid, and niacin as well as 800 to 1000 mcg of folic acid and 10 mg of pyridoxine (vitamin B_6) daily is reasonable. The recommendations for folic acid, vitamin B_{12}, and vitamin B_6 continue to be reevaluated in light of the information concerning the amino acid intermediate homocysteine. Elevated levels of homocysteine have been demonstrated to be a risk factor for cardiovascular disease and can be present in CKD patients. High doses of folic acid, and in some studies vitamins B_6 and B_{12}, have been shown to normalize homocysteine levels and therefore may have a cardioprotective effect. The efficacy of high-dose supplementation of these B vitamins and the appropriate dosages are yet to be determined in the dialysis population. Vitamin C supplementation is limited to 60 mg/day. Higher doses of vitamin C should be avoided to prevent accumulation of oxalate, an ascorbic acid metabolite. Supplemental vitamin A should be avoided because of the potential toxicity related to the decreased kidney degradation of retinol-binding protein in kidney failure. Routine supplementation with a specially formulated vitamin is common in CKD patients undergoing maintenance dialysis.

What About the Need for Trace Minerals?

Trace mineral requirements are not well defined for dialysis patients, and at present, routine supplementation is not appropriate. Zinc deficiency may be present in some dialysis patients, although the best method of measuring stores is yet to be determined in this population. In patients who exhibit signs of zinc deficiency, such as hypogeusia (loss of sense of taste), delayed wound healing, or alopecia, a time-limited trial of zinc supplementation may be reasonable. Selenium is another trace metal, and investigation is ongoing into the possible role of selenium deficiency in promoting comorbid conditions, such as cardiovascular disease and cancer, in the dialysis population. The optimal method of assessing the selenium status and appropriate dosing remain to be defined.

How Is Iron Deficiency Assessed?

Iron deficiency is a common finding in dialysis patients receiving human recombinant erythropoietin and concomitant iron for erythropoiesis. Before the use of erythropoietin, iron overload was common in this population as a result of multiple blood transfusions. (Each unit of transfused blood contains approximately 200– 250 mg of iron.) Routine assessments of iron stores by serum ferritin and percent transferrin saturation (iron content divided by the total iron-binding capacity) should be included in any erythropoietin therapy protocol.

A low mean corpuscular volume may be a late indicator of iron deficiency. If deficiency is present, intravenous iron administration or oral iron supplementation is warranted. Increasing the iron content of the diet generally does not provide adequate replacement after iron deficiency is identified. Various oral forms of iron are available but may cause GI upset. Guidelines for administering intravenous iron and erythropoietin therapy are described in Chapter 17.

Do People on Dialysis Have to Control Fat Intake?

Dyslipidemia, typically seen as hypertriglyceridemia combined with low high-density lipoprotein cholesterol and normal total serum cholesterol, is the most common lipid abnormality found in dialysis patients. Some patients may present with elevated serum cholesterol, defined as serum cholesterol greater than 200 mg/dL. For these people, it may be appropriate to prescribe a low-cholesterol, low-fat diet.

Obesity may exacerbate hypertriglyceridemia. Therefore, in obese dialysis patients, weight control may be beneficial in helping to control triglyceride levels. A regular aerobic exercise program may also be beneficial in helping control both cholesterol and triglyceride levels. Carnitine, discussed later in this chapter, and fish oil supplements have also been shown to help lower triglyceride levels.

What About Sugar and Carbohydrates?

Restriction of sugar and carbohydrates is not appropriate or necessary for most people undergoing dialysis. Exceptions are people with diabetes and those who are overweight or have hypertriglyceridemia that may respond to total calorie restriction. Often sugars and other carbohydrates need to be increased to provide adequate calories in the diet.

How Is the Nutritional Status Monitored?

It is important to evaluate serum albumin levels and body weight in patients at least monthly. One category of assessment tools is anthropometric measurements, which include height, weight, ideal or desirable body weight, weight changes, and other measurements, such as triceps skinfold (to assess fat stores) and midarm muscle circumference (to measure somatic protein stores). A second category is biochemical data. Serum albumin correlates with the protein status in stable hemodialysis patients in the absence of a nephrotic syndrome or liver disease, although the levels are influenced by the volume status. Data from the US Renal Data System indicate that low serum albumin levels, as indicative of the overall nutritional status, are associated with increased mortality in hemodialysis patients. Serum albumin levels appear to be a less reliable indicator of the nutritional status in PD patients and do not correlate well with the mortality risk in these patients. Other biochemical parameters, such as serum transferrin levels, serum insulin-like growth factor 1 concentration, prealbumin levels, and low serum creatinine with low creatinine kinetics, have been used to assess the nutritional status, although each parameter has limitations.

Subjective data, such as food diaries or diet recall obtained by a skilled interviewer, can provide valuable information. A method called subjective global assessment has been used to quantify the nutritional status and includes physical assessment, functional impairment, GI symptoms, and anthropometric indices. Assessment of the patient's weight over the past 6 months, level of appetite, subcutaneous fat, and muscle mass are scored. The higher the score, the better is the nutritional status and the lower is the level of morbidity and mortality. The goal is to recognize and treat malnutrition before it becomes severe and debilitating, thus making it difficult to treat.

What Is Urea Kinetic Modeling?

Urea kinetic modeling (UKM) is used to prescribe and monitor dialysis therapy and to assess protein intake. Although there is no consensus regarding optimal methods for performing UKM and determining the results in the dialysis community, formal UKM has become a standard of practice for both hemodialysis and PD programs. UKM is usually performed using a computer because the mathematical computations are elaborate. Blood urea nitrogen (BUN) levels before and after a given dialysis treatment (some methods also include predialysis BUN levels from the subsequent dialysis treatment) are entered into the computer, and for patients who urinate, residual urea clearance is included. Information about the dialysis treatment (blood flow, dialysate flow, dialyzer clearance data, length of treatment, and interdialytic interval) and patient-specific data (predialysis and postdialysis weight, height, sex, and hematocrit) are also incorporated in the calculations.

What Do the Results of Urea Kinetic Modeling Mean?

One result derived from UKM is the Kt/V, which refers to the following:

$K =$ Dialyzer clearance for a given dialysis treatment and, if applicable, measurement of any residual urine urea clearance
$t =$ Length of time for a given dialysis treatment
$V =$ Volume of distribution of urea for a given patient that equates with total body water

The goal for delivered Kt/V is thought to be, at minimum, 1.2 for thrice-weekly dialysis for both adults and children. The goal Kt/V for other than thrice-weekly dialysis is a minimum of a delivered dose of 2.1 (NKF, 2015). Levels less than 1.2 may indicate inadequate dialysis and are associated with increased morbidity and poor prognosis on dialysis. Whether the Kt/V can be too high and whether higher levels of Kt/V improve morbidity and mortality remains to be evaluated.

What Other Methods Are Available for Estimating the Adequacy of Dialysis?

Percent urea reduction or urea reduction ratio (URR) is another method used to assess dialysis adequacy. A 65% reduction in BUN levels during a given dialysis treatment roughly correlates with a Kt/V of 1.2 for patients undergoing dialysis three times a week. URR is not a substitute for formal UKM because it does not reflect the contribution of residual kidney function or protein catabolic rate (PCR) and does not provide a means of evaluating the validity of the results.

How Is the Urea Reduction Ratio Calculated?

$$URR = 100 \times (1 - Ct/Co)$$

where Ct = Postdialysis BUN

Co = Predialysis BUN

What Is the Protein Catabolic Rate?

Protein catabolic rate refers to a given patient's protein intake expressed in grams of protein per kilogram normalized body weight, assuming that the patient is stable (i.e., neither anabolic nor catabolic). The goal PCR is between 0.8 and 1.4 g protein per kilogram and is probably optimal at the upper end of the range.

What Is the Basis for Interpreting the Results of Urea Kinetic Modeling?

Interpretation was originally based on the National Cooperative Dialysis Study (NCDS) published in 1983, in which an attempt was made to correlate patient outcome with the amount of dialysis delivered. Both hospitalization and morbidity increased with high BUN levels in the presence of inadequate protein intake. The NCDS data later underwent mechanistic analysis by Gotch and Sargent, from which the concept of Kt/V was derived. Since then, the generally accepted goals for Kt/V have continued to be reevaluated and revised upward.

What About Urea Kinetic Modeling for Peritoneal Dialysis?

Studies comparable to the NCDS are not available in the PD population. Guidelines are available for determining urea clearance and weekly creatinine clearance as well as PCR for this treatment modality. For continuous ambulatory peritoneal dialysis (CAPD), the delivered dose of PD should be a Kt/V of at least 1.7 per week and total creatinine clearance of at least 60 L/wk/1.73 m² (NKF KDOQI Clinical Practice Guidelines for Peritoneal Dialysis Adequacy, 2006). Variables that can be manipulated to achieve the targeted clearance include exchange volume, cycle time, ultrafiltration volume, continuous versus intermittent therapy, and dwell time or drainage time.

Peritoneal equilibration testing (PET) is performed to assess the clearance capabilities of a given patient's peritoneal membrane and to determine the optimal PD regimen. See Chapter 19 for further information on PET.

What Are Oral Nutritional Supplements?

Patients with CKD who are not meeting their nutritional needs may be offered oral nutritional supplements (ONSs). These supplements may help to improve serum albumin levels and the nutritional status of patients as well as reverse weight loss and decrease the morbidity and mortality associated with low serum albumin levels and malnutrition. Specially formulated ONSs for CKD patients are available with reduced potassium and phosphorus and high caloric and protein contents. ONSs usually come in the form of a liquid, powder, or bar. Examples of ONSs include Nepro, ZonePerfect protein bars, Pro-Stat, and VitalProteinRx protein bars. Liquacel is one ONS that might be offered to patients intradialytically. Specific facility guidelines must be followed for the type and amount of supplement that may be distributed. Nutritional supplements are ordered by the physician, and the dietitian can help to make recommendations on the best product for each patient. Protein powders are often used and may be derived from egg, rice, soy, or whey. These powders do not have to be mixed with liquids but can be mixed with other foods so as not to increase the patient's fluid intake. The patient's response to ONS must be monitored for efficacy in improving nutritional status on a regular basis.

What Is Intradialytic Parenteral Nutrition?

Intradialytic parenteral nutrition is a form of nutrition support by which protein, fat, and carbohydrate can be given during dialysis treatment. Typically, a 1-L solution of amino acids, lipid solution, and dextrose is infused during a dialysis run through the venous drip chamber. This provides 800 to 1000 calories and 60 to 90 g of amino acids. The advantage is that nutrients can be provided with concomitant removal of the volume, and a central line is not necessary because the dialysis access serves as the line of administration. Although this method cannot meet a patient's entire nutritional needs, it can provide supplemental nutrition for patients who are unable to take adequate intake by mouth, for whom enteral feeding is not an option, and for whom a central line is contraindicated. Approximately 90% of the amino acids infused are retained during this process. The potential side effects include hyperglycemia and reactive hypoglycemia.

What Can Be Done for Constipation?

Constipation is a common problem for people undergoing dialysis and is often related to medication taken for phosphate binding and iron preparations. The usual recommendations for this problem that are given to people not undergoing dialysis, such as increasing fluid intake, consuming relatively large amounts of bran products, and eating foods such as prunes and other fruits and vegetables, may not be appropriate for dialysis patients. Medications including stool softeners or substances such as sorbitol, which draws fluid into the intestinal tract, may be necessary to alleviate constipation. In chronic kidney failure, stool output is a major route of potassium excretion, allowing for 30 to 40 mEq/day of potassium excretion. In patients with hyperkalemia that cannot easily be accounted for by increased potassium intake, constipation should be considered as a possible etiological factor.

How Does the Diet Differ for Patients on Peritoneal Dialysis?

The diet for patients undergoing CAPD, continuous cycling PD, and other PD modalities differs from that of patients undergoing hemodialysis in several ways.

Protein

Protein needs are higher for PD patients as a result of dialysate protein losses in the dialysate that average about 9 g/day. Protein levels of 1.2 to 1.3 g per kilogram of body weight are prescribed and are often difficult to achieve, although there is evidence that some patients maintain a positive nitrogen balance on lower protein intakes. As with hemodialysis, the general recommendation is that at least 50% of the protein should be derived from high biological value sources; however, it is possible to maintain good protein nutriture with a carefully planned vegetarian diet. Protein supplements may be used when the needs cannot be met by high-protein foods alone.

Calories

Although caloric needs are the same for both hemodialysis and PD patients, those undergoing PD absorb 150 to 1000 calories per day from the dextrose in the dialysate. This may provide a particular advantage in patients with energy malnutrition or may be problematic in obese or hypertriglyceridemic patients. PD may create a full feeling in the abdomen resulting in a decreased appetite or cause early satiety.

Sodium and Fluid

Typically, dietary sodium and fluid can be liberalized for the PD patient compared with the same patient undergoing hemodialysis because the dextrose content of the dialysis solution can be adjusted with each exchange to remove varying volumes of fluid. A sodium intake of 4 g and a fluid intake guided by thirst can often provide acceptable fluid management, provided that dialysis can be adjusted to maintain euvolemia.

Potassium

Potassium control tends to be less of a problem in PD patients in part because the constant glucose infusion combined with endogenous insulin production drives potassium intracellularly. Supplemental potassium may be indicated in approximately 10% of PD patients. Hyperkalemia may be present in others.

Phosphorus

Control of serum phosphorus presents a challenge for PD patients. An obligatory higher phosphorus intake is often necessary to achieve an adequate dietary protein intake because foods that are high in protein tend to be high in phosphorus. The requirements for phosphate binding medications may therefore be higher.

Vitamins and Other Minerals

The need for these other nutrients is generally thought to be the same as that of hemodialysis patients.

What Is the Diet for a Patient with Acute Kidney Injury?

There is no set diet for AKI because the nutritional requirements vary considerably depending on the comorbid conditions, degree of kidney compromise, presence of anuria or oliguria, and whether the patient is receiving dialysis. The inflammatory process and physiologic stress which is often seem with AKI precipitates protein wasting and negative nitrogen balance (Gilbert & Weiner, 2018). High mortality rates continue to be associated with AKI, and protein-calorie malnutrition is thought to be one predictor of outcome. Although aggressive nutritional support has yet to be demonstrated to improve outcome, protein and caloric intake should be provided to meet the increased needs associated with hypercatabolism. Protein requirements may be 1.0 to 1.2 g/kg protein per kilogram per day if not receiving dialysis or 1.2 to 1.4 g/kg protein per kilogram per day if receiving dialysis. Increased loss of amino acids and proteins may occur in patients receiving continuous renal replacement therapy and PD (Gilbert & Weiner, 2018). If oral nutrition is not possible, enteral feeding is recommended.

Both essential and nonessential amino acids should be used in most situations requiring parenteral nutrition. Caloric requirements vary considerably and can be best determined in the intensive care unit setting using indirect calorimetry.

Do the Various Treatment Modalities Influence the Provision of Parenteral Nutrition?

Yes. The use of continuous arteriovenous or venovenous hemofiltration with or without dialysis allows for provision of the large volumes of fluid necessary to give adequate amounts of parenteral nutrition in hypercatabolic AKI patients. Renal replacement therapy, however, also contributes to the catabolic state because the loss of nutrients (amino acids), and high-flux membranes increase these losses in comparison with low-flux membranes. In addition, membrane characteristics, in particular bioincompatibility, may further enhance catabolism.

Can the Patient with Chronic Kidney Disease Use Herbal Remedies?

In recent years, people have become increasingly aware of alternative therapies in medicine and diet. Supplementing diets with herbs, vitamins and minerals, and other supplements may provide some health benefits; however, these products must be used with caution in CKD patients. Declining kidney function causes changes in the pharmacokinetics of many medications, leading to altered absorption, distribution, metabolism, and excretion. These changes necessitate dosage adjustments to prevent the patients from being exposed to toxic levels of certain medications. Recommendations from KDIGO suggest that herbal remedies should not be used in CKD because some are known to be nephrotoxic (KDIGO, 2013). There are no good-quality safety or efficacy data for many of these compounds. Many believe that these remedies are safe because they are labeled as "natural" and not viewed as drugs. Unfortunately, some of these remedies and natural products can have a detrimental effect on the kidneys and other organs of the body. AKI secondary to interstitial nephritis is associated with the use of certain Chinese herbal drugs, Aristolochia in particular. Juice from the noni plant *(Morinda citrifolia)*, which is promoted to increase mental clarity and improve physical performance, contains excessive potassium and should not be ingested by CKD patients. Ingestion of star fruit has been associated with harmful outcomes in CKD patients, causing neurologic symptoms, seizures, and intractable hiccups.

In the United States, herbal remedies are not regulated by the Food and Drug Administration. Therefore, consumers must trust that the manufacturer has prepared and advertised its product in good faith. Some herbal remedies have a direct toxic effect on the kidneys, and some may affect the electrolyte balance, blood pressure control, and anticoagulation. Some products may interfere with the efficacy of antirejection medications used in transplant patients. It is critical to question patients regarding their use of herbal supplements and alternative therapies because they are sometimes reluctant to reveal this information because they do not consider these supplements to be medications. Assessing herbal remedy use should become part of the nursing assessment performed in CKD patients. Health care workers should become familiar with herbal remedies and their effects on the kidneys and CKD patients. CKD patients should be encouraged to discuss the use of any herbal remedy with their nephrologist before use. Potassium and phosphorus are two minerals that should be limited in patients on dialysis. It is recommended that a physician be consulted for specific management of patient related medication management.

What About the Needs of Pediatric Patients?

The basic concepts of diet management apply to pediatric patients with chronic kidney failure, with one key exception: meeting the needs of protein, calories, and other nutrients to facilitate growth and development and electrolyte management. The NKF released an update to the Clinical Practice Guidelines for Nutrition in Children with CKD in 2008. The goals focus on maintaining an optimal nutritional status with near-normal growth patterns, avoiding uremia toxicity and metabolic abnormalities, and reducing chronic illness and mortality in adulthood. Additional focus has been placed on the presence of overnutrition in this population and the dietary and lifestyle practices that play a contributing role.

CHAPTER 15

LABORATORY DATA: ANALYSIS AND INTERPRETATION

What Are Normal Laboratory Values, and How Are They Interpreted in the Patient with Chronic Kidney Disease?

Review of the laboratory reports is included in the overall patient assessment. Any deviations from normal should be further evaluated according to the acceptable values for a dialysis patient. For example, creatinine and blood urea nitrogen (BUN) levels may not fall within the normal range because of chronic kidney disease (CKD). However, the dialysis personnel should follow a protocol that defines when BUN and creatinine levels exceed the acceptable range for a person undergoing dialysis and take appropriate action. Deviations from the acceptable range of laboratory values should be reported to the dialysis physician for appropriate intervention. Interventions may include a change in the dialysis prescription, medication, or both. See Table 15.1 for laboratory values in end-stage renal disease.

What Is Albumin?

Albumin is a type of protein that provides a good measure of the nutritional status of an individual. It is also the protein with the highest concentration in plasma. Albumin carries smaller molecules in the blood, such as medications, bilirubin, and calcium. Albumin helps to hold fluid in the blood vessels and is a good reflection of the patient's protein stores and nutritional status. It is a well-known and powerful predictor of morbidity and mortality in CKD patients. The normal levels range from 3.5 to 5.4 g/dL. A serum albumin level of 4.0 g/dL or greater is desired for CKD patients.

What Are the Symptoms of Low Albumin?

Low albumin levels, or hypoalbuminemia, cause edema as fluid shifts from the blood vessels into the tissues. Other symptoms of hypoalbuminemia include weight loss, fatigue, muscle wasting, and hypotension.

Why Are Dialysis Patients at Risk for Low Albumin Levels?

Albumin levels are greatly influenced by diet. Dialysis patients are well known to have poor nutrition because uremia causes a loss of appetite. Lack of knowledge regarding adequate protein intake, difficulties with cooking or shopping for food, nausea, and loss of appetite for protein-rich food are all barriers to good nutrition in dialysis patients. Some patients lose albumin in their urine, and peritoneal dialysis patients are at a high risk of reduced levels because albumin is transported across the peritoneal membrane.

Why Do We Monitor Albumin Levels So Closely?

Hypoalbuminemia affects one third of all hemodialysis patients and is linked to a higher risk of morbidity and mortality, particularly when the serum albumin level is below 3.8 g/dL (Sridhar & Josyula, 2013).

What Is the Relationship Between Albumin and C-Reactive Protein Levels?

C-reactive protein (CRP) is a protein produced in response to infection, inflammation, and tissue trauma and is used as a marker of inflammation. Elevated serum CRP levels are associated with low serum albumin levels in dialysis patients. A combination of the two factors has been identified as placing dialysis patients at a higher risk of developing heart disease and inflammation of the blood vessels. CRP is present in the sera of normal individuals at levels between 0 and 3 mg/L. Serum levels greater than 3 mg/L indicate an increased risk of a cardiovascular event. Serum CRP levels increase dramatically during infection or injury. Other factors associated with an increase in CRP levels in CKD patients include surgery, bioincompatible membranes, periodontal disease, high-flux dialysis, impure dialysate, arthritis, and uremia. The levels may increase 100 times or more during bacterial or viral infection. CRP levels peak 2 to 3 days after an acute infection and begin to decrease 1 to 2 weeks after the infection subsides. This is why CRP is useful as an early marker of infection, inflammation, or injury. Infection and inflammation have been identified as drivers of hypoalbuminemia that help to precipitate EPO resistance (Nissenson & Fine, 2017). The National Kidney Foundation (NKF) Kidney Disease Outcomes Quality Initiative (KDOQI) guidelines suggest CRP levels greater than 5 to 10 mg/L as being indicative of inflammation (NKF, 2006). Other recommendations include the frequent monitoring of CRP levels and assessment for sources of infection or inflammation in CKD patients.

Are Dialysis Patients At Risk for Aluminum Toxicity?

Aluminum is a light metal found in cookware, beverage cans, antacids, cosmetics, antiperspirants, aluminum-containing phosphate binders, and contaminated water. The kidneys are the main organs for the filtration and excretion of aluminum in the body. Most aluminum is protein bound, so it is not easily diffusible through the glomerulus. Deposition of aluminum in the bone, tissues, and brain can be seen with elevated levels.

Table 15.1 Laboratory Values in End-Stage Renal Disease[a]

NORMAL VALUE	NORMAL FOR PEOPLE ON DIALYSIS	FUNCTION	DIET CHANGES
Sodium			
135–145 mEq/L	135–145 mEq/L	Found in salt and many preserved foods. A diet high in sodium causes thirst. When patients drink too much fluid, it may actually dilute their sodium, and serum levels will appear low. If patients eat too much sodium and do not drink water, sodium may be high. Too much sodium and water raise blood pressure and can cause fluid overload, pulmonary edema, and congestive heart failure.	*High:* Check the fluid status. If the fluid gains are high, tell the patient to eat fewer salty foods. If the fluid gains are low, make sure that the patient is gaining approximately 1.5 kg between dialyses (or <4% body weight) and is not dehydrated (this is rare). *Low:* If the fluid gains are high, tell the patient to eat less salt and drink less fluid. Check the fluid status; the patient is probably drinking too much fluid. Limit weight gain to less than 4% of the body weight between runs and ask the patient to eat fewer salty foods and limit daily fluid intake to 3 cups (720 mL) plus the volume of 24-hr urine output.
Potassium			
3.5–5.5 mEq/L	3.5–5.5 mEq/L	Found in most high-protein foods, milk, fruits, and vegetables. Affects the activity of muscles, especially the heart. High levels can cause the heart to stop. Low levels can cause symptoms such as muscle weakness and atrial fibrillation.	*High:* Ascertain that no other causes, such as GI bleeding, trauma, or medications, are creating high potassium levels. Tell the patient to avoid foods with more than 250 mg/serving and limit the daily intake to 2000 mg. Consider lowering the potassium levels in the dialysate bath. Recheck the blood level on next treatment. *Low:* Add one high-potassium food/day and recheck the blood level. Consider raising the potassium level in the dialysate bath if the diet changes are not working.
Urea Nitrogen (BUN)			
7–23 mg/dL	50–100 mg/dL	Waste product of protein breakdown. Unlike creatinine, this is affected by the amount of protein in the diet. Dialysis removes urea nitrogen.	*High:* The patient is probably underdialyzed. Check eKt/V. Check nPNA. *Low:* Underdialysis is also a cause. BUN levels may decrease if the patient is not eating because of uremic symptoms. Also decreases with loss of muscle.

Table 15.1 Laboratory Values in End-Stage Renal Disease (*Continued*)

NORMAL VALUE	NORMAL FOR PEOPLE ON DIALYSIS	FUNCTION	DIET CHANGES
Creatinine 0.6–1.5 mg/dL	Less than 15 mg/dL	A normal waste product of muscle breakdown. This value is controlled by dialysis. Patients have a higher amount because they are not dialyzing 24 hrs a day, 7 days a wk, as they would with normal kidney function.	Dialysis normally controls creatinine levels. Low creatinine levels may indicate good dialysis or low body muscle. Check the clearance of urea during dialysis (Kt/V) to assess dialysis adequacy. A patient who is losing weight will break down more muscle, so creatinine levels may be higher. The patient may need to eat more protein and calories to stop weight loss.
URR N/A	Above 65% (or 0.65)	A measure of urea reduction that occurs during dialysis treatment. Postdialysis BUN levels are subtracted and divided by predialysis BUN levels to give a percentage.	No diet changes, but catabolism or anabolism will affect values as with Kt/V and equilibrated clearance of urea during dialysis (eKt/V).
eKt/V N/A	Above 1.2	A mathematic formula that attempts to quantify how well a patient is dialyzed. Represents the clearance of urea by the dialyzer multiplied by the minutes of treatment and divided by the volume of water the patient's body holds.	No diet changes. *High:* Higher values are associated with better outcomes. *Low:* Values below 1.2 are associated with increased morbidity and mortality.
Kt/V	Above 1.4 for hemodialysis Above 2 for peritoneal dialysis	Not adjusted for urea equilibration. See above.	No diet changes. See above.
nPNA N/A	0.8–1.4	A calculation used to assess the rate of protein turnover in the body. Assumes that the patient is not catabolic because of infection, fever, surgery, or trauma. A good indicator of stable protein intake when combined with dietary history and albumin. The term "normalized" means that values have been adjusted to the patient's "normal" or ideal weight.	*High:* The patient may need to decrease protein intake. Have the patient consult a nutritionist. The patient may be catabolic. The patient may be eating large amounts of protein. *Low:* The patient may need to increase protein intake. If the patient is putting out urine, a small urine volume can produce a big difference in the results. Have the patient keep a 48-hr urine collection.

Continued on following page

Table 15.1 Laboratory Values in End-Stage Renal Disease (*Continued*)

NORMAL VALUE	NORMAL FOR PEOPLE ON DIALYSIS	FUNCTION	DIET CHANGES
Albumin 3.5–5 g/dL (bromcresol green) 3–4.5 g/dL (bromcresol purple)	3.5–5 g/dL Above 3.4 g/dL	A good measure of health in dialysis patients. The protein is lost with all dialysis. If albumin levels are below 2.9 g/dL, fluid will "leak" from the blood vessels into the tissue, causing edema. When fluid is in the tissue, it is more difficult to remove with dialysis. Low albumin levels are closely associated with an increased risk of death in dialysis patients.	*Low:* Increase intake of protein-rich foods: meat, fish, chicken, eggs. A protein supplement may be needed. IV albumin corrects short-term problems with oncotic pressure but does not change serum albumin levels.
Calcium 8.5–10.5 mg/dL	8.5–10.5 mg/dL	Found in dairy products. Dialysis patients' intakes are usually low. Active vitamin D is needed for absorption. The calcium value multiplied by the phosphorus value should not exceed 59 or calcium will deposit in soft tissues. Because it is bound to albumin, calcium can be falsely lower if albumin is low. Ionized calcium is a more accurate test in this case.	*High:* Check with the doctor if the patient is taking calcium supplement or a form of active vitamin D These should be temporarily stopped. *Low:* If albumin levels are low, suggest an ionized calcium be drawn. The patient may need a calcium supplement between meals and active vitamin D. Check with the physician.
Phosphorus 2.5–4.8 mg/dL	3–6 mg/dL	Found in milk products, dried beans, nuts, and meats. Used to build bones and helps the body produce energy. Acceptable levels depend on a variety of factors, including serum calcium, PTH levels, and the level of phosphorus in the diet. If calcium and PTH levels are normal, a slightly higher-than-normal level of phosphorus is acceptable.	*High:* Limit milk and milk products to 1 serving/day. Remind patient to take phosphate binders as ordered with meals and snacks. Noncompliance with binders is the most common cause of high phosphorus levels. *Low:* Add 1 serving of milk products or other high-phosphorus food per day or decrease phosphate binders.
PTH Intact (I-PTH) 10–65 pg/mL	150–600 pg/mL	A high level of PTH indicates that calcium is being pulled out of bones to maintain serum calcium levels. This syndrome is called secondary hyperparathyroidism. Leads to osteodystrophy. Pulsed doses of oral or IV vitamin D usually lower PTH.	*High:* Check whether the patient is taking oral or IV active vitamin D. Contact the patient's physician regarding therapy. If the patient has no symptoms (high phosphorus, bone pain, fractures), treat less aggressively. *Low:* No treatment available.
Aluminum 0–10 mcg/L	Less than 40 mcg/L	Patients taking aluminum hydroxide phosphate binders may develop aluminum toxicity, which can cause bone disease and dementia. The levels should be checked every 6 mo.	*High:* Discontinue aluminum hydroxide treatment.

Table 15.1 Laboratory Values in End-Stage Renal Disease (*Continued*)

NORMAL VALUE	NORMAL FOR PEOPLE ON DIALYSIS	FUNCTION	DIET CHANGES
Magnesium 1.5–2.4 mg/dL	1.5–2.4 mg/dL	Magnesium is normally excreted in urine and can become toxic for dialysis patients. High levels may be caused by antacids or laxatives that contain magnesium such as milk of magnesia or Maalox.	No dietary changes, except use of nontoxic methods such as fiber to aid in constipation relief. If magnesium is used as a phosphate binder, the levels will need to be checked more often.
Ferritin *Male:* 20–350 mcg/L *Female:* 6–350 mcg/L	300–800 mcg/L with EPO 50 mcg/L without EPO	This is how iron is stored in the liver. If iron stores are low, RBC production is decreased.	*Low:* Iron in food is not well absorbed. Most patients need an IV iron supplement. Patients should not take oral iron at the same time as phosphate binders.
CO_2 22–25 mEq/L	22–25 mEq/L	Dialysis patients are often acidotic because they do not excrete metabolic acids in their urine. Acidosis may increase the rate of muscle and bone catabolism.	*Low:* Review eKt/V, BUN levels, and nPNA. Oral sodium bicarbonate may be given to raise CO_2, but it presents a significant sodium load to the patient.
Glucose 65–114 mg/dL	Same for nondiabetic patients Less than 300 mg/dL (patients with diabetes)	Because the kidney metabolizes insulin, low blood sugar levels caused by a longer half-life of insulin are possible. For patients with diabetes: high blood sugar levels may increase thirst.	Most people need 6–11 servings of breads and starches or cereals per day and 2–4 servings of fruit per day to provide energy. Patients with diabetes should avoid concentrated sweets unless the blood sugar level is low.

[a]This guide is to help in understanding laboratory reports. In this table, the normal values are for people with good kidney function. The acceptable values for dialysis patients are also given. Many factors affect blood values. Diet is only one of these. Underlying disease, adequacy of treatment, medications, and complications may all affect laboratory values.

BUN, Blood urea nitrogen; *CO_2,* carbon dioxide; *DHT,* dihydrotachysterol; *EPO,* erythropoietin; *GI,* gastrointestinal; *IV,* intravenous; *N/A,* not applicable; *nPNA,* normalized protein nitrogen appearance; *PTH,* parathyroid hormone; *RBC,* red blood cell; *URR,* urea reduction ratio.
Developed by Katy G. Wilkens MS, RD, Northwest Kidney Centers, Seattle, WA.

Aluminum toxicity was once prevalent among dialysis patients because they were exposed to aluminum from the water used in dialysis treatment and from the oral intake of aluminum-based binders. The use of aluminum-based phosphate binders is now generally avoided because of the harmful effects of aluminum accumulation in patients. The clinical consequences of aluminum toxicity involve symptoms in the brain, bone, and blood. These may or may not occur concurrently. High serum aluminum levels are associated with progressive neurologic symptoms, such as behavioral changes, slurred speech, and memory loss, that occur very subtly over time. Gastrointestinal (GI) irritation, loss of energy and appetite, anemia, and constipation are also associated with elevated aluminum levels. Dementia may be seen with advanced toxicity. Elevated aluminum levels may also cause epoetin alfa–resistant anemia and aluminum-induced bone disease. Normal serum levels range from 0 to 6 mcg/L, and the NKF KDOQI Clinical Practice Guidelines for Bone Metabolism and Disease in Chronic Kidney Disease (2003) recommend dialysate concentration of aluminum be maintained at less than 10 mcg/L, and baseline levels of serum aluminum should be less than 20 mcg/L.

WHAT IS THE TREATMENT FOR ALUMINUM TOXICITY?

Aside from removing the sources of exposure, the chelating agent deferoxamine mesylate (Desferal) may be used to remove excess aluminum. To chelate means to remove a heavy metal, such as lead, mercury, or aluminum, from the bloodstream. When administered, deferoxamine mesylate will form complexes with aluminum, which can then be removed from the blood during dialysis treatment. See Chapter 17 for additional information on deferoxamine.

How Does Potassium Work Inside the Body?

Potassium is the major intracellular cation and the second most abundant cation in the body. All but 2% of the total body potassium is within the cells of the body. Potassium is necessary for many cellular functions; neuromuscular control; skeletal, cardiac, and smooth muscle activity; and intracellular enzyme reactions. Potassium is influenced by the acid–base balance as potassium ions are shifted out of the cell and replaced with hydrogen ions in acidosis. The majority of excess potassium in the body is excreted by the kidneys in urine.

What Causes Hypokalemia?

Hypokalemia indicates serum potassium levels less than 3.5 mEq/L and may be caused by excessive GI losses, such as vomiting and diarrhea, diuretic use, laxative use, excessive sweating, poor diet, and burns. The symptoms of hypokalemia include weakness, fatigue, and abnormal heart rhythms.

How Is Hypokalemia Treated?

Dietary intake of potassium may need to be increased and intravenous (IV) potassium may be given if a rapid rise in serum potassium levels is needed. Dialyzing the patient on a higher potassium bath will minimize the diffusion of potassium and help maintain the serum levels. Hypokalemia can be a dangerous problem if left untreated.

What Is Hyperkalemia?

Hyperkalemia indicates serum potassium levels greater than 5.5 mEq/L and is usually the result of excessive dietary intake of high-potassium foods. The expected level for a dialysis patient is 3.6 to 5.0 mEq/L. Other causes of increased serum potassium are catabolic states, tissue or crush injury, blood transfusions, GI bleeding, hemolysis, missed dialysis treatments, and acidosis. The symptoms include abdominal cramps, shortness of breath, dizziness, diarrhea, muscle weakness, hypotension, electrocardiogram changes, arrhythmias, and cardiac arrest. The rapidity of the change in potassium levels rather than the actual serum measurement has a greater influence on the degree of symptoms produced.

What Is the Treatment for Hyperkalemia?

A variety of treatment options exist for hyperkalemia. Sodium bicarbonate or glucose and insulin may be given intravenously to help drive the excess potassium into the cell. Sodium polystyrene sulfonate (Kayexalate) is a cation exchange resin that may be given orally or by retention enema. It works by exchanging two sodium ions for one potassium ion and allowing potassium to be eliminated in the stool. Oral Kayexalate is more effective than retention enema.

The fastest and most efficient way to lower the total body potassium is hemodialysis. The dialysate potassium may be lowered to allow greater diffusion of potassium from the blood into the dialysate. It is important to exercise caution when performing dialysis in patients on digoxin therapy because toxicity may develop as serum potassium levels are lowered. Potassium levels should always be monitored more frequently for patients on a lower potassium dialysate. Most dialysis providers have specific policies and guidelines to follow when a patient is dialyzing on a lower or higher potassium bath.

Is Magnesium Ever a Problem for the Patient with Chronic Kidney Disease?

Magnesium is a mineral and the second most abundant cation in the intracellular fluid and the main storage site is the bone and muscle. Most magnesium is eliminated in the stool, but the kidneys are responsible for some of the excretion. Magnesium is responsible for neuromuscular activity and activates various enzymes involved in carbohydrate and protein metabolism. Magnesium is found in foods and medications, such as antacids, laxatives, and phosphate binders. Hypo- or hypermagnesemia may be experienced with CKD.

Low magnesium levels (hypomagnesemia) may be caused by malnutrition, malabsorption syndrome, chronic diarrhea, certain diuretics (loop and thiazides), and antibiotics, such as amphotericin B and neomycin. Symptoms of low magnesium include twitching, tremors, spasms, confusion, restlessness, dysrhythmias, and seizures. Magnesium deficiency is sometimes accompanied by hypokalemia and hypocalcemia and may increase the risk of a cardiovascular event. A magnesium deficiency may also contribute to osteoporosis.

Elevated magnesium levels (hypermagnesemia) may occur with dehydration, dialysate magnesium content, and use of magnesium-based antacids or laxatives. Elevated levels of magnesium will cause excessive perspiration, respiratory paralysis, hypotension, muscle weakness, loss of deep tendon reflexes, sedation, and loss of consciousness (Feehally & Floege, 2019). Patients should be advised regarding the use of magnesium-containing antacids and laxatives. The normal magnesium level ranges from 1.6 to 2.4 mEq/L.

How Is the Calcium Level Affected in the Patient with Kidney Disease?

Calcium is the most abundant mineral in the body, with 99% located in the bones and teeth. Calcium is necessary for blood clotting, bone growth and health, and conduction of neuromuscular impulses. Calcium may be ionized or nonionized. Only ionized calcium is free to be used by the body and represents 50% of the calcium in the body. The remaining calcium is bound to proteins. Calcium is maintained within a narrow therapeutic range in the body with the help of the parathyroid hormone (PTH, parathormone) and calcitriol (1,25-dihydroxycholecalciferol).

Patients with CKD normally have lower serum calcium levels because calcium absorption is hindered by the suppression of 1,25-dihydroxycholecalciferol (vitamin D) production, decreased phosphorus excretion, and increased phosphorus retention. Normal calcium levels range from 8.5 to 10.5 mg/dL.

Why Do We Monitor the Phosphorus Levels of the Patient with Chronic Kidney Disease?

Phosphorus is normally excreted by the kidneys and accumulates in CKD patients. Studies show an increased risk of morbidity and mortality from cardiovascular disease and vascular calcification in CKD patients on maintenance dialysis who have higher serum phosphorous levels (Askar, 2015). As kidney failure progresses, the ability of the kidneys to filter phosphorus decreases. High phosphorus levels are usually the result of decreased glomerular filtration coupled with excessive dietary intake. The normal phosphorus range is 2.5 to 4.8 mg/dL for CKD patients. The treatment for hyperphosphatemia is phosphate binders, which bind phosphorus in the GI tract, allowing it to be excreted through the intestines. Patients can keep their phosphorus levels within a therapeutic limit by monitoring and limiting their dietary intake of high phosphorus foods and remembering to take their phosphate binders with all meals and snacks. Dietary instruction should be provided related to foods and food groups high in phosphorus as well as guidance on how to determine which foods have additives containing inorganic phosphorus as a preservative.

What Role Does the Parathyroid Hormone Play in Maintaining Calcium Levels?

The parathyroid gland is located on the posterior surface of the thyroid gland located in the neck (Fig. 15.1). PTH is secreted by the parathyroid gland and helps to regulate calcium and phosphorus levels. PTH helps the body to absorb calcium and eliminate phosphorus. Low serum calcium levels stimulate PTH secretion. PTH secretion stimulates the movement of calcium out of the bones, increases calcium absorption from the small intestine, and minimizes calcium loss in the urine. Untreated hyperphosphatemia and hypocalcemia may lead to persistent and prolonged secretion of PTH in an attempt to raise calcium levels in the blood. Chronically elevated phosphorus levels will cause secondary hyperparathyroidism, which can cause bone disease known as renal osteodystrophy. In addition to renal osteodystrophy, when both serum calcium and phosphorus are elevated, metastatic calcifications can form that deposit in the soft tissues of the body, such as the lungs, corneas, joints, and skin. Vascular calcifications increase the risk of cardiovascular disease in CKD as arteries lose their elasticity. Vascular stiffening and arteriosclerosis also contribute to adverse outcomes, including cardiac events, and all cause cardiovascular mortality (Palit & Kendrick, 2014). Elevated phosphorus levels need to be controlled with the use of phosphate binders and nutritional education regarding phosphorus restrictions. The expected PTH range is 150 to 600 pg/mL for CKD patients on dialysis (NKF, 2012).

What Is the Relationship Between Calcium and Phosphorus?

Phosphorus is a major intracellular anion. Eighty percent of the body's phosphorus is present in the bone. Phosphorus acts as a urinary buffer in maintaining the acid–base balance, helps to maintain cell wall integrity, and is involved in transferring energy to cells in cellular metabolism. Calcium and phosphorus have an inverse relationship. When the phosphorus level is high, the calcium level is low.

What Is the Importance of the Calcium–Phosphorus Product?

Maintaining the calcium–phosphorus product between 40 and 60 mg/dL is essential for avoiding bone disease. The calcium–phosphorus product is determined by multiplying the value of the calcium level by the value of the phosphorus level. For example, if the patient's calcium level is 10 mg and the phosphorus level is 9 mg, the patient would have a

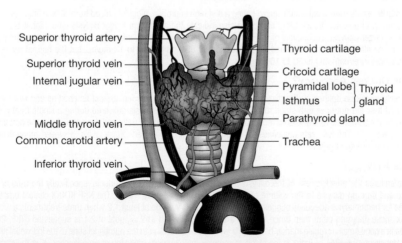

Superior thyroid artery

Superior thyroid vein

Internal jugular vein

Middle thyroid vein

Common carotid artery

Inferior thyroid vein

Thyroid cartilage

Cricoid cartilage

Pyramidal lobe ⎤ Thyroid
Isthmus ⎦ gland

Parathyroid gland

Trachea

Fig. 15.1 The thyroid and parathyroid glands. (From National Institute of Health: National Cancer Institute SEER Training Modules: https://training.seer.cancer.gov/index.html.)

calcium–phosphorus product of 90. A high product places the patient at risk for developing calcification in the soft tissues and coronary arteries. The KDOQI clinical practice guidelines for bone metabolism and disease in CKD recommend that the calcium–phosphorus product should be maintained at less than 55 mg/dL. Individual values of serum calcium and phosphorus, elevated together, should be used to guide clinical practice rather than the mathematical construct of the calcium–phosphorus product (Ca $\times$ P) (NKF, 2012).

WHY DO WE MONITOR THE HEMATOCRIT AND HEMOGLOBIN SO CLOSELY OF THE PATIENT WITH CHRONIC KIDNEY DISEASE?

A hemoglobin and hematocrit test is a laboratory study used to evaluate anemia and to prescribe a therapeutic dose of epoetin alfa. Both hematocrit and hemoglobin are typically low in CKD patients because of decreased erythropoietin production. Hematocrit is the percentage of red blood cells (RBCs) in whole blood, and hemoglobin measures the oxygen-carrying capacity of RBCs. Low levels of hematocrit are caused by decreased production of RBCs, blood loss from dialysis treatment, and shortened survival time of RBCs. Low hematocrit values are associated with fatigue, shortness of breath, chest pain, palpitations, and cold sensations. The normal hematocrit range for kidney disease patient on an erythropoiesis-stimulating agent (ESA) is approximately 30% to 36%.

Hemoglobin is an iron-containing protein that carries oxygen from the lungs to all of the body's tissues. The hemoglobin test is most often used to assess for the presence of anemia. The hemoglobin test is a reliable measure of anemia as is not influenced by time or temperature. The hemoglobin is not susceptible to false low readings from dilutional factors such as fluid overload as compared to the hematocrit. The Food and Drug Administration, the NKF Kidney Disease Outcomes Quality Initiative (NKF KDOQI), and the Kidney Disease Improving Global Outcomes (KDIGO) International Society of Nephrology all have minor differences in their approaches to the treatment of the anemia in CKD and when to initiate or stop ESA administration. The target hemoglobin range for CKD patients on an ESA is approximately 10 to 12 g/dL.

Two additional proteins help determine iron availability: (1) ferritin, which is a protein that stores the iron until it is needed, and (2) transferrin, whose saturation indicates the amount of iron immediately available for RBC production. Guidelines for anemia in CKD patients recommend that to achieve and maintain the target hemoglobin level, sufficient iron should be administered to maintain a transferrin saturation of 20% to 40% and a serum ferritin level of 100 ng/mL or higher (Macdougall & Eckardt, 2019).

WHAT IS THE RETICULOCYTE HEMOGLOBIN COUNT, AND WHY IS IT MEASURED?

Reticulocyte hemoglobin count (CHr) is a sensitive indicator of iron deficiency and a diagnostic tool that can monitor the efficacy of IV iron therapy. Reticulocytes are the most recent RBCs released into the bloodstream, and they circulate for only 1 to 2 days. CHr provides an assessment of the availability of iron to the RBCs most recently produced by the bone marrow. Because CHr is a more sensitive and specific marker of iron status at the reticulocyte level, determining the dose of IV iron therapy on the basis of this index should improve hemoglobin levels in CKD patients.

WHAT IS UREA NITROGEN, AND WHY IS IT MONITORED?

Urea is the nitrogenous end product of protein and amino acid catabolism. Urea nitrogen is filtered as a waste product in the kidneys and leaves the body in the urine. Urea nitrogen is monitored to determine if the kidneys are functioning normally. Urea nitrogen is also monitored to determine whether kidney disease is progressing.

WHY DO DIALYSIS PATIENTS HAVE ELEVATED BLOOD UREA NITROGEN LEVELS?

Increased BUN results from renal insufficiency, eating a diet high in protein, digesting blood from GI bleeding, dehydration, infection, injury, or elevated temperature and could also indicate the need for a longer dialysis time, higher blood flow rate, or larger dialyzer. High levels of BUN produce symptoms of fatigue, insomnia, irritability, dry and itchy skin, nausea, and an altered sense of taste and smell. The normal BUN range is 7 to 18 mg/dL, but the normal range for dialysis patients (pretreatment) is 60 to 100 mg/dL.

WHAT IS DIALYSIS ADEQUACY?

Optimal dialysis can be defined as the dialysis treatment that makes patients feel almost as good as and live almost as long as if they did not have end-stage renal disease. The amount of dialysis delivered during a single treatment is measured by the computed Kt/V and urea reduction ratio (URR). The higher the delivered dose of dialysis, the better will be the patient outcome. The NKF sets guidelines for recommended acceptable adequacy levels; however, many dialysis clinics set more stringent goals.

WHAT IS KT/V$_{UREA}$?

Kt/V$_{urea}$ measures the effectiveness of the dialysis treatment in removing waste products, specifically the ratio of urea clearance and time on dialysis to the volume of urea distribution (total body water). The NKF KDOQI clinical practice guidelines for hemodialysis adequacy suggest that the delivered Kt/V$_{urea}$ be at least 1.2 when three treatments a week are given. For those dialyzing other than thrice weekly, a targeted delivered Kt/V$_{urea}$ goal of 2.1 is suggested (NKF, 2015).

Urea is a good small molecule marker because its levels correlate well with the nutritional state of the individual and with protein catabolism. The Kt/V$_{urea}$ index is the result of complex mathematical modeling of urea kinetics. K is the dialyzer clearance of urea (mL/min), t represents the dialysis time (in minutes), and V indicates the volume of distribution of urea in the body fluid. V_{urea} is not a real volume that can be measured. It is derived from pharmacokinetic modeling and involves more than one fluid pool and the rates of transfer between them. These cannot be measured directly. Chapter 19 discusses dialysis adequacy goals specific to peritoneal dialysis because they differ from the goals of hemodialysis adequacy.

What Is the Urea Reduction Ratio?

The URR measures the reduction of urea in the dialyzed patient from predialysis to postdialysis. The URR reflects the delivered dose of dialysis. The KDOQI clinical practice guidelines for hemodialysis adequacy suggest a delivered dose of at least 65% when three treatments a week are given. The latest NKF clinical practice guidelines advocate to phase out this method of assessing dialysis adequacy in favor of more precise methods such as Kt/V (NKF, 2015).

What Factors Affect Dialysis Adequacy?

The NKF identifies the following factors as instrumental in adversely affecting the prescribed dose of dialysis:
Compromised urea clearance caused by the following:
- Access recirculation
- Inadequate blood flow from the vascular access
- Inaccurate estimation of dialyzer performance
- Inadequate dialyzer reprocessing
- Clotted dialyzer fibers
- Errors in blood and dialysate flow rates caused by miscalibrated equipment
- Inadequate blood and dialysate flow rate
- Dialyzer leaks
Reduced treatment time caused by the following:
- Premature discontinuation of treatment
- Incorrectly calculated time on dialysis
- Failure to account for interruption in treatment
Laboratory or blood sampling errors caused by the following:
- Dilution of BUN sample with saline
- Drawing predialysis BUN after initiation of dialysis
- Laboratory error
- Drawing postdialysis BUN before the end of dialysis treatment
- Drawing postdialysis BUN more than 5 minutes after the end of dialysis

When Should Serum Glucose Levels Be Monitored in Patients with Diabetes?

Serum glucose (Chemstick or Accucheck) assessment should be performed at the beginning of dialysis. Unstable diabetic patients need more frequent checks. Serum glucose levels less than 50 mg/dL may require a bolus of 50 mL of 50% dextrose to prevent hypoglycemic shock. Elevated glucose levels may require a dose of regular insulin to prevent diabetic coma (see Chapter 16).

What Is Creatinine?

Creatinine is a protein produced by muscles and is measured to determine kidney function. The amount produced by any person is relatively constant, and the serum volume is determined by the rate of removal by the kidney. The amount of creatinine produced is relative to the muscle mass. Older adults have lower creatinine levels because of decreased muscle mass. Serum creatinine levels increase with declining kidney function. Normal creatinine levels range from 0.5 to 1.5 mg/dL. Serum creatinine levels are a more sensitive marker of kidney function because they are not influenced by diet or fluid volume. The expected range for CKD patients is 12 to 20 mg/dL.

What Does It Mean to Measure Creatinine Clearance?

Creatinine clearance is the amount of blood cleared of creatinine per unit of time and is normally expressed in milliliters per minute. The normal creatinine clearance range is approximately 85 to 135 mL/min. With CKD, there is a decline in creatinine clearance. The normal values may vary slightly from laboratory to laboratory or from textbook to textbook.

What Is the Glomerular Filtration Rate?

The glomerular filtration rate (GFR) is a measure of kidney function and a more sensitive marker of kidney impairment than serum creatinine. The GFR varies with age, sex, and body size. The normal GFR in young adults ranges from approximately 120 to 130 mL/min/1.73 m^2. The GFR declines with age and with the onset of kidney failure. Renal replacement therapy is needed when the GFR falls below 15 mL/min/1.73 m^2.

What Is the Role of Cystatin C in Estimating the Glomerular Filtration Rate?

Cystatin C is a low-molecular-weight (13,359 Da) serum protein produced at a constant rate and filtered out of the blood by the kidneys. Cystatin C is completely reabsorbed by the tubules and generated at a constant rate by all cells of the body. It is minimally affected by height, weight, age, sex, diet, inflammatory state, or lean body mass and is therefore recognized as a useful marker of kidney damage. An accurate estimate of the GFR is crucial to diagnose, stage, and manage

CKD. Estimation of the GFR by combining serum creatinine and cystatin C levels may provide a more accurate measure of the true GFR. Cystatin C measurement can be used when the traditional GFR is inconclusive or needs to be confirmed. Because cystatin C measurements are not influenced by muscle mass, it may be a good assessment for patients who are overweight, for older adults, and for those who have large muscle mass, such as body builders. The usefulness and efficacy of cystatin C as a marker of the GFR is still being explored, using cystatin C alone or with the addition of creatinine and adding age, race, and sex with or without creatinine (NKF, 2015).

DIABETES AND CHRONIC KIDNEY DISEASE

More than 30.3 million people, or 9.4% of the population, in the United States have diabetes (National Diabetes Information Clearing House, 2017). Diabetes mellitus continues to be the leading cause of chronic kidney disease (CKD) in this country with an estimated 7.2 million adults undiagnosed.

WHAT IS DIABETES MELLITUS?

Diabetes mellitus is a chronic metabolic disease in which the body's natural ability to produce enough insulin is defective, leading to the progression of elevated glucose levels in the blood. It is first important to understand how the body produces glucose. When you eat foods containing sugars and carbohydrates, the body breaks down these substances into a special sugar known as glucose. Glucose is used by the body to provide energy and to fuel cells. Insulin is a hormone produced by the beta cells in the pancreas. Insulin is what moves glucose from the blood to the liver, fat, and muscle cells. When there is a deficiency or absence of insulin, the cells do not have the energy needed to perform their processes.

WHAT ARE THE THREE TYPES OF DIABETES?

There are three types of diabetes: type 1 diabetes, type 2 diabetes, and gestational diabetes (diabetes during pregnancy).

Type 1 diabetes, formerly called juvenile diabetes or insulin-dependent diabetes mellitus (IDDM), is caused by the destruction of pancreatic beta cells. Pancreatic beta cells are the only cells in the body that produce the hormone insulin, which is essential for regulating blood glucose levels. This type of diabetes typically affects children or young adults but can occur at any age. Susceptibility to this disease is inherited, but the actual onset of the disease is caused by an environmental trigger such as a virus. The resulting autoimmune response leads to beta cell dysfunction.

The most common type of diabetes is type 2 diabetes and accounts for more than 95% of diabetes cases in the United States (National Diabetes Information Clearing House, 2017). In this condition, insulin production is present or reduced and the body's ability to use insulin becomes insufficient, a process called insulin resistance. Dietary control, exercise, and weight loss are important factors in lowering insulin requirements and increasing insulin use. Family history, obesity, hypertension, and smoking are major risk factors for this type of diabetes. African Americans, Latinos, and Asians are at a particularly higher risk for this type of diabetes. See Box 16.1 for criteria for testing.

HOW IS DIABETES TREATED?

Diabetes is best managed with a multidisciplinary approach in which the physician, nurse, and dietitian plan and implement a comprehensive system of care. Often these professionals specialize in diabetic care and work with the primary care physician. The endocrinologist determines the severity of the disease and assesses its effects. Other specialists, such as nephrologists, cardiologists, and ophthalmologists, are consulted periodically for assessment of organ damage and for treatment. Annual visits to an ophthalmologist are necessary for all patients with diabetes. A podiatrist should be consulted early to treat existing foot problems, assess the risk of future problems, and recommend appropriate footwear. The medical goal is to arrest tissue and organ damage by normalizing blood sugar levels. Monitoring of blood glucose values dictates the need for medication or dosage adjustments (Fig. 16.1). The dietitian creates a meal plan on the basis of the American Diabetes Association (ADA) guidelines and the individual's lifestyle preferences. In addition, all health care providers, certified diabetes educators, and dietitians teach and counsel the patient about the vital role that diet and exercise play in the patient's long-term outcomes. The nurse coordinates care, educates the patient and his or her family about all aspects of care, and assesses all parameters of the patient's health, including psychosocial adjustments, responses to medication, diet and exercise, foot care, and other follow-up assessments as needed.

HOW IS BLOOD SUGAR MEASURED AND WHAT IS THE NORMAL RANGE?

Four blood sugar tests are used to diagnose and monitor diabetes.
- Fasting plasma glucose (FPG) levels are measured after an 8-hour fast. Values greater than or equal to 126 mg/dL in repeated studies may indicate diabetes. Fasting is defined as no caloric intake for at least 8 hours.
- Random plasma glucose levels greater than or equal to 200 mg/dL are diagnostic if accompanied by classic signs and symptoms.
- The oral glucose tolerance test measures blood glucose levels after the patient drinks a 75-g glucose solution. A value of 200 mg/dL or higher confirms a diagnosis of diabetes. The term *impaired glucose tolerance* is used if the value is between 140 and 190 mg/dL.

A hemoglobin A_{1c} (HbA_{1c}) value greater than or equal to 6.5% is diagnostic for diabetes. This is a recently added measurement that should be performed in a laboratory using a method that is certified and standardized.

Box 16.1 Criteria for Testing for Diabetes or Prediabetes in Asymptomatic Adults

Consider in overweight (BMI $\geq$25 kg/m^2 or $\geq$23 kg/m^2 in Asian Americans) with one or more of the following risk factors:

First-degree relative with diabetes

African American, Latino, Native American, Pacific Islander

History of cardiovascular disease

Hypertension ($\geq$140/90 mm Hg or on antihypertensive medication)

HDL cholesterol <35 mg/dL and/or

Triglyceride level >250 mg/dL

Females with polycystic ovary syndrome

Physically inactive

BMI, Body mass index; *HDL,* high-density lipoprotein.
From American Diabetes Association: 2. Classification and diagnosis of diabetes: standards of medical care in diabetes—2019. *Diabetes Care* 42(suppl 1):S13–S28, 2019.

Health care providers teach patients or family members to perform a fingerstick blood glucose test for ongoing monitoring and evaluation. This test is not used to diagnose diabetes. As implied by the name, blood is obtained from a fingerstick, and the amount of glucose is measured by a handheld device called a glucometer.

Diagnosis requires two abnormal test results from the same sample or in two separate test samples. If the results are not diagnostic for diabetes but are near the threshold, the test should be repeated within 3 to 6 months (ADA, 2019).

WHAT IS HEMOGLOBIN A$_{1c}$?

The HbA$_{1c}$ value is the measurement of a patient's average blood glucose control during the previous 2 to 3 months. Elevated blood glucose levels cause hemoglobin to become saturated with glucose in the form of glycohemoglobin. Glycohemoglobin is present for the 120-day lifespan of the red blood cell (RBC). The average measurement of the glycolated part of hemoglobin is called hemoglobin A$_1$. In most laboratories, HbA$_{1c}$ is measured because it is the most prevalent form. Other laboratories measure the total glycohemoglobin as A$_1$. Glycohemoglobin A$_1$ values are 2% to 4% higher than HbA$_{1c}$ values, so it is imperative to know the standard of measurement used by the laboratory providing the service. This laboratory value is a good indicator of the patient's response to the current treatment plan with the prescribed diet and medication regimen because it measures long-term glycemic control. Studies are being conducted to develop tests to evaluate HbA$_{1c}$ and interpret its altered values in CKD patients. It is suspected that dialysis patients may have altered values because of the decreased RBC lifespan and use of exogenous erythropoietin (Ramirez, McCullough, Thumma, et. al, 2012).

The Kidney Disease Outcomes Quality Initiative (KDOQI) Clinical Practice Guidelines for Diabetes and CDK recommend a target HbA$_{1c}$ of 7.0% to prevent or delay the microvascular complications, including diabetic kidney disease (DKD) and other microvascular complications. A target HbA$_{1c}$ above 7.0% is recommended for those with a limited life expectancy, multiple comorbidities, or those at risk for hypoglycemia (National Kidney Foundation [NKF], 2012).

Estimated average glucose (eAG) is a newer term recommended by the ADA. Whereas A$_{1c}$ is reported as a percentage, eAG is reported in the same units (mg/dL or mmol/L) used by the patient's daily self-monitoring device. This value is more meaningful to patients and may facilitate improved patient glycemic control because they can relate more closely to this value. Values for HbA$_{1c}$ and glycosylated hemoglobin may be calculated here: https://professional.diabetes.org/diapro/glucose_calc.

WHAT IS HYPERGLYCEMIA?

Hyperglycemia means high blood glucose levels and is the cause of the vascular complications of diabetes. High blood glucose occurs when the body is unable to produce enough insulin or metabolize glucose efficiently. The signs and symptoms include frequent urination, excessive thirst, nausea and vomiting, weakness, confusion, and dehydration. When high glucose levels occur, treatment should be based on the appropriate clinical situation and may include change in the insulin plan, change in the oral medication plan, adjustments of diet and exercise habits, or treatment of acute illness. The NKF (2002) states that intensive treatment of hyperglycemia prevents albuminuria or can delay its progression.

WHAT IS HYPOGLYCEMIA?

Hypoglycemia means low blood glucose levels. The signs and symptoms include a rapid onset of headache, fatigue, anxiety, confusion, tachycardia, diaphoresis, and shakiness. Blood glucose levels are usually less than 70 mg/dL, although some patients become symptomatic at higher values. The treatment involves returning the blood glucose levels to normal by ingesting 15 to 20 g of quick-acting (simple) carbohydrates, such as quick-dissolving glucose tablets or gels, half a cup of juice, or regular soda. Intravenous glucose is used for treating patients who may be unconscious.

Both hyperglycemia and hypoglycemia can lead to seizures and unconsciousness, which constitute a life-threatening emergency. Before becoming comatose, the patient may appear to be very drunk.

IS THERE A CURE FOR DIABETES?

There is no cure for either type 1 or type 2 diabetes at this time. Diabetes prevention is being studied by identifying people at risk and instituting treatments designed to delay or prevent damage to the pancreas in type 1 diabetes or to the

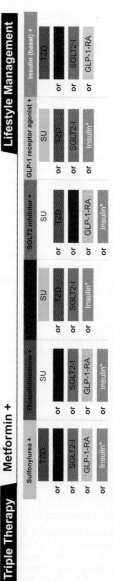

Start with Monotherapy unless:

- A1C is greater than or equal to 9%, consider Dual Therapy.
- A1C is greater than or equal to 10%, blood glucose is greater than or equal to 300 mg/dL, or patient is markedly symptomatic, consider Combination Injectable Therapy.

Monotherapy | Metformin — Lifestyle Management

EFFICACY*	high
HYPO RISK	low risk
WEIGHT	neutral/loss
SIDE EFFECTS	GI/lactic acidosis
COSTS*	low

If A1C target not achieved after approximately 3 months of monotherapy, proceed to 2-drug combination (order not meant to denote any specific preference – choice dependent on a variety of patient- & disease-specific factors):

Dual Therapy | Metformin + — Lifestyle Management

	Sulfonylureas	Thiazolidinedione	SGLT2 inhibitor	GLP-1 receptor agonist	Insulin (basal)
EFFICACY*	high	high	intermediate	high	highest
HYPO RISK	moderate risk	low risk	low risk	low risk	high risk
WEIGHT	gain	gain	loss	loss	gain
SIDE EFFECTS	hypoglycemia	edema, HF, fxs	GU, dehydration, fxs	GI	hypoglycemia
COSTS*	low	low	high	high	high

If A1C target not achieved after approximately 3 months of dual therapy, proceed to 3-drug combination (order not meant to denote any specific preference – choice dependent on a variety of patient- & disease-specific factors):

Triple Therapy | Metformin + — Lifestyle Management

Sulfonylurea +	Thiazolidinedione +	SGLT2 inhibitor +	GLP-1 receptor agonist +	Insulin (basal) +
TZD	SU	SU	SU	TZD
or SGLT2-I	or SGLT2-I	or TZD	or TZD	or SGLT2-I
or GLP-1-RA	or GLP-1-RA	or GLP-1-RA	or SGLT2-I	or GLP-1-RA
or Insulin*	or Insulin*	or Insulin*	or Insulin*	

If A1C target not achieved after approximately 3 months of triple therapy and patient (1) on oral combination, move to basal insulin or GLP-1 RA, (2) on GLP-1 RA, add basal insulin, or (3) on optimally titrated basal insulin, add GLP-1 RA or mealtime insulin. Metformin therapy should be maintained, while other oral agents may be discontinued on an individual basis to avoid unnecessarily complex or costly regimens (i.e., adding a fourth antihyperglycemic agent).

*If patient does not tolerate or has contraindications to metformin, consider agents from another class.

Fig. 16.1 Pharmacologic approaches to glycemic treatment. *DPP-4-i,* DPP-4 inhibitor; *fxs,* fractures; *GI,* gastrointestinal; *GLP-1 RA,* GLP-1 receptor agonist; *GU,* genitourinary; *HF,* heart failure; *Hypo,* hypoglycemia; *SGLT2-i,* SGLT2 inhibitor; *SU,* sulfonylurea; *TZD,* thiazolidinedione. (From American Diabetes Association: Pharmacologic approaches to glycemic treatment. *Diabetes Care* 40[suppl 1]:S65–S74, 2017.)

insulin receptors on the patient's cells in type 2 diabetes. A successful pancreas transplant can restore normal insulin production, but as with any organ transplant, the patient is immunosuppressed and at risk for the adverse effects of these medicines.

WHAT IS DIABETIC NEPHROPATHY?

Diabetic nephropathy or DKD is a kidney disease caused by diabetes. It is a complication of the small blood vessels that feed the kidneys and results from damage to the glomeruli. The pathological condition glomerulosclerosis involves fibrotic thickening of the glomeruli. It is thought to be caused by hyperfiltration and accumulation of glycosylated or "caramelized" proteins. As the disease progresses, the glomeruli lose their ability to filter blood effectively, resulting in the accumulation of waste products such as urea and creatinine in the body.

Diabetic nephropathy occurs in five stages:

Stage 1. Increased blood flow through the kidney (hyperfiltration) results in enlarged kidneys (renal hypertrophy). The estimated glomerular filtration rate (eGFR) is greater than or equal to 90 mL/min/1.73 m^2.

Stage 2. Hyperfiltration of the glomeruli damages the membrane, causing it to leak larger molecules that normally would not pass across. Leakage of albumin from the blood into the urine is known as microalbuminuria. As the loss of this and other proteins increases, clearance of waste products as urea and creatinine decreases. The eGFR is 60 to 89 mL/min/1.73 m^2.

Stage 3. Microalbuminuria exceeds 200 mcg/min. The eGFR is 30 to 59 mL/min/1.73 m^2.

Stage 4. The GFR decreases to between 15 and 29 mL/min/1.73 m^2, proteinuria is significantly increased, and the patient becomes hypertensive. This stage is called advanced clinical nephropathy.

Stage 5. End-stage renal disease (ESRD). The eGFR is less than 15 mL/min/1.73 m^2.

CAN DIABETIC NEPHROPATHY AND PROGRESSION TO CHRONIC KIDNEY DISEASE BE PREVENTED?

Diabetic nephropathy does not occur in all patients with diabetes and is more likely in patients with type 1 rather than type 2 diabetes. However, diabetic nephropathy continues to be the most common cause of ESRD in the United States. Studies have shown that strict glycemic control can significantly reduce the development and rate of progression of diabetic nephropathy. With an intensive regimen of blood glucose monitoring, insulin and/or oral hypoglycemic agent administration, and adherence to a program of diet and exercise, the majority of patients can maintain normal blood glucose levels.

Progression of diabetic nephropathy can be delayed by the use of an angiotensin-converting enzyme inhibitor. This class of drugs is usually prescribed to control hypertension but is useful for both purposes in patients with diabetic nephropathy. It is given in stage 1 to control hyperfiltration. The National Kidney Foundation (NKF) KDOQI 2012 guidelines recommend screening patients with diabetes for DKD. This screening should include measurements of microalbuminuria or the urinary albumin-to-creatinine ratio, measurements of serum creatinine, and estimations of the GFR. The cadence for screening differs for types 1 and 2 diabetes:

- In type 1 diabetes: 5 years after diagnosis; then annually
- In type 2 diabetes: at diagnosis; then annually

WHEN SHOULD A DIABETIC PATIENT WITH NEPHROPATHY START DIALYSIS?

Initiation of dialysis depends on the individual needs and condition of the patient, but a clear indicator is low creatinine clearance combined with symptomatic edema. Patients with diabetes develop symptoms of uremia earlier than their nondiabetic counterparts. For this reason, it is usual to begin dialysis when the creatinine clearance rate is between 10 and 15 mL/min; however, dialysis may be started at a clearance rate of up to 20 mL/min. Hypertension is very difficult to manage in patients with a clearance rate less than 10 mL/min. Blood pressure control is important in the management of diabetic retinopathy, as well as cardiovascular and peripheral vascular disease.

FOR PATIENTS WITH DIABETES, IS HEMODIALYSIS BETTER THAN PERITONEAL DIALYSIS?

There are advantages and disadvantages to both modalities of treatment. The health care team and the patient must choose the treatment that best suits his or her lifestyle, taking into consideration the comorbidities and medical history.

Advantages of in-center hemodialysis include frequent medical surveillance and smaller losses of protein into the dialysate. Disadvantages include a higher risk of vascular access complications, risk of predialysis hyperkalemia, and an increased incidence of hypotension during dialysis.

Peritoneal dialysis may offer better glycemic control, especially if intraperitoneal insulin is used; it also offers better cardiovascular tolerance and potassium control and does not require vascular access. Some patients have difficulties with glycemic control because of the high peritoneal exposure and potential absorption of intraperitoneal glucose. The contraindications are all of the usual problems of peritoneal dialysis magnified. Examples include increased episodes of peritonitis caused by a reduced immune response to infection, protein loss, and increased intraabdominal pressure complications such as gastroparesis.

Finally, the inability to perform peritoneal dialysis because of poor eyesight or poor fine-motor control requires the patient to be dialyzed in center if he or she does not have an assistant at home.

Can Patients with Diabetes Receive a Transplant?

Living related donor transplantation is the treatment of choice for patients with diabetes because it offers a higher rate of survival than dialysis. Many younger patients with type 1 diabetes receive combined kidney–pancreas transplants that offer the additional benefit of normal insulin production. However, many patients are not considered transplant candidates because of advanced age or atherosclerosis. A thorough evaluation is required, and cardiac surgery is often necessary before listing the patient for a deceased donor transplant. A higher percentage of transplanted patients with diabetes undergo limb amputation than do their dialysis counterparts. Infection and peripheral vascular disease may be exacerbated by steroid use. However, the increased length of survival after transplantation probably accounts for the development of these complications in this patient population.

Why Do Patients with Diabetes Require More Dialysis Than Those without Diabetes?

Diabetes affects every cell, tissue, and organ of the body, as does uremia. Patients with diabetes who also have CKD present a unique challenge. According to the current mortality data, only one in five such patients who begin dialysis will be alive in 5 years. Patients with diabetes with autonomic neuropathy are at risk for underdialysis because of hypotension during the first hour of dialysis. Diseased cardiovascular and autonomic nervous systems cannot adequately respond to the intravascular volume changes that occur with ultrafiltration. Dialysis blood flow is frequently lowered to treat this hypotension, along with the administration of extra saline. Symptomatic hypotension sometimes leads to the early termination of treatment, which affects the adequacy of dialysis and leaves the patient with fluid overload, further stressing the cardiovascular system. Peripheral vascular disease contributes to vascular access problems, with subsequent inadequacy of dialysis. Because of steal syndrome and previous graft failures, many patients with diabetes can only dialyze with catheter access.

Why Do Some Dialysis Patients Say That They Are "No Longer Diabetic" After They Start Dialysis?

Kidney failure caused by diabetes has the paradoxical outcome of making the available insulin last longer because it cannot be broken down and excreted as efficiently. Patients with uremia frequently eat much less and therefore need less insulin. Patients with type 1 diabetes will always require some insulin unless they undergo a successful pancreas transplant. Patients with type 2 diabetes, however, frequently no longer need additional insulin or oral medications. If they lose weight, their own insulin will be used better. Oral hypoglycemics, especially the long-acting ones, can cause severe hypoglycemia in hemodialysis patients. These drugs are excreted by healthy kidneys and are not dialyzable.

How Does Hemodialysis Affect Patients?

The chemical composition of the dialysate is designed to be compatible with normal blood values. It has been determined that a dextrose level of 200 mg/dL is optimal for all patients. For those with diabetes, this level prevents hypoglycemia and alleviates hyperglycemia.

Are Insulin and Oral Hypoglycemic Agents Dialyzable?

Insulin is the most common hypoglycemic agent for patients with diabetes who are on dialysis. Insulin and most oral hypoglycemic agents are not dialyzable. The exceptions include metformin (Glucophage) and glyburide (Diabeta). These drugs are contraindicated for use in ESRD patients.

How Is Hypoglycemia Managed During Hemodialysis?

Hypoglycemia must be verified by monitoring blood glucose levels. The signs and symptoms of hypoglycemia can be confused with hypotension. Changes in a patient's schedule to accommodate dialysis treatment may interfere with eating routines and medication administration, placing the patient at risk for a hypoglycemic episode. Some patients require a snack or some apple juice. However, the blood volume diverted to the abdomen for digestion may increase the patient's risk of hypotension. Profound hypoglycemia may require a physician's order for intravenous dextrose infusion.

How Is Hyperglycemia Managed During Hemodialysis?

If hyperglycemia is verified by monitoring blood glucose levels, the physician may order rapid-acting insulin (Humalog, Novolog, or Apidra). Hyperglycemia can be a sign of infection, and the patient must be assessed and treated if an infection is present. Aggressive treatment of hyperglycemia is based on the clinical status of the individual and is discouraged in patients with ESRD because of the higher risk of hypoglycemia. Heparin doses may need to be increased if unusual incidences of clotting associated with hyperglycemia occur.

Is It More Difficult To Maintain Good Health in Patients with Diabetes Than in Nondiabetic Dialysis Patients?

Statistics show a higher mortality rate for patients with diabetes who are undergoing dialysis. Cardiovascular disease is the leading cause of death followed by sepsis and voluntary withdrawal from dialysis. The progression of atherosclerosis is accelerated in patients with diabetes undergoing dialysis, making them more prone to cardiovascular complications, such as hypertension, angina, gangrene, and myocardial infarction. Hyperglycemia coupled with uremia delays wound healing and compromises immunity. Gastrointestinal neuropathy resulting in constipation as well as sudden, uncontrollable diarrhea can be a source of great distress to patients with diabetes. Gastroparesis may cause regurgitation and aspiration.

What Is Gastroparesis?

Gastroparesis, or delayed stomach emptying, is a disorder in which the movement of food from the stomach to the small intestine is slowed or even stopped. Diabetes is the leading cause of gastroparesis and usually occurs as a consequence of autonomic neuropathy. Delayed gastric emptying is evidenced by difficulty in swallowing, heartburn, nausea and vomiting, abdominal pain, feelings of fullness after eating, and erratic blood glucose levels. Treatment includes eating small, low-fat, low-fiber meals; use of drugs such as metoclopramide (Reglan) and cisapride (Propulsid) to improve gastric motility; and improved glycemic control.

Do Individuals with Diabetes Have More Vascular Access Problems Than Nondiabetic Patients?

Along with atherosclerotic peripheral vascular disease, calcification of the vascular tree further limits the quantity and quality of blood vessels normally used to create a vascular access. Patients with diabetes undergoing dialysis do not experience more episodes of sepsis with their vascular access but do require more hospitalization and have poorer prognosis. Patients with diabetes also have a higher rate of graft thrombosis.

How Should Patients with Diabetes Modify Their Diets When They Are Undergoing Hemodialysis?

Patients with diabetes already know about diet modification necessitated by errors in glucose metabolism. Now they must further modify their diets to accommodate renal failure and hemodialysis. Some patients hear about restrictions in the renal diet and think there is nothing left to eat. This is not true. Although they must make new adjustments to avoid the dangers of hyperkalemia and bone disease, it is imperative that they eat well to meet the demands of dialysis, which increases the risk of malnutrition. Hemodialysis removes nutrients by depleting amino acids at the rate of 1 to 2 g/hr during treatment. Blood losses in the dialyzer and lines also contribute to protein loss. Dietary protein replacement should be at a minimum of 1.2 g/kg/day. A caloric intake of 35 kcal/kg is required to prevent the body from burning protein stores for energy. Generally, protein should make up about 20% of the diet, with the rest being fat (30%, preferably monounsaturated) and carbohydrate (50%). Diets should be tailored to the patient's preferences and customs. The dietary goal is to make eating pleasurable while meeting the nutritional needs. Highly refined carbohydrates such as candy, cake, and pie can be incorporated into the diabetic renal diet as long as they are factored into the overall dietary plan. High-calorie, low-nutrient foods must be limited but are not forbidden. The goal is to maintain good glycemic control. Fluid control may be a challenge, as hyperglycemia may increase thirst.

If Patients with Diabetes Undergoing Dialysis No Longer Need Medication for Blood Sugar Control, Should Their Blood Sugar Still Be Checked?

Daily blood glucose checks are important to confirm good glycemic control. More frequent checks are made if the patient is not feeling well. An elevated blood glucose level may indicate the presence of infection.

What Assessments Are Critically Important for Patients with Diabetes Undergoing Dialysis?

Although patients with diabetes comprise 9.4% of the US population, 60% of all lower limb amputations are performed in this population (National Diabetes Information Clearing House, 2017). Frequent and careful assessment of the feet and legs of patients with diabetes undergoing dialysis should be performed to identify potential problems associated with skin breakdown or infection. Early detection and prompt treatment may prevent serious complications.

Can Diabetic Foot Problems Be Prevented?

Absolutely! Regular foot inspections should be done by a nephrology nurse, with referrals to a podiatrist for attention to potential problem areas, such as toenails, corns, and bunions, among others. Patients should never cut their own corns or calluses and should be warned never to use heating pads, hot water bottles, or unsupervised hot water soaks. Patients and caregivers must be educated about the basics of good foot hygiene. Prosthetic footwear to protect insensitive feet from trauma is a necessity. Medicare reimburses patients for orthotic shoe inserts and prescribed footwear.

CHAPTER 17

MEDICATION PROBLEMS AND DIALYSIS

Patients with chronic kidney disease (CKD) are at an increased risk of adverse drug events because of polypharmacy, multiple comorbid conditions, and pharmacokinetic and pharmacodynamic alterations (Sharif-Askari et al, 2014). It is estimated that nonadherence to medication may vary from 17% to 74% among patients with CKD and from 3% to 80% among patients on hemodialysis, depending on the methods used to assess nonadherence (Nielsen et al, 2017). To optimize drug outcomes, health professionals must be prepared to recognize and manage problems associated with medication use. Table 17.1 lists several problematic reactions to medications that clinicians encounter when providing care to patients on dialysis and other patients with renal impairment.

All these problem areas are complex and require consideration of multiple factors unique to each situation, including patient characteristics (e.g., severity of renal impairment, acuity or chronicity of kidney failure, comorbidities, age, nutritional status), drug properties (e.g., pharmacokinetics, pharmacodynamics, dose, route), and dialysis procedures (e.g., treatment type, equipment, duration). CKD impacts the effects of medications such as prolonging their effects, slowing elimination, and increasing serum drug levels, all of which increase the risk of side effects and toxicity. The purpose of this chapter is to emphasize the pharmacologic principles common to managing these problem areas and to provide a brief overview of each problem area.

How Do Drugs Cause Renal Impairment?

The incidence drug-induced acute kidney injury (AKI) is as high as 60% and is more common in those with underlying kidney dysfunction and cardiovascular disease (Shahrbaf & Assadi, 2015). There are several reasons why the kidneys are particularly vulnerable to damage by drugs. The kidneys constitute only 0.4% of body weight but receive 20% to 25% of total blood flow. This disproportionate blood flow exposes the kidneys excessively to drugs in the blood. In addition, drugs become concentrated as the tubular filtrate passes through the nephron and water is reabsorbed. Tubular transport systems further concentrate drugs in the filtrate. Enzymes in the kidney may metabolize drugs to metabolites that are nephrotoxic. In renal insufficiency, the remaining functional nephrons are even more susceptible to nephrotoxins.

Other predisposition to nephrotoxicity from drugs is volume depletion, congestive heart failure, CKD, sepsis, and is highest in people with diabetes and CKD.

The most commonly implicated pharmacologic nephrotoxins are antimicrobials (acyclovir, aminoglycosides, amphotericin B, cephalosporins, pentamidine, sulfonamides, tetracycline, vancomycin), radiocontrast agents used for radiologic studies, chemotherapy agents and immunosuppressants (cyclosporine, cisplatin, tacrolimus), angiotensin-converting enzyme (ACE) inhibitors, and nonsteroidal antiinflammatory drugs (NSAIDs). Because of the development of new agents (e.g., lower osmolar radiocontrast agents), changing drug use patterns (e.g., decreased use of aminoglycosides) and the shift of care from inpatient to outpatient settings, NSAIDs and ACE inhibitors are increasingly predominant causes of transient AKI. In chronic outpatient settings, CKD can occur because of combinations of analgesics, which consist of either aspirin or an NSAID combined with acetaminophen, caffeine, and/or codeine. Although the agents specifically cited here are the most frequent causes of kidney damage, numerous other medications from diverse drug categories can cause kidney damage. The risk is greatest in individuals who already have poor renal perfusion. Whenever a patient evidences renal impairment, careful analysis of the drug profile for potential drug nephrotoxicity should be conducted. Nephrotoxins should be avoided in patients in any stage of CKD or used with appropriate dosage adjustments and meticulous monitoring.

How Can Kidney Damage From Such Drugs Be Minimized or Avoided?

Naturally, drugs with a potential to cause kidney damage should be avoided or used cautiously in patients at high risk for renal impairment. Conditions that predispose to kidney damage by drugs include use of multiple nephrotoxins, sodium or fluid depletion, preexisting kidney disease, and low renal blood flow in patients with diseases such as congestive heart failure and cirrhosis, advanced age, and diabetes mellitus (Rosner & Okusa, 2008). Often, drug-induced kidney damage is reversible if the drug is discontinued and supportive care is initiated before permanent effects occur. Intravenous (IV) saline may decrease damage by some nephrotoxins such as cyclosporine and cisplatin by diluting the concentration of the drug in the renal tubule. Misoprostol, a prostaglandin analog, may prevent NSAID nephropathy. Drugs with the least nephrotoxic potential should be selected. For example, acetaminophen, aspirin, nonacetylated salicylates, sulindac, or nabumetone may have less nephrotoxicity than other NSAIDs. Finally, drugs should be given in the lowest effective doses for the shortest possible duration.

How Does Chronic Kidney Disease Itself Alter Responses to Medications?

The changes that accompany CKD can alter drug responses through two major mechanisms: pharmacodynamics and pharmacokinetics. Medications chemically interact with receptors on cell membranes or on enzymes to cause their effects. These interactions are known as pharmacodynamics and can be thought of as what drugs do to the body. Adverse effects (also called side effects or toxic effects) occur when a drug or metabolite acts at receptors other than the target receptors or

Table 17.1 Problem Areas Involving Drugs

PROBLEM AREA	CORRESPONDING RESPONSIBILITY OF DIALYSIS PERSONNEL
Drugs can damage kidneys, initiating or worsening kidney failure.	Monitor the kidney function of patients taking drugs or drug combinations that can damage kidneys. Identify patients at high risk for kidney damage from drugs. Avoid or use with extreme caution drugs that damage kidney function in high-risk patients and in those with existing kidney disease. Initiate hydration and other documented measures to minimize nephrotoxicity.
Pharmacologic activity of drugs is altered by kidney failure.	Adjust dosages to compensate for altered pharmacokinetic and pharmacodynamic activity. Monitor for therapeutic failure, adverse effects, or toxicity of all drugs used. Anticipate more adverse effects in patients with renal impairment.
The amount of medication removed from the body during dialysis varies, depending on the characteristics of the drug and dialysis conditions.	Using references and formulas, estimate how much drug is removed by dialysis. Calculate dosage adjustments and postdialysis replacement dosages. Monitor clinical responses to calculated doses and alter the dosage as indicated.
Some poisons or drugs taken in overdose can be removed wholly or in part by dialysis.	Know which poisons and overdosed drugs can be removed by various dialysis procedures. Implement dialysis to treat poisoning and overdose, providing appropriate supportive care and observation during the procedure.
Medications may increase the risks associated with the dialysis procedure.	Know what medications the patient is taking. Monitor for excess effects of the medication.

when excess drug is present at the target receptor. Uremic substances in the blood or altered electrolyte concentrations resulting from kidney failure can modify the drug–receptor interaction, resulting in an altered drug effect. Altered receptor sensitivity is thought to be responsible for increased central nervous system (CNS) effects of narcotics, sedatives, and hypnotics, as well as for resistance to the effects of epinephrine and other catecholamines that occurs in uremic patients. Altered electrolyte and acid–base balances also affect the responses to medications such as antiarrhythmics, digoxin, phenothiazines, and antidepressants.

The magnitude and persistence of drug action depend on the duration and concentration of the drug in proximity to the receptor. This relationship between time and drug concentration is known as pharmacokinetics and can be thought of as how the body acts on the drug through the processes of absorption, distribution, metabolism, and excretion. How CKD affects pharmacodynamics is not well understood. On the other hand, many of the effects of altered pharmacokinetics in dialysis patients have been sufficiently studied to develop mathematical formulas for calculating drug dosages. Decreased renal excretion is the most obvious pharmacokinetic alteration resulting from renal dysfunction, but each of the other pharmacokinetic processes may also be altered.

WHAT FACTORS AFFECT THE ABSORPTION OF MEDICATIONS IN PATIENTS WITH CHRONIC KIDNEY DISEASE?

In uremia, the breakdown of urea in the gastrointestinal (GI) tract may increase the pH and slow the absorption of acid drugs, such as aspirin, iron preparations, and diuretics. Gastroparesis and GI responses to uremia (nausea, vomiting, and diarrhea) may significantly alter the absorption of oral medication. Antacids, which are commonly used to bind dietary phosphate in CKD patients, diminish the absorption of drugs by forming unabsorbable compounds with drugs such as digoxin, iron preparations, and some antibiotics (e.g., tetracyclines and fluoroquinolones). Drugs used to suppress gastric acid secretions, such as H_2 blockers (e.g., cimetidine, ranitidine, famotidine), antacids, and proton pump inhibitors (omeprazole, lansoprazole), affect the absorption of some drugs. For example, ketoconazole, which requires an acid environment for absorption, has reduced bioavailability in patients taking drugs that suppress gastric acidity, whereas oral penicillins, which are inactivated by gastric acid, have improved absorption in patients taking drugs that suppress acidity.

WHAT FACTORS AFFECT THE DISTRIBUTION OF MEDICATIONS IN PATIENTS WITH KIDNEY FAILURE?

When a drug is absorbed into the blood, some molecules bind to proteins in the plasma. Drugs that are highly bound to plasma proteins in the blood usually have a small volume of distribution (V_d) because most of the drug molecules are attached to plasma proteins, which normally cannot exit the blood vessels. Drugs that predominantly exit from the blood and bind to muscles or dissolve in fatty tissues in the periphery have a large V_d. In general, drugs with a small V_d have short half-lives because they are mostly retained in the plasma, which frequently passes through the liver and kidneys (and dialysis machine), where the drugs are eliminated. Conversely, drugs with a large V_d have longer half-lives and are less susceptible to removal by dialysis. Edema and ascites often increase the V_d and increase the half-lives of drugs that normally have small distribution volumes.

Binding of acidic drugs to the plasma protein albumin may be decreased in kidney failure as a result of either a decreased albumin concentration or decreased capacity of albumin to bind to drugs. Changes in protein binding can alter the V_d and drug effect because only free drugs are pharmacologically active. Decreased albumin binding in uremia is thought to contribute to CNS toxicity caused by acid drugs such as theophylline, phenytoin, penicillin, phenobarbital, and salicylates. Some alkaline drugs (e.g., lidocaine, phenothiazines, propranolol, quinidine, and tricyclic antidepressants) that bind to glycoproteins also undergo increased or decreased binding in kidney disease, but the clinical relevance of these changes is not as well studied as albumin binding.

What Factors Affect the Elimination of Medications in Patients with Chronic Kidney Disease?

Some drugs are cleared almost exclusively in their original chemical form by renal excretion; these drugs are said to be excreted unchanged. Other drugs undergo alterations of their chemical structures by enzymes, a process called biotransformation or metabolism. Most drugs are cleared by a combination of hepatic metabolism and renal excretion. Metabolites (the forms that drugs take after chemical alteration by metabolism) are usually more water soluble than the original drugs and are usually eliminated by the kidneys. Active metabolites retain the ability to bind to a receptor and elicit the same effect as the original drug. Inactive metabolites are usually insignificant because they do not stimulate the target receptor. Toxic metabolites are those that cause an adverse effect at a site different from the target receptor.

When a drug that is normally cleared unchanged by the kidneys is repeatedly administered to a patient with renal insufficiency, it begins to accumulate in the blood and may cause adverse effects. Increased portions of the drug may be eliminated by alternate routes, such as hepatic metabolism or through the lungs, bile, or sweat glands. Metabolites of drugs accumulate in patients with renal insufficiency, and active or toxic metabolites contribute to adverse effects. An example is normeperidine, a metabolite of meperidine, which causes stupor or seizures when it accumulates. Box 17.1 includes examples of drugs with active or toxic metabolites that may accumulate in kidney failure. Drugs with active or toxic metabolites are avoided in patients with renal failure if viable alternatives exist. When drugs with active or toxic metabolites are used in patients with kidney failure, decreased dosages may be required, and clinical monitoring must be vigilant. For example, patients with kidney impairment who take allopurinol for gout or cancer require lower dosages than those with normal kidney function because an active metabolite of allopurinol can cause exfoliative dermatitis when it accumulates in the body. Although far less important than active metabolites, inactive metabolites may also have consequences. For example, accumulation of inactive metabolites may cause interference with laboratory tests.

Impaired kidney function may also affect liver metabolism, decreasing the elimination of some drugs (e.g., morphine, clonidine) and increasing the metabolism of a few others (e.g., phenobarbital and phenytoin). Renal impairment alters metabolism through accumulation of uremic substances that can induce (speed up) or inhibit (slow down) drug-metabolizing enzymes in the liver. Insulin is metabolized by enzymes in the kidney, so it is more slowly cleared in patients with severe kidney disease. Liver metabolism is dependent on genetic inheritance, diet, environmental pollution, and concurrent administration of other medications; thus, the effects of renal dysfunction are likely to be highly variable from drug to drug and from person to person. The effects on renal elimination are more predictable: the greater the proportion of a drug or its active metabolites eliminated by the kidneys, the more likely that altered dosing will be required for patients with kidney impairment and those undergoing dialysis.

How Does Dialysis Affect the Pharmacokinetics of Drugs and Poisons?

The kidneys eliminate drugs through several processes. Although dialysis is not a substitute for all of these renal processes, some drugs are removed by dialysis. Dialysis may also affect other pharmacokinetic parameters. For example, changes in total body water from predialysis to postdialysis will affect the V_d of some drugs. The characteristics of drugs that promote their removal by dialysis are as follows: (1) small molecular size, (2) small V_d, (3) water solubility, and (4) low protein binding. If protein binding exceeds 90%, the drug will be negligibly eliminated by dialysis. Drugs are more likely to be removed when the dialysis membrane is highly permeable and has a large surface area and when the blood flow

---

Box 17.1 Examples of Drugs with Active or Toxic Metabolites

Acetaminophen	Diazepam	Metronidazole
Allopurinol	Enalapril	Nitroprusside
Amiodarone	Fluoxetine	Procainamide
Azathioprine	Glyburide	Propoxyphene
Buspirone	Levodopa	Quinidine
Cefotaxime	Meperidine	Triamterene
Cimetidine	Methyldopa	Verapamil

rate and dialysate flow rate are high. Peritoneal dialysis generally provides little drug removal because the dialysate flow rate is slower than that with other methods; however, a greater amount of protein-bound drug can be removed because of the large protein losses seen with this mode. Continuous therapy with hemofiltration or continuous hemodialysis for critically ill patients can remove substantial fractions of drugs. Removal of drugs by hemofiltration procedures is determined by the ultrafiltration rate and degree of protein binding. Treatment of drug overdoses and poisoning can be treated with renal replacement therapies. The pharmacologic substance to be removed must meet several criteria: have a low molecular weight ($<$500 Da), low degree of protein binding, be water soluble, and have a low volume of distribution (Mirrakhimov, Barbarya, Gray, et al, 2016). Similarly, poisons with high protein binding or a large V_d are not dialyzable. Although many standard references classify a drug as dialyzable or not dialyzable, dialyzability is not an all-or-nothing characteristic. Some drugs are virtually entirely removed by dialysis; others have negligible removal. Many drugs fall somewhere in the middle. The type of dialysis equipment and length of dialysis greatly influence whether a drug is removed. Classification of dialyzability as "yes" or "no" is based on an expert's opinion of whether removal is clinically significant, that is, sufficient to remove an overdose, or whether the patient will require dose replacement.

How Should Drugs and Dosages Be Selected for Patients with Kidney Impairment or Chronic Kidney Disease?

Drug selection for patients with kidney impairment requires consideration of the effect of the drug on kidney function, electrolyte balance, and uremia. Agents that would worsen the disease state or increase the metabolic load are avoided or used with caution. A drug that increases the metabolic load burdens the failing kidney with chemicals that accumulate in kidney disease, such as urea, sodium, potassium, or acids. For CKD patients, these substances must be removed by dialysis and may affect the patient's well-being or cause serious adverse effects, such as cardiac arrhythmia from hyperkalemia. Drugs with nephrotoxic properties are also used with caution in patients with renal impairment. Meticulous monitoring should be incorporated into the care plan for patients with renal impairment who take medications that are nephrotoxic or increase the metabolic load. Medications should be avoided for self-limiting conditions and those that can be managed by nonpharmacologic methods. Whenever possible, a single agent that can manage several conditions should be selected. For example, in the absence of contraindications such as renal stenosis, an ACE inhibitor would be a prudent choice for patients with both hypertension and congestive heart failure. Well-studied established agents are usually preferred over newly marketed drugs. All other therapeutic considerations being equal, drugs with reliable laboratory assays for drug levels are advantageous because the drug-level data can enhance clinical monitoring.

The need for and extent of dosage modification in patients with renal impairment depend on the pathophysiology of the disease process and its severity, as well as the pharmacology of the drug. The guidelines for dosage reductions of many drugs can be found in standard drug references such as the *Physicians' Desk Reference,* drug handbooks, and package inserts. Many nephrology textbooks and other sources provide summary tables that include pharmacokinetic parameters in CKD (e.g., V_d, clearance, half-life), recommended dosage adjustments for various levels of kidney function, and guidelines for postdialysis replacement doses. The physician would determine any dosage modifications that might be necessary. Each of the following five steps of dosage selection is defined and discussed in subsequent sections:

- Assessment of relevant patient variables
- Determination of loading dose
- Determination of maintenance dose
- Determination of postdialysis replacement dose
- Monitoring of drug levels and clinical response

What Are the Unique Assessment Requirements Related to Drug Dosing in Chronic Kidney Disease?

Patients with kidney failure require an estimation of the residual kidney function and determination of the ideal body weight in addition to the standard assessments of drug allergies, previous drug history, comorbidities, concurrent medications, and baseline laboratory and clinical findings that precede the initiation of a new drug in any patient. Because weight may fluctuate between dialysis procedures and because daily dosage requirements usually correspond to the lean body weight rather than the actual weight in obese or edematous patients, ideal or lean body weight should be calculated. A variety of lean body weight calculators are available through an internet search.

In addition to assessing residual renal function, the efficiency of extrarenal mechanisms for drug elimination, especially liver function, should be evaluated because concurrent hepatic impairment may necessitate more stringent dose reduction.

Can Drugs Affect the Dialysis Procedure?

Several groups of drugs can affect the dialysis procedure. Many dialysis patients use antihypertensive medications that can contribute to hypotension during the dialysis procedure. Epoetin therapy is associated with a decrease in the prolonged bleeding time seen in some CKD patients and may increase heparin requirement during dialysis in some patients. In controlled clinical trials of CKD patients comparing higher hemoglobin targets (13–14 g/dL) with lower targets (9–11.3 g/dL), Epogen and other erythropoiesis-stimulating agents (ESAs) increased the risk of hemodialysis vascular access thrombosis and other thromboembolic events in the higher target groups (Amgen, 2012). Patients taking anticoagulants or antiplatelet medications should be monitored for bleeding or prolonged bleeding with cannulation of the vascular access or after needle removal.

ANTIANEMICS

Patients with CKD and patients undergoing maintenance dialysis are anemic and have considerably lower hematocrit values. Causes include (1) failure of production, or inhibition of action, of erythropoietin, a hormone produced by the kidney that stimulates the bone marrow to produce red blood cells (RBCs); (2) a shortened life span of RBCs; (3) impaired iron intake; (4) blood loss caused by platelet abnormalities, including a tendency to bleed from the nose, gums, GI tract, uterus, or skin; and (5) blood loss related to the dialysis procedure itself.

How Does Dialysis Influence Anemia?

Anemia can be a complex problem with CKD as the disease progresses, most notably in stages 3 to 5. After hemodialysis is initiated, incomplete blood recovery after dialysis, dialyzer leaks, and frequent blood sampling contribute to anemia.

These patients still have considerably fewer RBCs than normal and become dyspneic and tire easily. Other symptoms attributable to anemia include poor exercise tolerance, weakness, sexual dysfunction, anorexia, and an inability to think clearly.

What Is an Erythropoiesis-Stimulating Agent?

Erythropoiesis-stimulating agent is a broad term to describe drugs that assist in stimulating the production of erythropoietin in the body. Examples of ESAs include epoetin alfa (EPO) (Epogen, Procrit) and darbepoetin alfa (Aranesp).

EPO is a recombinant form of the hormone erythropoietin that is produced by normal, healthy kidneys. Epogen was introduced in 1989 and has revolutionized the treatment of CKD-associated anemia. Darbepoetin alfa also is an erythropoiesis-stimulating protein.

How Is Epoetin Alfa Given?

Epoetin alfa is given either intravenously or subcutaneously, usually three times per week at the end of a regular dialysis treatment. Patients on alternate modalities may have a different dosage schedule, route, or frequency.

What Are Some Causes of Suboptimal Response to Epoetin Alfa Therapy?

The 2006 National Kidney Foundation (NKF) Kidney Disease Outcomes Quality Initiative (KDOQI) Clinical Practice Guidelines for Anemia of Chronic Kidney Disease identify iron deficiency as the most common cause of inadequate response to EPO therapy. Some patients will fail to achieve target hemoglobin levels despite ESA therapy. Ten conditions are cited as potential causes for a patient's nonresponse. The five most common conditions are infection and inflammation, underdialysis, chronic blood loss, osteitis fibrosa, and aluminum toxicity. The remaining five causes are less common and should only be considered after the first four have been ruled out as causes. They are hemoglobinopathies (such as sickle cell anemia), folate and vitamin B_{12} deficiency, multiple myeloma, malnutrition, and hemolysis.

The 2007 revision of the NKF KDOQI anemia guidelines recommended that the target hemoglobin level should range from 11 to 12 g/dL and should not exceed 13 g/dL for CKD-ND (not on dialysis) and dialysis patients receiving ESAs. Hemoglobin levels in the KDOQI target range of 11 to 12 g/dL are associated with improved outcomes, including increased energy and activity levels and a better quality of life, as well as a decreased risk of hospitalization and mortality. The US Food and Drug Administration (FDA) recently suggested more conservative guidelines for treating anemia in CKD patients and for the use of ESAs. The FDA cites an increased risk of cardiovascular events such as stroke, myocardial infarction, thrombosis, and death as the reason for the change in the recommendations. These new guidelines have become part of the boxed warning and suggest that health care professionals should carefully evaluate when to begin ESA therapy and how to monitor dosing in CKD patients. The FDA now recommends using the lowest dose of ESA sufficient to minimize the need to transfuse the patient.

For Patients with Anemia of Chronic Kidney Disease Who Are Not on Dialysis

- Consider starting ESA treatment only when the hemoglobin level is less than 10 g/dL and when certain other considerations apply.
- If the hemoglobin level exceeds 10 g/dL, reduce or interrupt the dose of ESA.

For Patients with Anemia of Chronic Kidney Disease Who Are on Dialysis

- Initiate ESA treatment when the hemoglobin level is less than 10 g/dL.
- If the hemoglobin level approaches or exceeds 11 g/dL, reduce or interrupt the dose of ESA (US FDA, 2011).

What Are the Complications of Epoetin Alfa?

The major complication of EPO is an elevation of blood pressure because of increased blood viscosity secondary to the increased RBC mass. This usually occurs during the initial 12 weeks of therapy while the hematocrit is rising and is treated with antihypertensive medications and fluid removal via dialysis. Blood pressure should be closely monitored and controlled.

As the hematocrit rises, the efficiency of dialysis falls somewhat because the RBCs do not release their toxins (e.g., creatinine, potassium) very readily as they pass through the dialyzer. Close attention to blood chemistry is essential in patients receiving EPO, and some adjustment of the dialysis prescription may be necessary.

When Should Transfusions Be Given?

Blood is not routinely administered to dialysis patients. If the patient suffers a large blood loss from a dialyzer leak or from hemorrhage, the blood should be replaced. If the patient becomes short of breath or excessively fatigued or has angina, transfusion will often relieve the symptoms. In general, increasing the dose of EPO to improve anemia is more desirable than transfusion.

What Are Some of the Complications of Transfusions?

The most common complications of transfusions include the following:
- Incompatibility reactions caused by major or minor blood group incompatibility may occur. Chest or back pain, chills, and fever occur soon after blood transfusion is started. If this occurs, transfusion should be stopped immediately. A blood specimen should be drawn from the patient for evidence of hemolysis and for a recheck of type and cross-matching. Chills or fever should be treated symptomatically. IV steroids may be used if the symptoms are severe.
- Allergic reactions to leukocytes, platelets, or protein in the donor blood may occur. Manifestations include chills, fever, or skin eruptions that develop approximately 30 to 60 minutes after the start of transfusion. These are treated by slowing the rate of infusion. An antihistamine, such as diphenhydramine (Benadryl) at 20 to 50 mg, or steroids should be given intravenously if the symptoms are severe.
- Infections caused by hepatitis A, B, or C; cytomegalovirus; Epstein-Barr virus; or human immunodeficiency virus (HIV) may be transmitted by blood. The onset occurs from 1 to 4 months after transfusion.
- Preformed antibodies may result from minor incompatibility or allergic reactions. These are particularly important in patients awaiting a kidney transplant because of the potential decrease in the pool of potential compatible donors for organ transplantation.
- Iron overload that may lead to organ damage.
- Hyperkalemia may result from potassium load of lysed RBCs and absorption of existing cells.

What Can Be Done to Minimize Anemia?

Iron deficiency is a major contributing factor to the anemia associated with CKD. Adequate iron intake is essential if the patient's iron stores are depleted before starting EPO. Maintenance iron therapy is needed in most patients to ensure adequate iron stores and an optimal response to EPO. Oral iron supplements are rarely adequate. These often cause GI upset, nausea, gas, vomiting, or anorexia. IV iron, such as iron dextran, can be given depending on the adequacy of iron stores. In patients on EPO, iron deficiency is almost inevitable because iron is used rapidly under EPO stimulation of RBC production and is continually lost from the patient. Patients on EPO may benefit from the regular administration of small doses of parenteral iron. Folic acid and vitamin B_{12}, both of which are important for RBC formation, are water soluble and could be theoretically depleted by dialysis. Although there is little evidence of serious deficiencies in these vitamins, it is usual practice to give a supplement, particularly of folic acid. Good dietary intake of protein is important.

When Is Epoetin Alfa Administered?

Epoetin alfa is administered intravenously during hemodialysis to stimulate RBC production. Predialysis hematocrit may be used to monitor anemia and determine EPO administration. Each dialysis unit should follow its written and approved protocol. The amount of EPO required is determined by the hematocrit, hemoglobin, and individual patient response. Adequate iron stores and folic acid are required for erythropoietin to be effective. (A serum ferritin level of 200–500 ng/mL is considered optimal as per the KDOQI guidelines for hemodialysis patients.) Although EPO is given mostly intravenously during hemodialysis, KDOQI suggests that the subcutaneous route of administration is as effective as or more effective than the IV route. The Anemia Work Group recommends subcutaneous EPO as the preferred route of administration. When given subcutaneously, the site of injection should be rotated. Most hemodialysis patients prefer the IV route because of the discomfort caused by subcutaneous administration.

When Is Iron Therapy Required?

Two factors determine the need for iron therapy: first, the serum iron value is divided by the total iron binding capacity and multiplied by 100. This is called transferrin saturation, or TSAT, and correlates with the amount of iron available for erythropoiesis. (An optimal TSAT is greater than 20%. A TSAT of less than 20% indicates absolute iron deficiency, and a TSAT of more than 50% indicates a risk of iron overload according to the NKF KDOQI guidelines.)

How Is Iron Administered?

Iron is administered orally, intravenously, or both. Oral iron should not be taken with phosphate binders, which diminish its effect. When oral iron is prescribed, the patient should be instructed to always take the medication with food to avoid GI distress. Patients will usually need to supplement oral iron with the IV form at intervals to maintain adequate stores for erythropoiesis. IV iron is given during hemodialysis. The dosage is determined by the patient's laboratory values and type of iron preparation. The KDIGO guidelines recommend a trial of IV iron therapy if the TSAT is 30% or less, and the ferritin is 500 ng/mL or less (KDIGO, 2012). Iron dextran (Infed) was used most commonly before the newer iron products Ferrlecit (sodium ferric gluconate) and Venofer (iron sucrose injection) became available. These newer forms of IV iron have been shown to cause a lower incidence of anaphylaxis than previous generations of IV iron. A test dose is recommended before administering iron dextran products, but other irons do not require a test dose. Various side effects may occur from the administration of IV iron, ranging from hypotension (which is usually related to the rate of administration) to cramping, nausea, headaches, and hypersensitivity reactions. IV iron should always be administered according to the manufacturer's instructions.

CAN A PATIENT RECEIVE TOO MUCH IRON?

Iron overload or hematochromatosis may occur from multiple transfusions, excessive iron intake via diet or medications, use of iron therapy for anemia not related to iron deficiency, or in patients with certain genetic markers predisposing them to iron overload. Nausea and vomiting, diarrhea, and elevated liver enzymes may be present.

ANTIHYPERTENSIVES

WHAT IS HYPERTENSION?

Blood pressure greater than 140/90 mm Hg is classified as stage I hypertension. Hypertension is commonly seen in CKD patients and can be a cause or result of the disease. Hypertension can be attributed to volume overload, increased renin secretion, uremic toxins, dietary sodium, and secondary hyperparathyroidism. Hypertension can cause left ventricular hypertrophy and other cardiac complications. Both nonpharmacologic and pharmacologic treatment options must be used to manage hypertension associated with CKD. A variety of antihypertensive medications are available to treat patients. It is not unusual for patients to be prescribed more than one antihypertensive for treatment.

The National Heart, Lung, and Blood Institute classifies two levels of hypertension: stage 1 and stage 2 (Table 17.2).

Antihypertensive medications are divided into different categories because their mechanisms of action vary by drug. Most of these medications are used for hypertension control; however, some of the medications are used to treat heart failure, angina, and cardiac dysrhythmias and to delay the progression of kidney disease in CKD patients not on dialysis. Antihypertensive medications can produce complications such as hypotension, hyperkalemia, and increased creatinine levels so frequent patient monitoring is necessary.

WHAT ARE THE GOALS OF ANTIHYPERTENSIVE THERAPY IN PATIENTS WITH CHRONIC KIDNEY DISEASE?

Hypertension is common in CKD patients and can worsen cardiovascular disease (CVD), leading to the acceleration of further kidney damage. KDOQI recommends the use of antihypertensive therapy to lower blood pressure, reduce CVD risk, and slow the progression of kidney disease in patients with or without hypertension.

WHAT ARE THE DIFFERENT TYPES OF ANTIHYPERTENSIVE MEDICATIONS?

Angiotensin-Converting Enzyme Inhibitors

Angiotensin-converting enzyme inhibitors work by blocking an enzyme in the body that is responsible for converting angiotensin I to angiotensin II, causing the blood vessels to narrow (vasoconstriction). When the blood vessels are relaxed, blood pressure is lowered. ACE inhibitors also lower the amount of salt in the body, which assists in decreasing the blood pressure. ACE inhibitors have renoprotective effects and are thought to prevent the progression of kidney disease in compromised patients.

Angiotensin-converting enzyme inhibitors do cause a number of side effects, including dry persistent cough, increased serum creatinine, rash, increased serum potassium, and angioedema. Examples of ACE inhibitors include quinapril

Table 17.2 Categories of Blood Pressure Levels in Adults[a] (in mm Hg)

CATEGORY	SYSTOLIC (TOP NUMBER)	DIASTOLIC (BOTTOM NUMBER)
Normal	Less than 120	Less than 80
Prehypertension	120–139	80–89
Hypertension		
Stage 1	140–159	90–99
Stage 2	160 or higher	100 or higher

[a]For adults age 18 years and older who are not taking medicine for hypertension, do not have a short-term serious illness, and do not have other conditions (e.g., diabetes, kidney disease). When systolic and diastolic blood pressures fall into different categories, the higher category should be used to classify the blood pressure level. For example, 160/80 mm Hg would be stage 2 hypertension. There is an exception to this definition of hypertension: a blood pressure of 130/80 mm Hg or higher is considered hypertension in people with diabetes and chronic kidney disease.

From the National Heart, Lung, and Blood Institute: Diseases and conditions index, high blood pressure. Retrieved from http://www.nhlbi.nih.gov/health/dci/Diseases/Hbp/HBP_Whatls.html.

(Accupril), ramipril (Altace), captopril (Capoten), benazepril (Lotensin), fosinopril (Monopril), lisinopril (Prinivil, Zestril), and enalapril (Vasotec).

Angiotensin Receptor Blockers

Angiotensin receptor blockers (ARBs) are an alternative to ACE inhibitors. ARBs block the enzyme angiotensin II, which causes vasoconstriction. ARBs are as effective as but do not cause the cough sometimes associated with ACE inhibitors. Some potential side effects of ARBs are headache, angioedema, orthostatic hypotension, and hyperkalemia. Examples of ARBs include losartan (Cozaar), valsartan (Diovan), irbesartan (Avapro), eprosartan (Teveten), and candesartan (Atacand).

Beta-Blockers

β-blockers work by slowing the nerve impulses that travel through the heart. When this happens, the heart has less demand for blood and oxygen, which makes it work less hard, thereby decreasing the blood pressure. Bradycardia, fatigue, cold hands and feet, weakness, dizziness, dry mouth, wheezing, and swelling of the hands and feet are side effects that might occur from taking a β-blocker.

β-blockers include carvedilol (Coreg), nadolol (Corgard), propranolol (Inderal), metoprolol (Lopressor, Toprol-XL), acebutolol (Sectral), atenolol (Tenormin), and pindolol (Visken).

Calcium Channel Blockers

Calcium channel blockers slow the rate at which calcium passes into the heart muscle and vessel walls. This relaxes the vessels and allows blood to flow more easily through them, thereby lowering the blood pressure. The side effects of calcium channel blockers are headache, lower leg and ankle edema, fatigue, nervousness, bradycardia, and stomach discomfort. Examples of calcium channel blockers include amlodipine (Norvasc), diltiazem (Cardizem, Cardizem CD, Cardizem SR, Dilacor XR, Tiamate, Tiazac), felodipine (Plendil), nifedipine (Procardia), and verapamil (Calan SR, Covera-HS, Isoptin, Isoptin SR).

Diuretics

Diuretics are recommended as the first line of treatment for hypertension. They are usually recommended as one of at least two medications to control hypertension. Diuretics work by restricting the reabsorption of water, promoting diuresis, and removing excess sodium and water from the body. This reduction in total body water reduces the blood pressure. Several different types of diuretics work on different areas of the kidneys.

The side effects include frequent urination, weakness, increased thirst, and reduced levels of some electrolytes in the blood (potassium, sodium, and magnesium). Examples of diuretics include *thiazide diuretics* such as hydrochlorothiazide (Hydrodiuril) and chlorothiazide (Diuril), *potassium-sparing diuretics* such as spironolactone (Aldactone), *loop diuretics* such as furosemide (Lasix) and ethacrynic acid (Edecrin), and *others* such as chlorthalidone (Hygroton, Thalitone) and bumetanide (Bumex). When the GFR falls to less than 30 mL/min/1.73 m^2, tradition suggests switching from thiazide diuretics to loop diuretics. Diuretics should not be prescribed in patients who are anuric (without a urine output) because they are ineffective unless significant residual kidney function is present (Sinha & Agarwal, 2018).

ARE THERE DRUGS USED TO INCREASE BLOOD PRESSURE?

Midodrine is a drug used to treat hypotension and can be useful for some patients with intradialytic hypotension. The medication is administered 15 to 30 minutes before dialysis and again midway if needed for blood pressure support (Reilly, 2014). Care must be taken to observe for hypertension. Midodrine is excreted by the kidneys and is also removed by dialysis.

CATION EXCHANGE RESIN

WHAT MEDICATION IS USED TO TREAT HYPERKALEMIA?

Sodium polystyrene sulfonate (Kayexalate) is used in the treatment of hyperkalemia. Kayexalate is a cation exchange resin that replaces potassium ions for sodium ions, mostly in the large intestine. This exchange or lowering of serum potassium levels may take hours to days, so this is not an effective method for treating severe hyperkalemia. Kayexalate is administered either orally or by retention enema. Some CKD patients take Kayexalate regularly to control hyperkalemia. The side effects of this medication may include constipation, diarrhea, nausea, vomiting, hypokalemia, hypomagnesemia, and hypocalcemia because it is not selective for potassium alone. Kayexalate should be used with caution in heart failure patients because of the sodium load that is precipitated with its use. Patiromer is another cation exchange resin used to treat patients with acute or chronic hyperkalemia. Patiromer is given orally once daily and is sodium free. Hypomagnesemia is a possible side effect of the medication, so blood levels should checked regularly, and a magnesium supplement may be prescribed.

INTRADIALYTIC PARENTERAL NUTRITION

Intradialytic parenteral nutrition is a form of nutritional support for patients with hypoalbuminemia and consists of an emulsion of amino acids, lipids, and dextrose. See Chapter 14 for more information.

PHOSPHATE BINDERS

Disturbances in calcium and phosphorus metabolism are common in patients who develop CKD gradually and are often apparent even before dialysis is required. During the progression of kidney failure, there is a loss of the ability to excrete phosphate. Phosphate ions accumulate in the body fluids and lead to a reciprocal decrease in serum calcium. The parathyroid glands seek to maintain a normal concentration of calcium in body fluids and respond by increasing the production of parathyroid hormone (PTH). This causes calcium to be resorbed from the bones, resulting in a loss of bone density and strength. In addition, the active form of vitamin D, which is needed for normal bone metabolism, is manufactured in the kidneys and is deficient in CKD patients. Dialysis does not fully correct disordered calcium–phosphorus metabolism, and progressive osteodystrophy (a term for several bony manifestations) is a serious problem in many CKD patients (Table 17.3). CKD patients should be assessed for mineral and bone disorders as early as CKD stage 3 (Uhlig et al 2010).

WHAT IS THE FUNCTION OF ORAL CALCIUM AS A PHOSPHATE BINDER?

Oral calcium (usually as calcium carbonate), when taken with a meal, binds phosphorus in the GI tract so that it passes out with the stool, thereby preventing serum phosphorus from increasing. This helps control the calcium–phosphorus product. If oral calcium is taken too long after eating or on an empty stomach, it may contribute to making the patient hypercalcemic. If high serum phosphorus levels with low serum calcium levels are left untreated, the parathyroid glands become stimulated, resulting in a loss of calcium from the patient's bones.

HOW ARE PHOSPHATE BINDERS TAKEN?

Phosphate binders need to be taken with every meal and with snacks containing protein. It is best not to take phosphate binders when taking oral iron or antibiotics because the efficacies of these medications become compromised. Patient compliance with regular use of phosphate binders is problematic. A major factor contributing to noncompliance with phosphate binder therapy is the number of medications the patient takes on a regular basis. The addition of phosphate binders, which need to be taken with every meal, to the already sizable number of pills the patient must take is cumbersome. Some of the phosphate binders leave a chalky taste in the mouth and may cause constipation, which becomes another deterrent to compliance.

ARE THERE DIFFERENT TYPES OF PHOSPHATE BINDERS?

Several different types of phosphate binders are available to control excess phosphorus in the bloodstream. Aluminum-based phosphate binders (aluminum hydroxide [Alu-Cap]) were the first type of binders used for the treatment of the hyperphosphatemia of CKD. Aluminum-based binders are extremely effective for maintaining low serum phosphorus levels because of their high phosphorus-binding abilities. These binders, however, can cause high serum aluminum levels or aluminum toxicity. Aluminum-based binders are now therefore seldom used in the management of phosphorus control. Calcium-based binders (calcium acetate [PhosLo, Phosex] and calcium carbonate [Titralac, Calci-Chew]) are more commonly used and serve a dual role of decreasing serum phosphorus as well as supplementing calcium in patients with hypocalcemia. Attention must be given to the patient's monthly laboratory studies to ensure that he or she is not becoming hypercalcemic.

Sevelamer hydrochloride (Renagel), a phosphate binder, is both calcium and aluminum free. Sevelamer works in the GI tract, where a positively charged hydrogel binds with negatively charged phosphate from the diet. The formed complex does not cross the GI tract but is instead excreted in the feces. Because sevelamer contains no calcium, the patient will be able to achieve phosphorus control while maintaining the calcium–phosphorus product at an acceptable level. Sevelamer must be taken with every meal and when eating between meals. Velphoro (sucroferric oxyhydroxides) is another phosphate binder used to control serum phosphorus in CKD patients. Velphoro is attractive because it reduces pill burden because usually only one chewable tablet per meal is required as a maintenance dose. Velphoro contains iron and may cause discolored feces and diarrhea. Auryxia (ferric citrate) is a nonchewable, noncalcium, iron-containing, phosphate binder. Auryxia works as other binders by binding with phosphorus in the GI tract but does provide an added benefit of providing absorption and storage of iron. Ferritin should be monitored to avoid iron overload.

VITAMINS AND VITAMIN ANALOGS

WHAT ARE THE INDICATIONS FOR ADMINISTERING THE VITAMIN D ANALOG 1,25-DIHYDROXYVITAMIN D_3 (CALCITRIOL)?

Calcitriol is used to treat hypocalcemia and is effective in the control of secondary hyperparathyroidism in maintenance dialysis patients. It is the active form of vitamin D_3. Calcitriol increases calcium levels and has been shown to reduce elevated PTH levels, preventing secondary hyperparathyroidism and improving renal osteodystrophy.

HOW AND WHEN IS CALCITRIOL ADMINISTERED?

Calcitriol in the IV form (Calcijex) is administered as a bolus during hemodialysis treatment. An oral form of calcitriol (Rocaltrol) is also available.

Table 17.3 Common Medications and Nutritional Supplement for Patients with End-Stage Kidney Disease

Phosphate Binders
- Taken with meals and snacks to prevent dietary phosphorus absorption

Calcium carbonate	TUMS, Os-Cal
Calcium acetate	PhosLo, Phoslyra
Mg/Ca^{++} carbonate	MagneBind
Sevelamer hydrochloride	Renagel
Sevelamer carbonate	Renvela
Lanthanum carbonate	Fosrenol
Ferric citrate	Auryxia
Sucroferric oxyhydroxide	Velphoro
Aluminum hydroxide	AlternaGEL

Vitamins
- Increased need for water-soluble vitamins because of losses during dialysis
- Fat-soluble vitamins A and K are not supplemented
- Vitamin E may be supplemented

Dialysis Recommendations

Vitamin C	60 mg (not to exceed 200 mg daily)
Folic acid	1 mg
Thiamin	1.5 mg
Riboflavin	1.7 mg
Niacin	20 mg
Vitamin B$_6$	10 mg
Vitamin B$_{12}$	6 mcg
Pantothenic acid	10 mg
Biotin	0.3 mg

Brand names include Nephrocap and Nephro-Vite. An OTC vitamin B complex is comparable.

Erythropoiesis-Stimulating Agents
- Stimulate bone marrow to produce RBCs

IV or IM	Epoetin alfa (Epogen), darbepoetin alfa (Aranesp)

Iron
- Iron needs are increased because of ESA therapy

IV only	Iron dextran (InFed), sodium ferric gluconate (Ferrlecit), iron sucrose (Venofer), ferric carboxymaltose (Injectafer), ferumoxytol (Feraheme)

Activated Vitamin D
- Used for the management of hyperparathyroidism

PO or IV	Calcitriol (Rocaltrol/Calcijex), doxercalciferol (Hectorol), paricalcitol (Zemplar)

Calcimimetics
- Mimic calcium and bind to parathyroid gland

PO	Cinacalcet (Sensipar)
	Etelcalcetide (Parsabiv)

Calcium Supplements

Oral	TUMS, Os-Cal, Calci-Chew

Phosphorus Supplements
- May contain sodium and/or potassium

Oral	K-Phos Neutral, Neutra-Phos, Neutra-Phos-K

Cation Exchange Resin
- For the treatment of hyperkalemia

Oral or rectal	Sodium polystyrene sulfonate (Kayexalate)

Ca^{++}, Calcium; EPO, epoetin; IM, intramuscular; IV, intravenous; OTC, over-the-counter; PO, oral; SPS, sodium polystyrene sulfonate.
Developed by Fiona Wolf, RD, and Thomas Montemayor, RPh, Northwest Kidney Centers, Seattle, WA, 2010.

Are There Any Adverse Effects of Calcitriol Therapy?

Hypercalcemia can result from calcitriol treatment. Serum calcium and phosphorus must be evaluated on a regular basis to avoid hypercalcemia that could lead to generalized vascular calcification and soft tissue (eyes, skin, and heart) calcification.

Caution should be exercised to avoid hypercalcemia and should be investigated if indicated. A relative increased risk for all-cause mortality exists with calcium levels at 9.5 to 11.4 mg/dL. Therapy can be discontinued or held as determined by the physician and dosage adjustments should be based on trends rather than a laboratory value at a single point in time (NKF, 2010).

What Is Paricalcitol Injection?

Paricalcitol (Zemplar) is a synthetic vitamin D analog for the treatment of secondary hyperparathyroidism. Paricalcitol is given intravenously or orally to CKD patients to decrease PTH levels with minimal effects on calcium and phosphorus; however, the calcium–phosphorus product should continue to be monitored for elevation. Hypercalcemia promotes digitalis toxicity, so laboratory studies should be closely monitored in patients using digitalis. Paricalcitol should never be used in patients with vitamin D toxicity or hypercalcemia. It is an aggressive treatment for secondary hyperparathyroidism.

What Is Doxercalciferol?

Doxercalciferol (Hectorol) is a synthetic vitamin D analog used to suppress PTH and manage secondary hyperparathyroidism. Doxercalciferol is available in either the IV or oral form. Hypercalcemia, hyperphosphatemia, and oversuppression of the parathyroid gland are possible adverse effects associated with the use of this medication. Dosing is based on PTH levels along with serum calcium and phosphorus monitoring.

What is a Calcimimetic?

Calcimimetics are a class of drugs which reduce PTH as well as serum calcium and phosphorus levels. Calcimimetics suppress the secretion of PTH by making the calcium sensing receptors on the cells of the parathyroid gland more sensitive to extracellular calcium. Serum calcium, phosphorus, and PTH levels should be closely monitored. Symptoms such as tingling or prickly sensations, numbness around the mouth, irritability, spasms, seizures, hypotension, and bradycardia may indicate hypocalcemia. Sensipar (cinacalcet) is taken daily in pill form and Parsabiv (etelcalcetide) is administered intravenously during discontinuation of the hemodialysis treatment.

Is Deferoxamine Mesylate Used?

Deferoxamine mesylate (Desferal) is a chelating agent used to remove excessive metals from the bloodstream. It was originally formulated to treat iron overload. Deferoxamine has been found to be useful as an aluminum-chelating agent in dialysis patients and acts to remove aluminum from the tissues, so it can be dialyzed out or adsorbed by a special cartridge. The dosage of deferoxamine varies for different patients. The dosage is usually based on body weight and is ordered by the physician. Deferoxamine is usually mixed with 200 mL of normal saline and infused during the last 2 hours of dialysis treatment, three times a week. Deferoxamine should be withheld for 2 weeks after infusion of IV iron. Deferoxamine administration may cause visual and auditory disturbances when administered over prolonged periods at high doses. Flushing, urticaria, hypotension, tachycardia, and shock may occur during IV administration, so the patient must be carefully observed during administration.

ACUTE KIDNEY INJURY AND DIALYSIS

Acute kidney injury (AKI) is the contemporary name for what was formerly termed *acute renal failure*. The new name more accurately describes the process of all phases of acute injury to the kidney. The definition of AKI can be referred to as RIFLE, representing three levels of renal dysfunction. These levels are described in the following categories: risk of renal dysfunction, injury to the kidney, failure of kidney function, loss of function, and end-stage renal disease, with the last two representing outcome categories (Table 18.1). Dialysis is often necessary for the treatment of AKI. The most common indications include uremia, hyperkalemia, acidosis, fluid overload, and drug overdose.

What Is Acute Kidney Injury?

Acute kidney injury is the rapid deterioration of renal function. It is usually reversible if diagnosed and treated early. The signs and symptoms of AKI include a urine output of less than 400 mL/day (oliguria) or less than 20 mL/hr for an adult, an increase in blood urea nitrogen (BUN) and creatinine, hyperkalemia, and acidosis.

What Are the Types of Acute Kidney Injury?

Acute kidney injury can be divided into three categories: prerenal, intrarenal, and postrenal (Box 18.1) (see Chapter 4). Even though some diseases overlap into all three categories, they are separated for ease of explanation. Prolonged prerenal and postrenal injury can cause intrarenal injury, and patients with underlying CKD with any of the aforementioned are more prone to AKI (Rahman et al, 2012).

Prerenal

Prerenal failure accounts for approximately 70% of AKI cases. Prerenal events result in decreased blood flow to the kidney. Examples include congestive heart failure, hypovolemia, sepsis, myocardial infarction, prolonged hypotension, and vascular disorders of renal arteries or veins.

Intrarenal

Approximately 25% of AKI cases are caused by intrarenal factors. Any event that damages the kidney tissue, structure, or function is categorized as intrarenal AKI. This damage, which may involve the glomeruli, tubules, or both, interferes with the ability of the kidneys to carry out their normal functions. The most common cause of intrarenal failure is damage to the tubules. This is called acute tubular necrosis (ATN). ATN is caused by severely reduced blood flow, leading to prolonged ischemia, or by direct toxic insult to the tubular cells. In oliguric ATN, urine flow decreases to about 20 mL/hr, and BUN, serum creatinine, phosphate, and potassium levels increase. With nonoliguric AKI, the patient may maintain better fluid balance, but elimination of waste products is impaired. Ischemic injury to the kidneys can occur when the mean arterial pressure (MAP) drops below 60 mm Hg for more than 30 minutes. Massive hemorrhage, transfusion reaction, sepsis, cardiovascular collapse, or major trauma can cause ischemic renal injury.

Substances that injure the kidneys are called nephrotoxins. The most common are medications, such as antibiotics and nonsteroidal antiinflammatory drugs (NSAIDs). Other medications, including anesthetics and cancer chemotherapy agents as well as street drugs, are toxic to the kidney in varying degrees. Radiocontrast dyes used for intravenous (IV) pyelography, cardiac catheterization, and computed tomography are potentially nephrotoxic. Other nephrotoxins include hemoglobin (from red blood cell [RBC] hemolysis) and myoglobin from muscle breakdown (rhabdomyolysis) caused by crush injury, heatstroke, or seizure.

Postrenal

Postrenal causes account for approximately 5% of AKI cases. Postrenal failure is usually the result of obstruction in the flow of urine anywhere from the kidney to the urinary meatus. The obstruction can be functional or mechanical. Functional causes include diabetic nephropathy, medications such as ganglionic blocking agents that block the autonomic nerve supply to the urinary system, and neurogenic bladder subsequent to spinal cord injury or cerebrovascular accident. Tumors, stones, prostatic hypertrophy, and urethral strictures are some mechanical causes of postrenal failure.

Do Patients with Acute Kidney Injury Have Urine Output?

Some patients with AKI have significant urine output; this is referred to as nonoliguric renal failure. Most patients progress through several stages from oliguria to anuria and polyuria, depending on the phase of AKI (Table 18.2).

Table 18.1 Risk, Injury, Failure, Loss, and End-Stage Renal Disease (RIFLE) Classification[a]

CLASS	GLOMERULAR FILTRATION RATE CRITERIA	URINE OUTPUT CRITERIA
Risk	Serum creatinine × 1.5 (GFR decrease >25%)	<0.5 mL/kg/hr × 6 hr
Injury	Serum creatinine × 2.0 (GFR decrease >50%)	<0.5 mL/kg/hr × 12 hr
Failure	Serum creatinine × 3 (GFR decrease >75%)	<0.5 mL/kg/hr × 24 hr or anuria × 12 hr
Loss	Persistent acute renal failure = complete loss of kidney function and need for renal replacement therapy for >4 wk	
End-stage renal disease	End-stage renal disease and need for dialysis for >3 mo	

[a]For the conversion of creatinine expressed in conventional units to SI units, multiply by 88.4. The RIFLE class is determined on the basis of the worst of either the glomerular filtration criteria or urine output criteria. Glomerular filtration criteria are calculated as an increase in serum creatinine levels above baseline serum creatinine levels.
Modified from Cameron JL, Cameron AM: *Current surgical therapy: multiple organ dysfunction and failure,* ed. 12, Philadelphia, 2017, Elsevier.

Box 18.1 Causes of Acute Kidney Injury

Prerenal (Decreased Renal Perfusion)
- Hypovolemia
- Hemorrhage
- Shock
- Third spacing (edema, ascites)
- Burns
- Dehydration (gastrointestinal losses, overuse of diuretics)
- Decreased cardiac output
- Cardiogenic shock
- Dysrhythmias
- Cardiac tamponade
- Congestive heart failure
- Myocardial infarction
- Thromboembolic obstruction of the renal vasculature

Intrarenal (Damage to the Nephron)
- Acute tubular necrosis
- Ischemic
- Prolonged prerenal acute kidney injury
- Transfusion reaction
- Rhabdomyolysis
- Nephrotoxic
- Prolonged postrenal acute kidney injury
- Antibiotics (aminoglycosides, carbenicillin, amphotericin B)
- Contrast media
- Heavy metals (lead, mercury)
- Carbon tetrachloride
- Insecticides, fungicides
- Cytotoxic drugs (certain chemotherapeutic agents)
- Hemolytic-uremic syndrome
- Inflammatory
- Acute glomerulonephritis
- Acute pyelonephritis

Postrenal (Obstruction)
- Benign prostatic hypertrophy
- Calculi (stones)
- Urinary tract infection
- Tumors
- Strictures
- Altered bladder contraction (neurogenic bladder from medication or injury/disease)

Modified from Banasik JL: *Pathophysiology,* ed. 6, St. Louis, 2019, Elsevier.

Table 18.2 Phases of Acute Kidney Injury

DEFINITION	APPROXIMATE TIME SPAN	CLINICAL FEATURES
Prodromal Phase Normal or declining during output	Depends on the degree of injury	Increased BUN and creatinine
Oliguric Phase <400 mL/day	10 days–8 wk	Hypervolemia Hyperkalemia Uremia Metabolic acidosis
Postoliguric Phase 1–5 L/day	1 wk–12 mo	Polyuria Fluid volume deficit

Modified from Banasik JL: *Pathophysiology*, ed. 6, St. Louis, 2019, Elsevier.

Prodromal Phase

This phase is identified with normal or declining urine output and BUN and creatinine beginning to rise. The cause of kidney injury, volume of toxin ingested, and degree of hypotension will determine duration of the prodromal phase. It is essential to record accurate daily weights as well as precise and detailed intakes and outputs.

Oliguric Phase

Oliguria is defined as a urine output of less than 400 mL/day. Oliguria is typically seen in this phase in the majority of patients, but some patients remain nonoliguric. Anuria is a urine output of less than 50 mL/day and is seen in those with severe injury. The longer oliguria or anuria continues, the less likely is the prospect of returning to normal urine output. Proper management of fluid volumes is essential as hypervolemia will be present. Patients should be monitored for fluid volume overload symptoms such as jugular vein distention, weight gain, and hypertension. It is important to monitor glomerular filtration rate (GFR) and for the development of uremic symptoms.

Postoliguric Phase

This phase begins when the urine output reaches 1 L/day. The renal indices may stabilize and then begin to approach normal with a gradual return of renal function. The 24-hour urine volume can increase to as much as 4 to 5 L. Accurate evaluation of the patient's status to avoid dehydration leading to hypoperfusion of the kidneys is mandatory. Laboratory values are closely monitored with the expectation that they will return to normal in the late phase of AKI.

This period begins with the stabilization of serum chemistries and gradual return of normal kidney function. This phase may last from 3 to 6 months. Return to a normal GFR, if it occurs, may take up to 1 year.

WHAT ARE THE CLINICAL PRESENTATIONS OF ACUTE KIDNEY INJURY?

The clinical presentations of AKI include all of the symptoms, signs, and findings of rapidly developing uremia (see Chapter 5) and can vary with the cause and severity of the kidney injury and associated comorbidities. Symptoms may include listlessness, confusion, fatigue, anorexia, nausea, vomiting, weight gain, or edema (Raham & Smith, 2012).

WHAT BIOCHEMICAL CHANGES ARE PRESENT IN ACUTE KIDNEY INJURY?

The damaged kidneys are unable to excrete the products of normal body metabolism. Serum urea and creatinine levels are elevated, and electrolyte levels are altered. An increased hydrogen ion concentration causes acidosis and low serum pH. Hyperkalemia, hypokalemia, hypocalcemia, hyperphosphatemia, hypermagnesemia, and low bicarbonate levels may be observed.

HOW IS ACUTE KIDNEY INJURY TREATED?

Many treatment options are available depending on the cause of renal failure, severity of symptoms, and overall condition of the patient. Options include hemodialysis, isolated ultrafiltration (UF), peritoneal dialysis, continuous renal replacement therapy (CRRT), and charcoal hemoperfusion.

What Differences Between Acute and Chronic Renal Failure Should Be Evaluated by the Caregiver When Assessing Patients with Acute Kidney Injury?

- Comparison of the previous GFR and creatinine. Absence of previous renal impairment is suggestive of AKI.
- A thorough history to evaluate symptoms over several months, which may suggest renal insufficiency before hospitalization
- Evaluation of kidney ultrasound and scans showing the size and condition of the kidney
- Anemia, a sign of chronic kidney disease
- Long-term bone disease, which supports the idea of chronic kidney disease versus AKI (Ashley & Morlidge, 2008)

What Are the Indications for Treatment?

The most common indications for acute dialysis include the following:

Uremia

Acute dialysis is initiated when a patient becomes symptomatically uremic (see Chapter 5) regardless of BUN or creatinine levels. Dialysis may be started prophylactically when BUN reaches 100 mg/dL even if the patient has few or no symptoms.

Pulmonary Edema

Acute pulmonary edema is a life-threatening complication of AKI that necessitates immediate dialysis. Acute pulmonary edema can result from fluid overload directly attributable to AKI, an acute myocardial infarction, or overzealous fluid administration. Pulmonary edema can also result from a poor ejection fraction, and it is prudent to be aware of these results if available.

Hyperkalemia

Hyperkalemia is a result of the damaged kidney's inability to secrete potassium and the release of intracellular potassium (because of acidosis and tissue breakdown). Hemodialysis is effective in lowering potassium and is initiated when rapid reduction in plasma potassium is indicated. Peritoneal dialysis is an acceptable treatment option, although its effects are slower than that of hemodialysis. Hyperkalemia can be managed in an emergency, while waiting for hemodialysis, by IV administration of glucose and insulin in combination with IV sodium bicarbonate. These shift extracellular potassium into the cell, where it cannot cause cardiac arrhythmia. Calcium gluconate may be given intravenously to reduce myocardial irritability. A sodium polystyrene sulfonate cation exchange resin (Kayexalate) can be administered by mouth or by enema when a slower correction of potassium is acceptable or during the initial management of hyperkalemia.

Acidosis

Metabolic acidosis is caused by the inability of the kidneys to excrete hydrogen ions and reabsorb bicarbonate. Acidosis can be treated temporarily with IV sodium bicarbonate. Hemodialysis may be required because of the added sodium, which increases the risk of volume overload.

Neurologic Changes

Toxic effects of uremia can result in central nervous system changes. Headache, insomnia, and drowsiness are early symptoms; confusion, convulsions, and coma may occur later. Dialysis is indicated when any of these serious symptoms are seen and preferably before they occur.

Drug Overdoses and Poisonings

Dialysis is indicated for the treatment of some drug intoxications. Drugs normally excreted by the kidneys or water-soluble drugs of low molecular weight will diffuse rapidly across cellulosic dialysis membranes. Such drugs are readily removed with hemodialysis. Examples include ethanol, lithium, methanol, and salicylates. Water-soluble drugs with a high molecular weight, such as vancomycin and amphotericin B, diffuse across cellulosic membranes much more slowly and are less well removed. Hemodialysis is not useful if the intoxicant is protein bound (e.g., digoxin and acetylsalicylic acid) or lipid soluble (e.g., carbamazepine). However, both these types of intoxicants can be removed by hemoperfusion with a charcoal cartridge or plasma membrane filter.

Multiple Organ Failure

An increased incidence of AKI is seen with multiple organ failure. Studies have shown an increased incidence of AKI with an increased number of body system failures (Schrier, 2007).

What Type of Vascular Access Is Used for Acute Dialysis?

The most common access to circulation for acute dialysis is a double-lumen venous catheter. The catheter may be placed in the subclavian, internal jugular, or femoral vein. Insertion of a catheter into the subclavian or internal jugular vein must be followed by x-ray examination to determine correct placement and to rule out pneumothorax or hemothorax before the catheter is used (see Chapter 12). With advanced medical care, many patients remain in the acute phase for longer periods and therefore require a tunneled catheter to help prevent line sepsis (see Chapter 12).

Can an Arteriovenous Fistula or Graft Be Used for Acute Dialysis?

Patients with an arteriovenous (AV) fistula or graft may require acute dialysis, and the fistula or graft may be used after its patency is determined (see Chapter 12 for additional information).

How Often Are Patients Dialyzed?

The frequency of dialysis is determined by the patient's response to treatment. Patients may be hemodialyzed daily for a few days until BUN, serum creatinine, and potassium levels and acidosis are considered acceptable. Daily dialysis may be necessary for volume overload or if the patient is receiving parenteral nutrition.

What Complications May Occur with Acute Kidney Injury?

Cardiac and Pulmonary

Congestive heart failure is common. It is most often caused by hypertension, volume excess, or anemia. Pulmonary edema and infiltrates as well as respiratory failure are common with AKI. Monitoring cardiac output, central venous pressure, daily weight, intake and output, vital signs, pulse oximetry, clinical assessment, and Crit-Line (see Chapter 13) usage are essential.

Hypertension

Fluid removal by dialysis may correct hypertension. Antihypertensive medication may be necessary.

Hypotension

Hypotension may result from blood loss, stringent fluid restriction, sepsis, myocardial infarction, or pericarditis. To prevent additional kidney damage, the underlying cause of hypotension must be corrected to maintain adequate renal perfusion. Use of a vasopressor, such as dopamine, may be necessary.

Anemia

In AKI, the release of erythropoietin is decreased. The usual response to therapy with recombinant erythropoietin or epoetin alfa requires 3 to 4 weeks, so it is not immediately helpful. Uremic RBCs also have a shortened life span. Blood loss from the dialysis procedure and increased bleeding tendencies are often present (see Chapter 5 for additional information about complications).

Infection

This is one of the most serious complications. Patients must be monitored for dialysis line sepsis, blood cultures, elevated temperature, and any other signs of infection. Line sepsis must be addressed with utmost importance.

Electrolyte Imbalance

Hyperkalemia and hypokalemia are most often seen with AKI and must be addressed immediately so that the patient does not have cardiac complications. Hyperkalemia is related to potassium release from tissues. Another complication is hypokalemia, which is not as common but must also be addressed to prevent cardiac complications.

What Is the Most Serious Complication of Acute Kidney Injury?

Infection is the leading cause of death in patients with AKI. Uremia causes immune suppression, which predisposes patients to sepsis. Strict aseptic techniques must be used for all invasive procedures, including initiating and discontinuing dialysis, starting an IV line, and caring for the bladder catheter. "Acute renal failure is a major cause of morbidity and mortality, particularly in the hospital setting. Despite improvements in renal replacement therapy (RRT) techniques during the last several decades, AKI places the patient at an increased risk of ESKD, pulmonary complications, and cardiovascular events. The severity of AKI is positively correlated to patient morbidity and mortality" (Brown et al, 2016).

Are There Special Considerations When Dialyzing a Patient for the First Time?

An infrequent syndrome known as "first-use" syndrome results from an allergic type of reaction to new dialyzers and is characterized by itching, hypotension, chest and back pain, and breathing difficulties. In severe cases, cardiopulmonary arrest may occur. Symptoms usually manifest during the first 15 to 30 minutes of dialysis. Cuprophan dialyzers are most often implicated. Cellulose acetate and modified cellulosic and synthetic membranes (polysulfone, polyamide, and polyacrylonitrile) are less likely to cause first-use syndrome.

What Is the Treatment for First-Use Syndrome?

When the symptoms are severe, blood must not be returned to the patient, and the dialyzer must be discarded. The physician should be notified, and assessment of the symptoms, particularly the cardiopulmonary status, should be performed. Use of a more biocompatible membrane may be necessary. When the symptoms are less severe, symptomatic treatment (e.g., nasal oxygen or oral diphenhydramine [Benadryl]) is adequate, and the physician should be notified. In this situation, dialysis can continue because the symptoms usually subside after the first hour.

ARE THERE SPECIAL PRECAUTIONS WHEN DIALYZING PATIENTS WITH ACUTE KIDNEY INJURY?

Patients requiring acute dialysis are generally critically ill with multisystem failure. Thorough and accurate assessment of the patient is essential before initiating dialysis (see Chapter 13). The nephrology nurse must be highly cognizant of changes, be prudent in assessing and monitoring the patient's vital signs, and respond appropriately.

Maintaining a MAP of less than 60 mm Hg is critical for continued perfusion of the already insulted kidney. Use of Crit-Line to assist in determining the intravascular volume must be monitored to preserve vascular flow to the kidneys.

Controlled anticoagulation with heparin may be necessary to minimize clotting of the dialyzer; however, dialysis can be performed with little or no heparin. Careful monitoring of the clotting time may be necessary to prevent complications related to heparinization during hemodialysis. Most often, heparinization is based on hemoglobin levels, hematocrit, platelet count, prothrombin time/international normalized ratio, and the patient's overall status and assessment.

The physician determines the anticoagulation technique. The "tight" or "no heparin" technique may be used for patients at high risk for bleeding. "No heparin" dialysis requires a blood flow rate between 250 and 300 mL/min; otherwise, significant dialyzer clotting will occur. The dialyzer is flushed every 20 to 30 minutes with 100 mL of normal saline so that it can be easily examined visually for clotting as well as proteins and clotting factors can be removed from the dialyzer membrane surface. Before the start of dialysis, this extra volume is calculated into the required fluid loss to achieve the planned fluid removal goal. The risk of clotting the dialyzer, resulting in an average blood loss of 150 mL, must be weighed against the risk of administering an anticoagulant to a high-risk patient.

Patients in an intensive care unit (ICU) are attached to a cardiac monitor. It is important to watch for arrhythmias during dialysis because they may be treatment related. However, it is common to see some aberrant or premature ventricular beats during dialysis.

WHAT IS CRIT-LINE?

The Crit-Line monitor is a device which measures the inverse relationship of red cell blood volume to plasma volume. Crit-Line provides the clinician with real-time information about blood volume changes during dialysis with respect to plasma volume refilling and depletion. It helps to determine the intravascular volume noninvasively. Crit-Line is attached to the arterial end of the dialyzer and uses technology similar to that of the SaO_2 monitor. The monitor gives a continuous read-out of hemoglobin levels, hematocrit, oxygen saturation, and blood volume changes. Crit-Line is a helpful and noninvasive tool. This monitor should be used along with all other physical assessments and with the physician's orders to determine the fluid removal rate.

WHAT MEASURES MAY BE TAKEN DURING ACUTE DIALYSIS TO COUNTERACT HYPOTENSION?

Abnormalities causing hypotension must be identified and corrected as much as possible. These usually involve the intravascular volume, cardiac output, or vasomotor tone. Although patients are often overhydrated and edematous, some may have hypotension because of a low intravascular volume and require infusion of normal saline or dextrose and water. Patients who do not respond to normal saline infusion may require colloid or hyperosmolar products such as albumin. These colloids will increase the oncotic pressure and attract fluid from the extracellular space into the vascular space. Hypotension resulting from a decreased RBC mass due to hemorrhage or other causes may require transfusion of RBCs. When hypotension is caused by a low cardiac output, cardiotonic drugs, particularly inotropic agents (dopamine) and antiarrhythmic medications (amiodarone and Cardizem), may be helpful. It may be appropriate to reduce the blood flow rate to between 150 and 200 mL/min to yield an apparent decrease in the cardiac output. The physician will need accurate assessment data about the duration of dialysis, blood flow rate, UF estimate (or weight), blood pressure readings, and all medications administered to determine the most appropriate treatment. Note that dialysis efficiency is reduced when the blood flow is lowered; in other words, there is a decrease in urea reduction, Kt/V, and creatinine clearance. If hypotension is caused by poor vasomotor tone, patients may be maintained above their ideal weight to promote vascular filling and normotensive blood pressure. Use of Crit-Line assists in determining the intravascular volume and should be used along with other intensive care tools to treat hypotension.

WHAT MEASURES ARE APPROPRIATE FOR HYPERTENSION?

Most hypertension in acute dialysis patients is related to fluid excess and responds to UF. If it is not controlled through fluid removal, the physician may prescribe an antihypertensive medication. Patients taking antihypertensive agents may be subject to hypotensive episodes. Administration of antihypertensive agents may need to be deferred before hemodialysis if ordered accordingly by the physician.

WHAT IS DISEQUILIBRIUM SYNDROME?

Disequilibrium syndrome is a complex of signs and symptoms ranging from headache, restlessness, and impaired mental concentration to confusion, twitching, and jerking, occasionally culminating in a grand mal seizure. It may occur during or soon after dialysis.

WHAT CAUSES DIALYSIS DISEQUILIBRIUM?

Disequilibrium is thought to be related to cerebral edema. The blood–brain barrier has a selective effect on the transfer of solutes and water between the plasma and the brain. During dialysis, the plasma solute concentration is reduced more rapidly than the brain solute concentration, and the plasma becomes hypotonic relative to the brain cell water, causing water to shift from the plasma to the brain.

WHEN SHOULD DISEQUILIBRIUM BE ANTICIPATED?

Disequilibrium is most common in more severely catabolic patients or in those with severe azotemia (BUN greater than 200 mg/100 mL).

WHAT ARE THE WAYS TO PREVENT OR MINIMIZE DISEQUILIBRIUM?

Prevention is best. Care must be taken not to lower the urea level too rapidly; it is best to perform short (2–3 hours) dialysis at 24-hour intervals for the first few treatments. A reduced blood flow rate of 150 to 200 mL/min may lessen the risk of dialysis disequilibrium by slowing the solute shift rate. Using a small dialyzer with lower clearance properties will help. Configuring the extracorporeal blood circuit with the dialysate flow concurrent rather than countercurrent to the blood flow is an easy method of decreasing the rapid removal of urea by reducing clearance throughout the treatment. Decreasing the dialysate flow rate will also lead to decreased urea removal. The physician may also prescribe IV administration of a high osmotic solution, such as 25% mannitol, at the beginning of treatment. Disequilibrium manifested by seizures and coma is unusual with frequent and less aggressive dialysis. Early detection of the potential for severe neurologic changes must be promptly reported to the physician.

PROCEDURES

Isolated UF is a process by which excess fluid is removed with little or no change in blood solute concentrations. Very small amounts of urea and creatinine are removed passively from the patient's serum along with the ultrafiltrate. The rate and amount at which the fluid can be removed depend in part on the amount of excess extracellular fluid present, the patient's intravascular volume, and cardiovascular stability.

WHAT ARE THE INDICATIONS FOR USING ISOLATED ULTRAFILTRATION?

Isolated UF is indicated to remove fluid when removal of the solute is not a priority. Isolated UF can be performed immediately before, after, or independently of hemodialysis treatment.

WHAT EQUIPMENT IS NEEDED FOR ULTRAFILTRATION?

Isolated UF is performed with the same dialyzer and tubing used for hemodialysis. The dialysate flow is turned off or placed in the bypass mode. The dialyzer membrane does not come in contact with the dialysate solution. With volumetric equipment, the set value for UF determines the fluid to be removed. A blood pump, air detector, blood leak detector, and pressure monitors are standard equipment needed to perform the procedure safely.

ARE THERE COMPLICATIONS WITH ISOLATED ULTRAFILTRATION?

Rapid fluid removal can cause hypotension and muscle cramps.

WHAT IS CONTINUOUS RENAL REPLACEMENT THERAPY?

Continuous renal replacement therapy is a gentle treatment primarily used to treat patients with AKI, particularly those with multiple organ failure. Such individuals tend to be hemodynamically unstable, have cardiac insufficiency, and tolerate hemodialysis poorly. Various hemofilters are available in a hollow-fiber or plate design and are characterized by a small contained blood volume and low resistance to flow. There is increasing evidence that CRRT improves the survival of patients with AKI.

WHAT TREATMENTS BESIDES HEMODIALYSIS ARE AVAILABLE TO TREAT ACUTE KIDNEY INJURY?

There are many alternatives to conventional hemodialysis. CRRT is the umbrella acronym for five approaches to this treatment, such as slow continuous ultrafiltration (SCUF), continuous arteriovenous hemofiltration (CAVH), continuous arteriovenous hemodialysis (CAVHD), continuous venovenous hemofiltration (CVVH), and continuous venovenous hemodialysis (CVVHD). SCUF, CAVH, and CAVHD were originally very popular because they do not require special equipment or the constant attention of the nephrology personnel. Currently, CVVH and CVVHD are being prescribed more often. Although the principles of CRRT are the same, special equipment is necessary for CVVH or CVVHD. The procedures are limited to the critical care setting for the treatment of AKI. A collaborative approach using the collective expertise of the critical care and nephrology personnel is strongly recommended.

Continuous arteriovenous hemofiltration requires both arterial and venous access but does not use a blood pump. If solute removal by convective transport is not sufficient, diffusive transport is added by using hemodialysis. CVVH and CVVHD do not require arterial access, with its attending problems, but instead use double-lumen catheters in major venous sites. In each person, flow is controlled with a blood pump (Fig. 18.1).

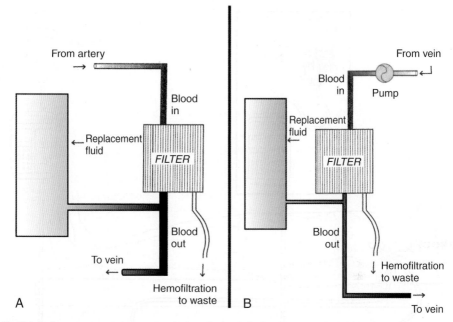

Fig. 18.1 Continuous renal replacement therapy using hemofiltration. **A,** Continuous arteriovenous hemofiltration. **B,** Continuous venovenous hemofiltration.

WHAT PROBLEMS OCCUR WITH THE USE OF CONTINUOUS RENAL REPLACEMENT THERAPY?

Procedures requiring arterial access, such as CAVH and CAVHD, carry the risk of damage to the artery itself, as well as the risk of hemorrhage if a connection is faulty or a leak develops in the blood circuit. Critically ill patients are often hypotensive, with blood flow rates inadequate for effective filtration. In addition, correction of electrolyte imbalance or fluid overload may be slower than desired. Clotting problems are frequent.

A blood pump is needed for systems using venovenous flow. Monitoring is required to avert drawing of air into the blood circuit and to watch for bleeding from a loose connection on the downstream side. Staff must be trained to perform this treatment and the system must be closely monitored.

WHAT IS SLOW CONTINUOUS ULTRAFILTRATION?

Slow continuous ultrafiltration is a gradual fluid removal method. As with isolated UF, little solute removal takes place; therefore, intermittent hemodialysis may be needed to treat azotemia and to maintain electrolyte balance. The amount of fluid removed is usually 2 to 6 L in a 24-hour period.

WHAT ARE THE INDICATIONS FOR SLOW CONTINUOUS ULTRAFILTRATION?

Many patients with AKI have a high rate of protein breakdown and require large volumes of total parenteral nutrition fluid. A few hours of hemodialysis may be inadequate to remove such large volumes of fluid, particularly in patients with hypotension and hemodynamic instability. SCUF allows slow continuous removal of the fluid, alleviating the large volume administered.

WHAT EQUIPMENT IS USED IN SLOW CONTINUOUS ULTRAFILTRATION?

A highly permeable hemofilter, similar to a dialyzer, is used in SCUF. SCUF can be performed without blood pump assistance by relying on the patient's cardiac output and MAP to provide adequate blood flow through the filter. Hydrostatic blood pressure forces the ultrafiltrate across the membrane, and it is collected in a drainage bag for disposal (Fig. 18.2). The length of tubing from the hemofilter to the fluid collection device creates a negative pressure that supports the UF rate. SCUF may also be performed with blood pump assistance from the Prisma machine.

DO PATIENTS REQUIRE HEPARIN DURING SLOW CONTINUOUS ULTRAFILTRATION?

Usually an initial bolus of 500 to 2000 units of heparin is injected followed by a continuous drip of 250 to 500 units/hr or 5 to 10 units/kg/hr. Clotting times are monitored. SCUF can be used without heparin by using normal saline flushes, but the risk of clotting the hemofilter is greatly increased.

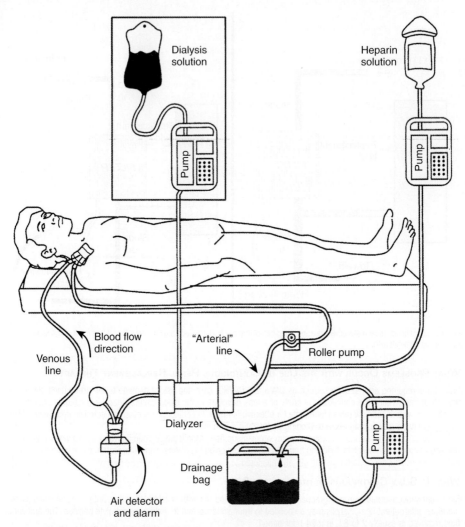

Fig. 18.2 Continuous venovenous hemodialysis (CVVHD) and (VV-SCUF). The equipment and circuit required for venovenous slow continuous ultrafiltration (VV-SCUF). The additional equipment required to perform CVVHD is shown in the *boxed area*. The "arterial" line also normally has a pressure transducer in-line (omitted from figure) between the roller pump and the dialyzer to monitor perfusion pressure. (From Lanken P, Lanken PN, Manaker S, Kohl BA, Hanson CW: *Intensive care unit manual*, Philadelphia, 2014, Elsevier.)

WHAT PROBLEMS ARE ASSOCIATED WITH SLOW CONTINUOUS ULTRAFILTRATION?

The most common problem associated with SCUF is failure to obtain the desired quantity of ultrafiltrate. The reasons are usually clotting of the hemofilter or reduced blood flow through the circuit. A problem with the patient's access, a kink in the tubing, or a decrease in the patient's arterial pressure can also result in a low UF rate.

WHAT IS CONTINUOUS VENOVENOUS HEMOFILTRATION?

Continuous venovenous hemofiltration (Fig. 18.3) is a form of continuous therapy similar to its predecessor, CAVH; however, a blood pump is used to control blood flow through the hemofilter. CVVH is a venous therapy and therefore uses the subclavian, internal jugular, or femoral vein as an access. Solute removal occurs through convection, and fluid removal is achieved using UF with the administered replacement fluid. The replacement fluid composition may vary and can be infused prefilter or postfilter to maintain the intravascular volume.

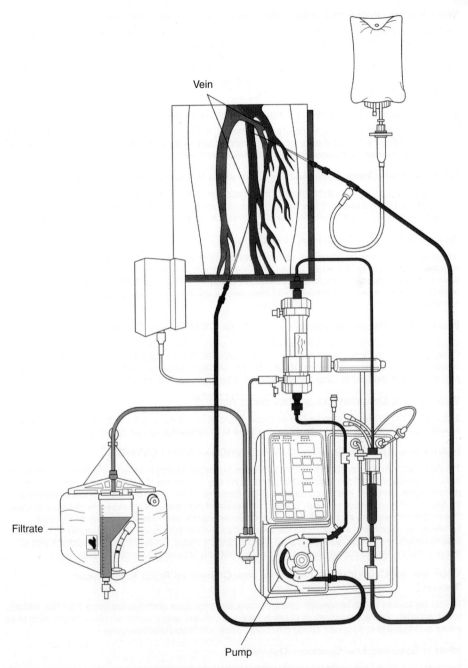

Fig. 18.3 Continuous venovenous hemofiltration. (Courtesy Baxter Healthcare, Renal Division, McGraw Park, IL.)

WHAT IS THE OBJECTIVE OF CONTINUOUS VENOVENOUS HEMOFILTRATION?

The objectives of CVVH are to provide CRRT, allow removal of solutes, balance fluids and electrolytes, and stabilize azotemia. Because this occurs evenly over time, this is a therapy of choice for patients who are unable to tolerate rapid fluid and solute concentration shifts similar to those that occur with hemodialysis.

What Are the Indications for Continuous Venovenous Hemofiltration?

Continuous venovenous hemofiltration is indicated when large volumes of fluid must be removed from hemodynamically unstable patients. CVVH is a recommended therapy to treat patients with AKI who exhibit cardiovascular instability. Other indications include fluid removal (carcinogenic shock), increased intracranial pressure (subarachnoid hemorrhage, hepatorenal syndrome), shock (sepsis, adult respiratory distress syndrome), and nutrition (burns). CVVH is also indicated for multiorgan failure and nonoliguric patients who require large volumes of IV fluids. CVVH is frequently employed in the care of critically ill and unstable pediatric patients.

What Equipment Is Used During Continuous Venovenous Hemofiltration?

The blood pump equipment includes an arterial pressure monitor, venous pressure monitor, and venous drip chamber with an air alert detector. Use of a blood pump replaces the patient's MAP as the driving force for the extracorporeal system, which is a significant advantage when treating a patient with decreased blood pressure.

What Are Some Other Advantages of Continuous Venovenous Hemofiltration?

Because a blood pump is used with this therapy, higher blood flow rates can be achieved, permitting higher UF rates and urea clearance. The increased blood flow also helps to reduce clotting of the hemofilter. CVVH has the ability to remove large-molecular-weight solutes because of the more porous nature of the hemofilter used in this treatment.

What Is Continuous Venovenous Hemodialysis?

Continuous venovenous hemodialysis (Fig. 18.3) is similar to CAVHD in principle, but as with CVVH, a blood pump is employed to control the blood flow rate. Unlike CVVH, CVVHD requires the dialysate running countercurrent to the blood flow through the extracorporeal circuit. The indications for CVVHD are the same as those for CAVHD. Intermittent hemodialysis would be an insufficient therapy for these patients, and they may be too unstable to tolerate aggressive hemodialysis.

What Are the Primary Advantages of CVVH or CVVHD Over CAVH or CAVHD?

Venovenous extracorporeal circuits do not require the use of an artery. A single double-lumen catheter can be used. Preferred sites include the subclavian and internal jugular veins. Blood flow through the hemofilter is consistent and controlled by the nurse, generally between 100 and 200 mL/min. The AV modalities (CAVH and CAVHD) require prolonged cannulation, which may lead to compromised blood flow to the extremities and infection.

What Are the Disadvantages of Venovenous Access?

Both CVVH and CVVHD require more bedside equipment that must be monitored by the critical care nurse. In-service education must be provided to assist the critical care nurse to be comfortable with the system.

Is Anticoagulation the Same for CAVH/CAVHD and CVVH/CVVHD?

The entire system must be constantly monitored for changes in pressure, clotting in the dialyzer or lines, and dark streaks in the dialyzer filters. These and frequent blood pump alarms may be warnings of a clotted system. Heparin is the primary anticoagulant used with all approaches of CRRT. Generally, a bolus of 500 to 2000 units is administered into the blood circuit upon initiation of therapy followed by a heparin infusion of 5 to 10 units/kg/hr. An alternative or adjunct therapy is to routinely flush the hemofilter and blood circuit with normal saline. This may prolong the life of the hemofilter. Trisodium citrate anticoagulation has been used successfully but requires additional monitoring of serum sodium, calcium, and bicarbonate levels to avoid compromising the patient. Citrate can be used in patients with an allergy to heparin. Venovenous circuits have fewer clotting problems because of the consistent blood flow.

What Are the Complications Associated with Continuous Renal Replacement Therapy?

Patient complications include hypotension, cardiac dysrhythmias, dehydration, electrolyte imbalance, blood loss, infection, and air embolism. Technical complications include blood leak, membrane rupture, clotted hemofilter, disconnection of the arterial or venous tubing, equipment malfunction, kinked tubing, and inexperienced personnel.

What Is Sustained Low-Efficiency Dialysis?

Sustained low-efficiency dialysis (SLED) is an AKI modality option that is becoming increasingly popular, particularly in the ICU setting. It is an acceptable compromise between intermittent hemodialysis and CRRT. It is also known as extended daily dialysis. This form of treatment delivers dialysis over a prolonged duration (8–12 hours) with modified blood and dialysate flow rates ($\leq$200 mL/min blood flow rate and 100–300 mL/min dialysate flow rate). Conventional dialysis machines preclude the need for costly CRRT machines, filters, and tubing. Hemodynamic stability is a benefit of SLED, allowing the patient to achieve the desired UF goal. SLED is an alternative for critically ill patients who have had poor outcomes on intermittent hemodialysis therapy. SLED is a slow and gentle therapy and assists with fluid and electrolyte control and solute clearance.

OTHER EXTRACORPOREAL TREATMENT MODALITIES

Techniques other than dialysis can remove metabolic wastes, toxic materials, or excess water. Some of these are very useful in the ICU for patients with complex problems or multiple organ failure.

WHAT ARE SOME OF THESE TECHNIQUES?

The following three basic modalities are in clinical use:
1. Hemofiltration
2. Hemoperfusion
3. Apheresis

HEMOFILTRATION

WHAT IS HEMOFILTRATION?

In conventional hemodialysis, diffusion or conductive transfer accounts for the major portion of solute movement across the membrane. The natural kidney actually uses UF or convective transfer in the process of glomerular filtration. Convective transfer across a synthetic membrane is also used to remove uremic wastes from the blood. This is the process of hemofiltration or diafiltration.

HOW EFFECTIVE IS HEMOFILTRATION?

Using polyacrylonitrile, polyamide, polysulfone, or polycarbonate membranes or hollow fibers, UF at a rate of more than 100 mL/min is possible at blood flow rates of 200 to 350 mL/min. If BUN levels are 50 mg/dL, that amount of BUN would also be removed in 1 minute. Removal of creatinine and medium- and large-sized molecules, such as β_2-microglobulin, with hemofiltration far exceeds that with conventional hemodialysis.

WHAT PROBLEMS MAY OCCUR WITH HEMOFILTRATION?

The following problems may occur with hemofiltration:
- Infusion of replacement fluid must be carefully and continually monitored to avoid underhydration or overhydration.
- Blood leakage can be a serious hazard when negative pressure is applied to the filtrate bag to enhance UF.
- The serum levels of various beneficial medications (antibiotics, cardiac drugs, anticonvulsants) may be adversely altered.
- Essential sterile replacement fluids are expensive.

WHAT ARE THE CLINICAL ADVANTAGES OF HEMOFILTRATION?

Several low-flow modalities of hemofiltration are useful for critically ill patients who need multisystem support. Hemofiltration offers the following clinical advantages:
- Hypotension is less of a problem than with hemodialysis even though a large volume of fluid is removed.
- Disequilibrium and other systems or findings of intracellular osmolar shift are rare.
- Large volumes of parenteral nutrition may be given; fluid balance is maintained at a stable level.
- Improved blood pressure control in hypertensive patients during periods between treatments has been attributed to better sodium and volume control and improved autonomic stability.
- Hemofiltration allows removal of harmful substances of large molecular size, such as myocardial depressant factors. These positive attributes of hemofiltration have resulted in the development of CRRT.

HEMOPERFUSION

In hemoperfusion, blood comes in direct contact with a sorbent material packaged in a cartridge or column. Most devices use 70 to 300 g of activated charcoal coated with a polymer film to reduce embolism by tiny carbon particles and to decrease platelet and cellular element build-up.

WHAT ARE THE INDICATIONS FOR USING HEMOPERFUSION?

Hemoperfusion is primarily used for drug overdose or toxic exposure of great severity. Activated charcoal binds most chemicals in the range of 100 to 20,000 Da. Most medications have molecular weights of 500 to 2000 Da. Hemoperfusion is more effective than hemodialysis for removal of most sedatives, theophylline, digoxin, and some pesticides and herbicides.

Charcoal may be used in association with deferoxamine chelation to remove excess aluminum or iron from body tissues.

WHAT ARE THE ADVERSE EFFECTS OF HEMOPERFUSION?

A transient decrease in platelets is frequent; it corrects within 24 hours in most instances. Some patients experience a decrease in white blood cell (WBC) count. Hemolysis or RBC damage is unusual. Hypotension is frequent because the poisoned patient is already very brittle. Heavy anticoagulation is needed, and postprocedural bleeding may be prolonged.

Is There a Limit to the Capacity of the Cartridge?

The adsorptive capacity of the cartridges is limited and difficult to determine in advance. The kinetics of adsorption is complex. Overall, mass transfer correlates with the fluid transfer rate and intraparticle transfer rate, which depend on the microcapillary size and solute diffusion. Clearance of some solutes may gradually decrease over time until the sorbent is filled; for other solutes, clearance may fall off rapidly even though considerable sorbent capacity remains.

APHERESIS

The term *apheresis* is a Greek expression that means "taking something away." Plasmapheresis has been conducted for a number of years to separate plasma protein components using special centrifuges. Synthetic hollow-fiber technology produces filters with selectively permeable capabilities to remove specific blood constituents (e.g., antibodies and immunoglobulins).

Plasmapheresis has been used experimentally for a variety of conditions, including transplant rejection, by reducing the antibody titer. Plasmapheresis removes the plasma portion of the blood that contains the antibody. The blood and albumin are returned to the patient, and the normal function of the immune system is unaffected. This technique is of definite value for patients with hyperviscosity syndrome, cryoglobulinemia, thrombotic thrombocytopenic purpura, myasthenia gravis crisis, Guillain-Barré syndrome, refractory idiopathic or autoimmune hemolytic anemia, multiple myeloma with renal failure, and Goodpasture syndrome.

What Types of Apheresis Therapies Are Available?

Several types of apheresis therapies are used according to the causative agent:

Plasmapheresis

Removal of the plasma portion of the blood to remove the harmful substance. Plasmapheresis has been conducted for a number of years to separate plasma protein components using special centrifuges.

Low-Density Lipoprotein Pheresis

This treatment is used to remove low-density lipoprotein from patients with familial hypercholesterolemia.

Photopheresis

This treatment is used to treat graft versus host disease, cutaneous T-cell lymphoma, and rejection in heart transplant patients.

Immunoadsorption with Staphylococcal Protein A-Agarose Column

This treatment is used to remove alloantibodies and autoantibodies.

Leukocytapheresis

This treatment is used to remove malignant WBCs in patients with high WBC counts as well as those with rheumatoid arthritis.

Thrombocytapheresis

This treatment is used to remove platelets in patients with symptoms from extremely elevated platelet counts.

Erythrocytapheresis

This treatment, also known as *red cell exchange (RCE)*, is used mostly in the treatment of patients with sickle cell disease. RCE removes the patient's sickled red cells and replaces them with allogenic nonsickled red blood cells to alleviate or control the disease (McPherson & Pincus, 2017). The American Society for Apheresis provides updated guidelines and recommendation for the treating and effectiveness of various diseases.

What Substances Can Be Removed by Either Dialysis or Hemoperfusion?

As a general rule, substances that are completely or almost completely excreted by the normal kidney will be removed by dialysis. Substances metabolized by the liver, or their byproducts, may not be removed by hemodialysis. Information about the site of metabolism and excretion of most drugs is often obtainable from the package insert or from pharmacology texts. The *Physicians' Desk Reference* is another quick resource. Various sites discussing treatment options for drug overdoses and poisonings can be found on the Internet, such as the Centers for Disease Control and Prevention Agency for Toxic Substances and Disease Registry's toxic substances web portal. Information available on this system is updated regularly and can be very useful. Regional poison centers have information on drugs or poisons. The intoxicating substance(s) should be identified and quantified as soon as possible. Quantitative results may often take several hours and are not available when needed most urgently.

What If the Substance Is Not Known or Cannot Be Readily Verified?

The decision to treat or not treat and by what modality is clinical judgment to be made by the physician. If the patient is severely ill and the circumstances suggest that one or more of the ingested substances is likely to be removable by hemoperfusion or dialysis, treatment should be started. This is because the duration of coma, morbidity, and mortality may be reduced by early treatment initiation.

For What Toxic Agents Is Dialysis Recommended as the Specific Treatment of Choice?

Alcohols, such as methyl alcohol and ethylene and propylene glycol (antifreeze), are easily dialyzed. Salicylates (aspirin), lithium carbonate, and aminophylline dialyze well. Certain mushrooms *(Amanita phalloides)* require immediate hemodialysis therapy. Early removal of toxins may prevent blindness, liver necrosis, renal failure, or death that can result from such poisons. Accidental therapeutic IV drug overdose of agents, such as theophylline, antibiotics, or mannitol, may require emergent dialysis to decrease the risk of serious complications.

Is Any Particular Type of Dialyzer Preferable for Poisonings?

In cases of poisoning, the objective is to remove as much of the offending agent as rapidly as possible. Therefore, a dialyzer with the largest surface area that the patient will tolerate should be used. The dialyzer of choice may be a device that can achieve a high-middle molecule clearance (i.e., 500–20,000 Da).

What Poisonings Are Best Treated by Charcoal Hemoperfusion?

Sedatives, including barbiturates, ethchlorvynol, and glutethimide, and many insecticides and herbicides are better removed by hemoperfusion than by hemodialysis.

What About Bloodstream Access for the Dialysis of Poisons?

If the patient does not already have a permanent vascular access, the most appropriate access is a temporary catheter placed in a large vein, such as the femoral, subclavian, or internal jugular vein. The greater the blood flow, the greater is the removal of toxins.

Does Peritoneal Dialysis Have Any Place in the Treatment of Poisoning?

Peritoneal dialysis is rarely appropriate in the treatment of poisoning and is only indicated if hemodialysis is not available or will be delayed. Peritoneal dialysis has a low clearance rate and takes longer to remove drugs than hemodialysis and hemoperfusion. However, if preparation for hemodialysis will be delayed and peritoneal dialysis can be instituted at once, it can be a temporary treatment option.

What Special Patient Problems May Be Encountered in the Dialysis or Hemoperfusion of Ingested or Intravenous Poisons or Drug Overdoses?

Such patients are generally critically ill, possibly with multisystem failure. Most are hemodynamically unstable. Specific patient problems may include the following.

Hypotension

This responds poorly to volume replacement; infusion of a pressor agent, such as dopamine, is frequently necessary. However, the effect of the pressor agent may be reduced by dialysis or hemoperfusion.

Respiratory Depression or Apnea

The patient may have an endotracheal tube or tracheostomy and may require ventilatory assistance equipment.

Severe Acid–Base Imbalance

Patients with alkalosis from drug intoxication may experience worsening of their condition with dialysis treatment. The amount of bicarbonate in the dialysate may have to be adjusted. Often custom dialysate is required with changes during the treatment.

DIALYSIS IN RELATION TO TRANSPLANTATION

Many patients receive dialysis as part of the plan for kidney transplantation (see Chapter 20). Dialysis may be initiated immediately before transplantation as a preparation for surgery, during surgery, or after transplantation as a supportive procedure because of technical complications or complications during rejection episodes. Patients who require dialysis during posttransplant dysfunction or acute rejection require special treatment considerations.

What is Posttransplant Kidney Dysfunction?

Posttransplant kidney dysfunction is a form of AKI seen occasionally in patients with living donor kidneys and more often in those with deceased donor kidneys. It is usually related to the length of the "warm and cold ischemia time." This is the time interval from kidney removal to its revascularization in the transplanted patient. The mechanism is similar to that of ATN. The kidney usually begins to function in about 10 days, although occasionally 3 to 4 weeks pass before quality urine is produced (see Chapter 20).

DIALYSIS PATIENTS WITH TRANSPLANT REJECTION

WHAT SPECIAL PROBLEMS OCCUR IN THE DIALYSIS OF POSTTRANSPLANT PATIENTS?

Maintenance of fluid balance is essential to the function of the transplanted kidney. Care must be taken not to be overly aggressive with fluid removal; the resulting hypotension could cause hypoperfusion of the new organ and lead to renal dysfunction. In the early postoperative period, such patients have all of the problems of recent major surgery. "No heparin" dialysis should be used to prevent bleeding at the operative site. Because of steroids, patients may be intensely catabolic, with BUN levels disproportionately high relative to serum creatinine levels. Hypertension may be aggravated by steroid treatment. Wound healing may be slow, and some drainage is common. Patients who have lost a transplant to severe rejection usually have been treated with steroids. Their tissues are often edematous and extremely friable. Patients with infections and rejection are almost always catabolic, edematous, and hypoproteinemic. Their cardiopulmonary and cardiovascular systems are often labile, and hypotension or cardiac dysrhythmias and pulmonary congestion should be anticipated.

CHAPTER 19

PERITONEAL DIALYSIS AND HOME DIALYSIS THERAPIES

Peritoneal dialysis (PD) is an alternative dialysis modality for patients with chronic kidney disease (CKD). The US Renal Data System (USRDS) reports that only 7% of the prevalent CKD patient population is on PD, and fewer than 10% of patients requiring maintenance dialysis are using any home modality (USRDS, 2017). Despite its safety and effectiveness, PD use has been in decline since the mid-1990s. PD is primarily a home dialysis therapy for stage 5 CKD, but although rare, it can also be a treatment option for the patients with acute kidney injury in the hospital setting. The range of home therapies for the patients with CKD includes PD and home hemodialysis (HD). Home therapy allows patients to remain somewhat independent in their own care and to have greater control over their schedules. Of all home therapy options, PD is the most commonly used. Increased emphasis has been placed on the use of home modalities because of the new bundling payment system. Home dialysis allows facilities to overcome capacity limits and maximize staff resources. The final Centers for Medicare & Medicaid Services (CMS) reimbursement bundle encourages the use of PD.

WHAT IS PERITONEAL DIALYSIS, AND HOW DOES IT WORK?

Peritoneal dialysis is a process during which the peritoneal cavity acts as the reservoir for the dialysate and the peritoneum serves as the semipermeable membrane across which excess body fluid and solutes, including uremic toxins, are removed (ultrafiltrate). The peritoneal membrane surface area is approximately equal to the body surface area (1.73 m^2). The peritoneum consists of the lining of the inner surface of the abdominal and pelvic walls, including the diaphragm (parietal peritoneum), as well as the covering of the abdominal organs (visceral peritoneum). In males, the peritoneum is a closed cavity, but in females, the fallopian tubes and ovaries open into the peritoneal cavity. Fig. 19.1 shows the location and the positioning of the dialysis catheter.

The peritoneal membrane is in contact with the rich blood supply to the abdominal organs. The dialysate is infused into the peritoneal cavity via a catheter, allowed to dwell for a predetermined amount of time, and then drained (effluent). This process is called an exchange. Dextrose is used in the dialysate to create an osmotic gradient that causes water to move into the peritoneal cavity from the bloodstream. The excess fluid is removed when the effluent is drained. Electrolytes and uremic toxins are removed by diffusion from an area of higher concentration (bloodstream) to an area of lower concentration (peritoneal cavity). Solute removal is further enhanced by "solute drag," created when a hypertonic dialysate is used, which increases ultrafiltration (UF) and causes additional low-molecular-weight solutes to be "dragged" along with the ultrafiltrate by convective transport.

WHAT SOLUTIONS ARE USED FOR PERITONEAL DIALYSIS?

The solutions used for PD should be biocompatible and preserve the peritoneal membrane structure and function as much as possible. Conventional solutions use glucose as the osmotic agent to cause UF and lactate as a buffer base to correct acidosis. Commercially available solutions approximate the composition of extracellular body water except for potassium because many patients tend to be hyperkalemic. The majority of solutions do not contain potassium. Potassium may be added (2–4 mEq/L) if necessary to correct hypokalemia. Oral potassium supplementation may also be prescribed. Dextrose provides the osmotic gradient between the plasma and dialysate that leads to fluid and solute removal. The more hypertonic the dialysate is (i.e., 1.5%, 2.5% and 4.25% dextrose), the greater the UF. After a 2-L exchange has dwelled for 4 hours, an average of 200 mL of ultrafiltrate will be obtained with a 1.5% exchange, and an average of 600 to 1000 mL will be obtained with a 4.25% exchange. Table 19.1 highlights some common compositions of PD solutions.

WHAT IS ICODEXTRIN?

Some PD solutions use different osmotic agents for UF and clearance. Icodextrin (Extraneal) is a PD solution that differs from standard dialysis solutions in that it does not contain dextrose. In standard PD dialysates, glucose is the osmotic agent. Icodextrin is a starch-derived osmotic agent made from a mixture of glucose polymers (polyglucose). This solution allows increased fluid removal from the bloodstream during PD as well as reduced net negative UF and increased small-solute clearance. Icodextrin is intended to be used for once-daily, long-dwell exchanges lasting 8 to 16 hours. The dialysate solution should be used for no more than one exchange in a 24-hour period. Icodextrin is contraindicated for those with glycogen storage diseases or an allergy to corn starch. The most common adverse effect from the use of icodextrin is a skin rash. Sterile peritonitis, hypertension, cold, headache, flulike symptoms, and abdominal pain are other possible side effects.

ARE THERE DIFFERENT WAYS TO PERFORM PERITONEAL DIALYSIS?

Peritoneal dialysis can be performed either manually or automatically with a cycler. The manual form of PD is called continuous ambulatory peritoneal dialysis (CAPD). In CAPD, four or more exchanges are performed each day, 7 days a week. Each exchange takes approximately 30 minutes. The patient connects to a tubing system, drains the effluent, and infuses new dialysate to dwell for a prescribed amount of time, usually 4 to 6 hours. The last exchange of the day dwells overnight

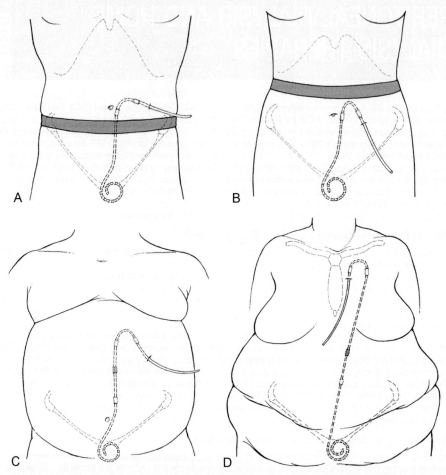

Fig. 19.1 Tenckhoff catheter used in peritoneal dialysis. **A,** Straight intercuff segment catheter with a laterally directed exit site emerging above a low-lying belt line. **B,** Preformed swan-neck intercuff arc bend catheter with a downwardly directed exit site emerging below a high-lying belt line. **C,** Extended catheter with an upper abdominal exit site for an obese rotund abdomen, lower abdominal skin folds, or incontinence. **D,** Extended catheter with a presternal exit site for severe obesity, multiple abdominal skin folds, intestinal stomas, or incontinence. (From Crabtree JH, Chow KM: Peritoneal dialysis catheter insertion. *Seminars in Nephrology 37*(1):17–29, 2017.)

and is then drained in the morning. Most patients use "bagless" CAPD in which they disconnect from the tubing system at the end of each exchange and retain a short transfer set or the capped catheter. Most CAPD tubing systems involve a Y configuration that enables the patient to "flush" any contaminants that might have been introduced while connecting to the system. Spiking the bag has been eliminated from most systems, thus reducing the potential for contamination by as much as 50%.

WHAT IS AUTOMATED PERITONEAL DIALYSIS?

Automated peritoneal dialysis (APD) is performed with a cycler, usually at night while the patient sleeps. Cyclers are programmed according to the physician's prescription to perform the following functions automatically: (1) measure the volume of dialysate to be infused, (2) warm the dialysate to body temperature before infusion, (3) time the frequency of exchanges, (4) count the number of exchanges, and (5) measure UF. Cyclers can be programmed for volumes of 50 to 3000 mL per exchange, have a last bag option to accommodate a unique diurnal (day) dwell (volume, percentage, additives), and have the capability to program one or more exchanges during daytime hours. All machines can be programmed to perform tidal PD. APD enables the patient to mix dextrose concentrations to achieve the desired UF (e.g., 2.5% mixed with 4.25% to achieve 3.3%). The machines used to perform APD have alarms for inflow failure, overheating, and inadequate drainage. Patients must be taught to set up and run the machine by a trained professional, such as a registered self-care home dialysis training nurse with at least 12 months of experience in providing care and an additional 3 months of experience in this modality.

Table 19.1 Typical Compositions of Common Peritoneal Dialysis Solutions

	Conventional Glucose-Based Solutions			ICODEXTRIN	LOW-GDP LACTATE-BUFFERED SOLUTIONS	LOW-GDP BICARBONATE-BUFFERED SOLUTIONS
	1.5%	2.5%	4.25%			
Na (mEq/L)	132	132	13	132	132	132
Cl (mEq/L)	96	96	96	96	96	96
Ca (mEq/L)	3.5[a]	3.5[a]	3.5[a]	3.5[a]	3.5[a]	3.5[a]
Mg (mEq/L)	0.5	0.5	0.5	0.5	0.5	0.5
Lactate (mEq/L)	40	40	40	40	40	40
Bicarbonate (mEq/L)	—	—	—	—	—	25
Glucose (mg/dL)	1360	2270	3860	–	1360-3860	1360-3860
pH	5.2	5.2	5.2	5.2	7.3	7.3
Osmolality (osmol/kg)	345	395	484	282	345-484	345-484
GDPs	+	++	+++	+	Very low	Very low

[a]Low calcium solutions are 2.5 mEq/L (1.23 mmol).
GDP, Glucose degradation product.
From Clarkson MR, Magee CN, Brenner BM: *Pocket companion to Brenner & Rector's The Kidney*, ed. 8, Philadelphia, 2010, Elsevier.

WHAT ARE THE DIFFERENT FORMS OF AUTOMATED PERITONEAL DIALYSIS?

Continuous Cycling Peritoneal Dialysis

In continuous cycling peritoneal dialysis (CCPD), three to five exchanges are performed nightly with a full diurnal dwell. The diurnal dwell improves the clearance of middle molecules.

Nocturnal Intermittent Peritoneal Dialysis

Three to five exchanges are performed nightly, but there is minimal or no diurnal dwell. Nocturnal intermittent peritoneal dialysis (NIPD) is indicated in patients who are unable to tolerate a diurnal dwell (e.g., those with hyperpermeability of the peritoneum to dextrose, resulting in absorption of the diurnal dwell) and in those with problems exacerbated by increased intraabdominal pressure, including hernias, low back pain, and cardiopulmonary compromise.

Intermittent Peritoneal Dialysis

Several frequent exchanges are performed three or four times a week, with the peritoneum left "dry" between treatments. Intermittent peritoneal dialysis (IPD) was widely used in the early 1970s but soon lost popularity because of concerns of insufficient small-solute clearances and growing proficiency with newer PD modalities such as CAPD. IPD is appropriate for patients with residual kidney function or for institutionalized patients. Also, IPD is used in economically underdeveloped countries because of the financial constraints imposed by daily PD.

Tidal Peritoneal Dialysis

An initial volume of the dialysate is infused followed by partial drainage of the effluent at the end of each exchange (leaving a constant reserve volume); finally, a "tidal" volume of fresh dialysate is infused. Tidal peritoneal dialysis (TPD) is intended to enhance clearance by maintaining continuous contact of the dialysate with the peritoneum and maintaining the dialysate/plasma (D/P) gradient. TPD may improve clearance by 20% but increases costs because of the need for additional dialysate.

Tidal peritoneal dialysis may also be used for patients who experience discomfort or "drain pain" at the end of the drain cycle because of the position of the PD catheter tip. By always maintaining a reserve of fluid, the tip is allowed to float, thus alleviating discomfort in sensitive individuals.

Urgent-Start Dialysis

Urgent-start PD has become an option for some patients with an urgent or unplanned need for dialysis within 48 hours to 14 days. This is sometimes seen with patients who have an unexpected progression of CKD, lack of predialysis education, or late referral to a nephrologist. Blake and Jain (2018) define urgent-start PD as "a strategy whereby patients with advanced CKD who urgently and unexpectedly need dialysis due to uremia or fluid overload are treated with PD rather than hemodialysis." Urgent-start PD can be initiated as soon as 48 hours after the placement of a PD catheter. The patient is then dialyzed with low fill volumes in the supine position for 1 to 2 weeks overseen by a trained nurse. Treatments typically take place in a dialysis center for 6 to 8 hours with fill volumes increasing based on patient tolerance. During the patient's time incenter, education and training on PD is provided to the patient, which facilitates transition to performing treatments independently in the home environment. Advantages to urgent start PD include avoidance of central venous catheter placement and preserved residual kidney function. To be successful, there must be adequate support in the dialysis center with trained and experienced nurses who have time allotted to care for, monitor, educate, and train the patient.

WHAT KINDS OF CATHETERS ARE USED FOR PERITONEAL DIALYSIS?

Catheters for both acute and chronic PD must transport fluid into and out of the peritoneal cavity as rapidly as possible and be biocompatible (maintain normal structure and function of the tissues near the catheter tract). Catheters manufactured for both acute and chronic PD are available in varied sizes to accommodate neonates to adults.

Catheters for acute PD can be placed at the patient's bedside and include rigid or soft silicone catheters. The patient should have an empty bladder, and the rectum should be free of stool at the time of insertion to minimize the risk of organ perforation. Placement may be by direct insertion with a trocar or guidewire or by use of a peritoneoscope. Dialysis may be initiated immediately after insertion. The risks associated with rigid catheters include bowel or organ perforation, dialysate leaks, peritonitis, discomfort, and inadvertent catheter loss. Silicone catheters, used for acute dialysis, are more comfortable and may be used for chronic dialysis if necessary. When an acute PD catheter is used immediately, the patient should be kept supine whenever the dialysate is in the peritoneal cavity to minimize the occurrence of dialysate leakage around the catheter.

Catheters used for chronic PD are usually placed surgically during a laparotomy or laparoscopically. The exit site should be directed in a downward or lateral direction and be located in the right or left midquadrant area, avoiding the belt line, scars, and skinfolds. Figure 19.2 shows modifications that can be made to allow a variety of exit site locations according to specific patient needs. Catheters are made of silicone or polyurethane with a radiopaque stripe for radiographic visualization. Intraperitoneal catheters may be straight or coiled, or T-fluted and have one or two cuffs. Coiled catheters are believed to minimize catheter migration out of the pelvis and have fewer outflow problems than straight catheters. Coiled catheters are also thought to improve patient comfort by keeping the tip of the catheter away from direct contact with the peritoneal membrane. Figure 19.3 shows the location of the catheter cuff and coiled catheter tip in the pelvis. The extraperitoneal portion of the catheter can be either straight or have a swan neck configuration with single or double cuffs. The most widely used catheter is the double-cuff, swan-neck, coiled Tenckhoff catheter (Skorecki et al, 2016).

Cuffs are made of Dacron polyester or velour and allow tissue ingrowth to stabilize the catheter. Cuffs are also intended to prevent migration of bacteria along the subcutaneous tunnel into the peritoneum. When placing double-cuffed catheters, the internal cuff is placed in the rectus muscle, and the external cuff is placed in the subcutaneous tissue proximal to the exit site. Implanted catheters (Fig. 19.4) consist of an intraperitoneal segment containing side holes and an

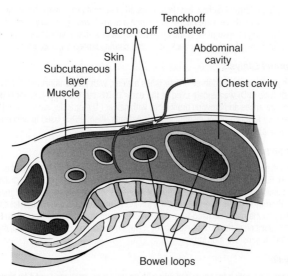

Fig. 19.2 Tenckhoff catheter modifications that provide for a variety of exit site locations according to patient-specific characteristics. (From Crabtree JH: Selected best practices in peritoneal dialysis access. *Kidney International* 103[suppl]:S27–S37, 2006.)

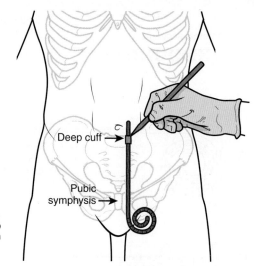

Fig. 19.3 Schematic drawing indicating the manner in which the catheter insertion site and deep cuff location are selected to achieve proper pelvic position of the coiled catheter tip. (From Crabtree JH: Selected best practices in peritoneal dialysis access. *Kidney International* 103[suppl]:S27–S37, 2006.)

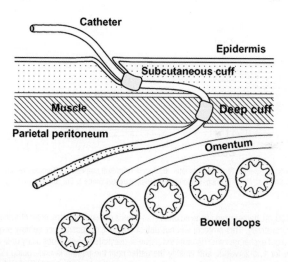

Fig. 19.4 Placement of double-cuffed Tenckhoff catheter. (From Crabtree JH, Chow KM: Peritoneal dialysis catheter insertion. *Seminars in Nephrology* 37(1):17–29, 2017.)

open tip for fluid flow; a subcutaneous segment that passes through the peritoneal membrane, muscles, and subcutaneous tissues; and an external segment that extends from the external cuff to the exit site. There are several versions of chronic catheters, including the Tenckhoff, column disk, Toronto Western, Swan neck, Cruz, and Moncrief-Popovich catheters (Fig. 19.5). The Tenckhoff catheter is the most commonly placed PD catheter. All versions include features intended to improve dialysate flow and decrease catheter complications.

WHAT IS MEANT BY CATHETER BREAK-IN?

Catheter break-in is the period after the chronic catheter is placed during which healing and tissue ingrowth into the cuff(s) occur. The goals are to promote healing and prevent complications such as dialysate leakage, infections, and catheter obstruction. Healing may take up to 6 weeks and includes scab formation, tissue granulation at the exit site, and sinus tract epithelialization. Full-volume dialysis, especially CAPD, should be avoided for at least 10 to 14 days to allow healing to occur. This healing period may necessitate the placement of a temporary HD access if the patient is severely uremic or fluid overloaded and in need of immediate dialysis. Postoperatively the patient should remain supine when possible and avoid activities that increase intraabdominal pressure, such as straining to defecate, excessive coughing, crying, and lifting. Treatment options during the postoperative period include the following:

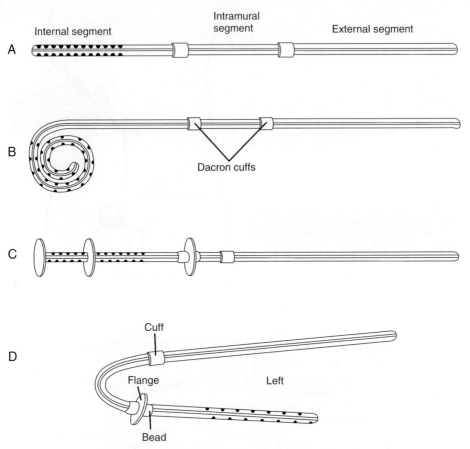

Fig. 19.5 Chronic catheters. **A,** Straight Tenckhoff catheter. **B,** Curled Tenckhoff catheter. **C,** Toronto Western catheter. **D,** Swan-neck (Missouri) catheter. (From Smith T: *Renal nursing,* Philadelphia, 1998, Harcourt Brace & Co. Bailliere Tindall.)

- Infusion of 25 to 100 mL heparinized saline solution (1–10 units of heparin per milliliter of saline) every 4 to 8 hours for 1 to 3 days postoperatively. This protocol will not detect catheter malposition or outflow problems.
- Low volume in and out exchanges with heparinized saline or dialysate several times a day until the effluent is no longer bloody, then daily for 1 to 2 weeks, and weekly thereafter until the patient is undergoing PD. A small volume of heparinized solution should remain in the peritoneum to inhibit the formation of fibrin (whitish protein formed in response to bleeding, inflammation, or infection) and prevent the development of adhesions. There is no systemic anticoagulation from the administration of low-dose intraperitoneal heparin.
- Low-volume dialysis in the patient who needs immediate dialysis but is unable to undergo HD. Frequent, low-volume exchanges (500–1000 mL) are performed using a cycler with the patient in the supine position. The volume is gradually increased to eliminate the signs and symptoms of uremia.

HOW IS EXIT SITE CARE PERFORMED?

The goals during the immediate postoperative period are to stabilize the catheter, promote healing, and prevent infection. The exit site dressing is generally not changed for 5 to 7 days postoperatively unless there is excessive drainage under the dressing (blood, exudate, dialysate). The first dressing change should be performed by trained dialysis personnel and then may be taught to the patient. It is recommended that masks be worn during dressing changes to avoid contamination with oral or nasal flora. Care should be taken to minimize manipulation of the catheter that may cause trauma to the exit site and may lead to infection. The skin around the exit site may be pink, similar to a healing scar, or it may have a brownish or purplish discoloration. During dressing changes, the exit site should be assessed for signs of infection (erythema, exudate, induration, tenderness), the subcutaneous tunnel should be palpated for tenderness, and the catheter and connections should be inspected for integrity. The exit site should be cleansed with an antibacterial soap and water and covered with a sterile nonocclusive dressing, such as gauze and tape, or an air-permeable adhesive sheet. Cytotoxic agents (e.g., 1% povidone–iodine, 3% hydrogen peroxide, and 0.5% sodium hypochlorite) may interfere with wound epithelialization during the immediate postoperative period and are used only when the exit site is well healed. The catheter should be secured to the patient's skin with tape or an immobilization device to avoid tension on the catheter and trauma to the exit site. The patient should avoid showers or tub baths until healed.

The goal of chronic exit site care is prevention of infection and thus peritonitis. The patient can be taught to perform routine exit site care once the exit site is well healed. Exit site care consists of daily cleansing with an antibacterial soap and water with careful rinsing and drying. An antibacterial solution (e.g., 1% povidone–iodine, 3% hydrogen peroxide, and 0.5% sodium hypochlorite) is then applied in a circular motion to the skin around the exit site based on the physician's order. The exit site should not be submerged in bathwater or hot tubs. Many programs allow swimming in chlorinated pools and oceans. After the healing period (4–6 weeks), a dressing may or may not be worn according to the patient or unit preference. It is extremely important to secure the catheter to the skin with tape or an immobilizing device to avoid trauma and infection should the catheter be accidentally tugged. The International Society for Peritoneal Dialysis (ISPED) provides recommendations for PD catheter care and training for both pediatric and adult populations. It is always best to follow the written policies and procedures of the specific program.

WHAT DOES PERITONEAL EQUILIBRATION TESTING MEASURE?

The clinical condition of the patient should be paramount when evaluating the adequacy of PD. An important element of evaluation is careful attention to both overt signs of uremia (laboratory values, fluid overload) and covert signs (sleep and concentration disturbances, anorexia, nutritional indices). Because PD is primarily a home therapy, patient compliance with the prescribed regimen must also be assessed in the evaluation of dialysis adequacy.

The efficiency of PD depends on the ability of the peritoneal membrane to ultrafiltrate fluid and solutes. Peritoneal solute clearance is determined by diffusion, which is driven by the concentration gradient between the dialysate and plasma and by the "solute drag" created by a hypertonic dialysate. Solutes and fluid may move from the intravascular compartment to the peritoneal cavity or from the peritoneal cavity to the intravascular compartment. Other substances lost in the effluent include protein (8.8–12.9 g/day), amino acids, water-soluble vitamins, trace minerals, and certain hormones.

Ultrafiltration and solute clearance in PD are influenced by (1) permeability of the peritoneal membrane, (2) volume of exchange, (3) dialysate glucose concentration, (4) dwell time, and (5) molecular size of the solute. Solute clearance is expressed as the D/P ratio at a given point in time during exchange. Equilibration is achieved when the D/P ratio approaches 1. Small solutes, such as urea (molecular weight, 60 Da), are highly diffusible and approach equilibration at 4 hours. Creatinine (molecular weight, 113 Da) moves more slowly toward equilibration and never reaches it during the typical 4-hour CAPD exchange.

Peritoneal equilibration testing (PET) is a standardized test of peritoneal membrane permeability used to estimate the solute transport characteristics, glucose absorption, and net UF. PET is done 1 month after initiation of dialysis and assists in prescribing therapy and making changes according to the current transport characteristics of the peritoneum. PET involves giving the patient an exchange of 2.5% dialysate and obtaining a serum sample at hour 2 and dialysate samples at hours 0, 2, and 4. Samples are analyzed for urea, creatinine, and glucose. Urea and creatinine are also analyzed from the long dwell (12 hours) obtained when the patient arrives for PET. Timing of the samples is important to help minimize inaccurate membrane classification.

The D/P ratios are calculated and plotted as graphs (Fig. 19.6). Decisions regarding the best dialytic therapy are made according to Table 19.2 based on the solute transport characteristics of the patient. The higher the D/P ratio for creatinine, the faster is the rate of transport for small solutes. The results of the D/P ratios for creatinine will determine

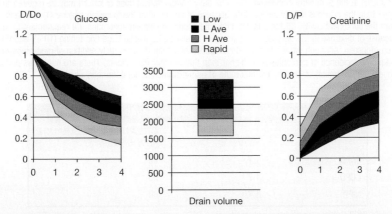

Fig. 19.6 Peritoneal equilibrium test. *D/Do,* Dialysate glucose concentration at indicated time/dialysate glucose concentration at time 0; *D/P,* dialysate to plasma. (Modified from Teitlbaum I, Burkhart J: Peritoneal dialysis. *American Journal of Kidney Diseases* 42(5):1082–1096, 2003; with permission of Elsevier.)

Table 19.2 Baseline Peritoneal Equilibration Testing Prognostic Value

		Predicted Response to CAPD	
SOLUTE TRANSPORT	UF	DIALYSIS	PREFERRED DIALYSIS PRESCRIPTION
High	Poor	Adequate	NIPD,[a] DAPD
Low average	Good	Adequate	Standard-dose PD[b]
		Inadequate[c]	High-dose PD[d]e
Low	Excellent	Inadequate[c]	High-dose PD[d] or

[a]Nocturnal intermittent peritoneal dialysis (NIPD) is intermittent peritoneal dialysis (IPD) performed every night for 8 to 12 hours using 10 to 20 L of dialysis solution. Daytime ambulatory peritoneal dialysis (DAPD) is ambulatory peritoneal dialysis performed only during daytime with three or four exchanges.
[b]Standard-dose peritoneal dialysis (PD) is standard-dose continuous ambulatory peritoneal dialysis (CAPD) using 7.5 to 9.0 L of dialysis solution per 24 hours or standard-dose continuous cycling peritoneal dialysis (CCPD) using 6 to 8 L of dialysis solution overnight and 2 L during daytime.
[c]Inadequate dialysis is likely in patients with a body surface area greater than 2.00 m^2.
[d]High-dose PD is CAPD using greater than 9 L of dialysis solution per 24 hours or CCPD using greater than 8 L of dialysis solution overnight or greater than 2 L during the daytime.
[e]Hemodialysis (HD) may be needed in patients with a body surface area greater than 2.00 m^2.
UF, Ultrafiltration.
From Twardowski ZJ: Clinical value of standardized equilibration tests in CAPD patients. *Blood Purification Journal* 7:95–108, 1989.

whether the patient has slow, slow average, average, fast average, or fast transport. A high PET score yields rapid waste clearance, poor UF of fluid, high glucose absorption, and high protein loss. A low PET score yields slow waste clearance, excellent UF of fluid, and decreased likelihood of protein loss.

Although PET helps to determine the transport characteristics of the peritoneum, 24-hour collections of urine (residual kidney function) and effluent (dialysis clearance) must be obtained at regular intervals to determine whether adequacy targets are being met. These collections are analyzed for urea and creatinine, and the weekly Kt/V and creatinine clearance are determined. The current adequacy targets recommended by the 2006 update of the National Kidney Foundation (NKF) Kidney Disease Outcomes Quality Initiative (KDOQI) are summarized in Table 19.3.

WHAT COMPLICATIONS ARE ENCOUNTERED IN PERITONEAL DIALYSIS?

Table 19.4 summarizes the common complications encountered in PD, including their causes, signs, symptoms, and interventions.

CAN PATIENTS WITH DIABETES BE TREATED WITH PERITONEAL DIALYSIS?

Peritoneal dialysis offers many advantages to patients with diabetes. PD maintains a steady physiological state without the drastic biochemical or fluid fluctuations seen with HD in patients with diabetes with cardiovascular instability or autonomic neuropathy. There is no need for a vascular access. Blood glucose is well controlled with intraperitoneal administration of regular insulin because the peritoneal cavity containing insulin provides a steady, gradual, and prolonged release of insulin in the peripheral circulation. The total daily intraperitoneal dose of insulin may be required to be much higher than the previous subcutaneous dose because of any or all of the following factors: (1) slow absorption of insulin from the peritoneal cavity, (2) the effect of dialysate dilution on insulin absorption, (3) requirement for extra insulin because of dextrose in the dialysate, (4) binding of insulin to the plastic bags and tubing (10%), and (5) hepatic degradation of insulin. Although intraperitoneal administration of insulin requires daily addition of medication to the dialysis bags, the incidence of peritonitis is no higher than that in other PD patients. There are numerous protocols for intraperitoneal administration of insulin, and this route of administration is not commonly used today.

Table 19.3 KDOQI Peritoneal Dialysis Adequacy Weekly Targets

	KT/V	CREATININE CLEARANCE (L/WK/1.73 M^2)
CAPD	1.7	60
CCPD	1.7	63
NIPD	1.7	66

CAPD, Continuous ambulatory peritoneal dialysis; *CCPD,* continuous cycling peritoneal dialysis; *KDOQI,* Kidney Disease Outcomes Quality Initiative; *NIPD,* nocturnal intermittent peritoneal dialysis.
From Twardowski ZJ: Clinical value of standardized equilibration tests in CAPD patients. *Blood Purification Journal* 7:95–108, 1989. S. Karger AG, Basel.

Table 19.4 Complications of Peritoneal Dialysis

COMPLICATION	CAUSE	SIGNS/SYMPTOMS	INTERVENTIONS
Peritonitis: infection of the peritoneal cavity	Invasion of the peritoneal cavity with microorganisms, usually because of a break in the closed system; may also enter along the outer surface of the catheter and through the bowel wall	Cloudy effluent; abdominal pain; nausea, vomiting, or peritoneal fluid cell count of >100 WBC and >50% neutrophils Culture results: gram positive, gram negative Multiple organisms Fungi	Prompt diagnosis and treatment; flush with 1.5% dialysate; IP antibiotics are as effective as IV antibiotics; coverage for both gram-positive and gram-negative organisms until causative agent identified; heparin added (0.5–1.0 unit/mL dialysate) to combat fibrin and adhesions
Exit site infection: purulent drainage and erythema of the skin at catheter exit point through the skin; may lead to peritonitis; catheter removal may be necessary for recurrent or resistant infection	Microorganisms in epidermal area; may be related to trauma, *Staphylococcus aureus* nasal carriage Causative organisms: *Staphylococcus epidermidis*, S. aureus, *Pseudomonas* spp.	Purulent drainage, with or without erythema of the skin at the catheter–epidermal interface; positive culture; induration; pain	Oral, IV, or IP antibiotics; exit site care increased to twice a day; duration of therapy unknown
Tunnel infection: inflammation along the subcutaneous tunnel-catheter tract	Migration of microorganisms along the tunnel	Erythema or thickening along the tunnel—"sausage" appearance; pain; may or may not be exit site drainage	IV or IP antibiotics; often leads to peritonitis; often results in catheter removal
Fibrin formation	Formed in response to inflammation because of decreased fibrinolysis of fibrinogen; increased during peritonitis	Whitish strands or clots seen in effluent or catheter; may lead to catheter obstruction if untreated	Heparin added to the dialysate to prevent fibrin production and adhesion formation (500–1000 units/L)
Hemoperitoneum	Menstruating women (retrograde menstruation); trauma; ovarian cysts; ovulation; peritonitis; postcolonoscopy or enema	Bloody effluent; 2 mL blood/L will result in blood-tinged effluent; effluent hematocrit of >5%, indicative of major bleeding; usually resolves spontaneously	In-and-out flushes with room-temperature dialysate (vasoconstriction); addition of heparin to prevent obstruction

Continued on following page

Table 19.4 Complications of Peritoneal Dialysis (*Continued*)

COMPLICATION	CAUSE	SIGNS/SYMPTOMS	INTERVENTIONS
Inflow/outflow problems	Obstruction of the catheter with fibrin, blood, omentum; catheter migration out of pelvis; entrapment of fluid in the abdominal cavity because of adhesions; constipation	The dialysate will not inflow or outflow; resistance when catheter is irrigated	Relief of constipation; radiography for internal kink, catheter position; inspect the catheter for external kinks; irrigation of the catheter with heparinized saline; irrigation with a thrombolytic; reposition or replace catheter; peritoneogram with contrast medium to identify loculation
Air in the peritoneum	Air entering the peritoneal cavity because of air in the system or loose connections	Shoulder pain; peritoneal eosinophilia	Drain patient in the knee–chest or Trendelenburg position; may need to resolve over time; tighten connections
Dialysate leak around the exit site or into the subcutaneous tissue	Increased intraabdominal pressure; delayed healing after catheter placement	Clear fluid from the exit site; abdominal, penile, scrotal edema	Dextrostix to document glucose; resuture acute catheter exit site; stop PD for 2 or more weeks to allow healing; decrease volume with APD in the supine position if unable to stop PD; stabilize the catheter; catheter replacement
Hernias	Increased intraabdominal pressure caused by presence of the dialysate in the peritoneum; seen in patients with congenital or acquired defects or previous abdominal surgeries	Swelling in inguinal, ventral, incisional, umbilical area; nonpainful, reducible	APD with minimal or no diurnal dwell; decreased exchange volume; surgical repair
Pain on inflow	Migration of the catheter; catheter resting against the pelvic wall; rapid infusion of the dialysate; hyperosmolarity of the dialysate; acidity of the dialysate	Pain when the dialysate is entering the peritoneum	Slower infusion of the dialysate: addition of $NaHCO_3$ to increase pH; local anesthetic (2% lidocaine, 3–5 mL/L dialysate IP); surgical revision or replacement of the catheter

APD, Automated peritoneal dialysis; *IP*, intraperitoneal; *IV*, intravenous; *NaHCO₃*, sodium bicarbonate; *PD*, peritoneal dialysis; *WBC*, white blood cells.

HOME DIALYSIS THERAPY: PERITONEAL DIALYSIS

WHO WOULD BE A GOOD CANDIDATE FOR PERITONEAL DIALYSIS?

Modality selection is best determined by the patient with her or his nephrologist. Predialysis education by a nephrologist, CKD nurse, renal case manager, or a neutral provider can provide guidance on modality options and requirements. Education should be objective and fact based so that the patient can make an informed choice and elect the modality that works for his or her unique lifestyle and health needs (Box 19.1).

HOW ARE PATIENTS SELECTED FOR PERITONEAL DIALYSIS AS A HOME DIALYSIS THERAPY?

Before a person is selected as a home PD patient, there must be thorough evaluation by the interdisciplinary dialysis team. The following areas need to be assessed:
1. Relative medical contraindications for PD, such as the following:
   - Abdominal adhesions
   - Concurrent abdominal disease, such as neoplasms
   - History of ruptured diverticulum
   - History of recurrent hernias
   - Documented inability of the peritoneal membrane to ultrafiltrate or diffuse solutes (PET results)
   - Opening between the peritoneal and pleural cavities
   - Body weight exceeding 70 kg without residual kidney function
   - Severe liver disease or polycystic kidney disease
   - Severe respiratory illness
2. Psychosocial evaluation, including the following:
   - Patient motivation for self-care
   - Lifestyle (job, school)
   - Educational background
   - Health beliefs
   - Support system within the family and community
   - Decision-making abilities of the patient
   - History of compliance with medical treatment
   - Distance from a dialysis center
   - Characteristics of the home (e.g., cleanliness; availability of water, electricity, and telephone; space for storage of supplies)
   - Availability of an alternate caregiver (spouse, sibling, parent, friend)
3. Physical characteristics and limitations of the patient, including the following:
   - Vision
   - Strength
   - Dexterity
   - Fine-motor coordination

COGNITIVE FUNCTIONING

It is important to keep in mind that a patient may be a candidate for a home modality even if barriers are assessed. A patient may have the ability to participate in a home modality if certain accommodations are made or if a self-care partner is identified. PD may be medically indicated in patients with cardiovascular difficulties. Home PD is particularly well suited to pediatric patients because it allows "normalization" of the lives of both the child and the family (normal school attendance, fewer dietary restrictions than HD, fewer needlesticks, steady-state body fluid and electrolyte status, independence, and so on).

Box 19.1 Candidate Considerations for Peritoneal Dialysis

Candidate Considerations
- Greater independence for travel and employment
- Fear of needles or blood
- Fragile cardiac status
- Lack of vascular access
- Flexible schedule

Quality of Life Benefits
- Fewer dietary restrictions
- Immediate Medicare coverage
- Greater blood pressure control
- More stable blood chemistries
- Preservation of residual kidney function

What Is the Match-D Method to Assess Treatment Choices for Home Dialysis?

Match-D is a tool developed to help nephrologists and other dialysis staff assess and identify patients who would be suitable candidates for either PD or HD home dialysis therapy. This tool was designed to sensitize clinicians to key factors that make the patient a good candidate for a home modality. The tool evaluates criteria that would indicate whether a patient is a good candidate, potential candidate, or absolute contraindication to a home dialysis therapy. The findings are discussed with the patient and family who can then make an informed decision. Use of the Match-D tool should increase the frequency of patients choosing the home dialysis option.

How Is a Patient Trained for Home Peritoneal Dialysis?

If possible, training is delayed for at least 2 weeks after the catheter is inserted to allow time for healing to occur and for the patient to recover physically and psychologically from surgery. Another family member should train with the patient for support and backup. It is important that the patient be trained by a primary nurse who has established a trusting relationship with the patient and family and can subsequently act as a liaison between the patient and dialysis team. Training is performed primarily on an outpatient basis. Patients are usually trained on CAPD before being trained on CCPD.

The content and method of presentation must be individualized to the patient's learning abilities. The content of training includes normal kidney function and the effects of kidney failure on body homeostasis; mechanism of PD; performance of aseptic technique; catheter and exit site care; monitoring of weight and blood pressure (BP); dialysis record keeping with weight, BP, and dialysis treatments performed; CAPD exchange procedure; use of cycler if on APD; decision making regarding the dialysate to be used to maintain dry weight and normalize BP; recognition of the signs and symptoms of infections (e.g., exit site, tunnel, peritonitis); importance of adequate PD treatment of peritonitis; medications; dietary counseling by the dietitian; ordering dialysis supplies; and management of complications.

There must be ample time for return demonstration of dialysis techniques and attainment of all training objectives before the patient is allowed to perform PD independently at home. At the completion of training, a home visit should be made by the primary nurse. Additional support is provided by having a PD nurse on call to assist the patient with problems encountered during off hours.

How Is the Quality of Care Monitored in Peritoneal Dialysis?

Quality assurance programs are required by The Joint Commission, formerly the Joint Commission on Accreditation of Healthcare Organizations, and the CMS, whose mandates are administered by the regional end-stage renal disease (ESRD) networks (see Chapter 26). The focus of quality assurance should be continuous improvement in the quality of care that patients receive.

The following are examples of quality assurance indicators:

- Incidence of infections, such as peritonitis and exit site or tunnel infections
- Incidence of catheter complications, such as pericatheter leaks, migration, obstruction necessitating catheter replacement, and holes or cracks in the catheter
- Patient morbidity (number of hospital days per year and causes for hospitalization) and mortality
- Attainment of adequacy targets
- Revision of policies and procedures to improve patient care

Peritoneal dialysis is a viable dialysis modality for both acute and chronic patients. Acute PD is appropriate for patients who cannot tolerate HD. Care must be taken in the selection of patients for chronic home PD to optimize the chances of success. Ongoing evaluation of patient satisfaction, compliance with treatment, incidence of complications, and adequacy of PD in removing uremic toxins and excess fluid must be undertaken, and adjustments must be made to ensure quality patient care.

What Are the Drawbacks of Peritoneal Dialysis?

Recently, concern has grown about the frequency of malnutrition and inadequate dialysis in PD patients. Protein malnutrition is frequent as a result of loss of amino acids and protein in the dialysate and because of appetite suppression resulting from inadequate dialysis and the glucose load absorbed from the dialysate. The latter often causes hypertriglyceridemia and the increased caloric intake results in weight gain, especially in patients who are overweight when they start PD. The other major concern is the adequacy of dialysis. Previously, most CAPD patients used four exchanges of 2 to 2.5 L daily, but it has become clear that many PD patients are receiving inadequate dialysis after losing their residual kidney function.

What Is the Most Frequent Complication of Peritoneal Dialysis?

The number of hospital days has decreased to 11.2 per patient year (PPY) for both patients undergoing HD and PD. From 2007 to 2016, hospital days PPY decreased from 15.5 to 12.2 for PD patients (USRDS, 2018). Structural changes to the peritoneum occur as a result of long-term PD and peritonitis can accelerate this process, which can lead to peritoneal fibrosis. Multiple episodes of peritonitis may cause membrane permeability changes, which may cause a decline in UF capabilities. Age, gender, level of education, diagnosis of diabetes mellitus, and hypoalbuminemia at the start of PD have been identified as predictors of peritonitis (Tian et al, 2016). Peritonitis continues to be the major complication of PD, and the ISPD 2016 guidelines recommend the overall peritonitis rate should be no more than 0.5 episodes per year (Li et al, 2016). The ISPD provides recommendations for PD-related infections and treatment (www.ispd.org). A peritonitis treatment decision algorithm covering treatment regimens for gram-negative and gram-positive organisms and the duration of therapy can be found on the ISPD's website. Peritonitis should always be considered when the patient has cloudy effluent or experiences abdominal pain.

What Are the Adequacy Guidelines for Peritoneal Dialysis?

The Clinical Practice Guidelines for Peritoneal Dialysis Adequacy, developed by the NKF and last updated in 2006, state that adequate peritoneal dialysis requires a Kt/V of at least 1.7 per week and a creatinine clearance of at least 60 L/1.73 m2 per week (see Appendix A for additional information on KDOQI). Even more dialysis is recommended for patients who are malnourished. Other possible indications to consider regarding an increased dose of dialysis[a] are as follows:

- Uremic neuropathy
- Uremic pericarditis
- Nausea or unexplained vomiting
- Sleep disturbances
- Restless leg syndrome
- Pruritus
- Uncontrolled hyperphosphatemia
- Evidence of volume overload
- Hyperkalemia
- Metabolic acidosis unresponsive to oral bicarbonate therapy
- Anemia

As a result, more CAPD patients are now using five exchanges daily, often with larger volumes of up to 3 L, and supplementing this regimen with overnight cycler dialysis. This may increase the time required by patients to perform the procedure, as well as the associated discomfort.

[a]National Kidney Foundation: 2006 Clinical Practice Guidelines for Peritoneal Dialysis Adequacy. Retrieved from http://kidneyfoundation.cachefly.net/professionals/KDOQI/guideline_upHD_PD_VA/pd_rec2.htm.

HOME DIALYSIS THERAPY: HEMODIALYSIS

For many patients with CKD, home HD is an excellent but underused alternative to dialysis in a center. Of all prevalent patients with ESRD in 2016 who received renal replacement therapy, only 2% used home HD (USRDS, 2018). This section briefly recounts the history of home dialysis in the United States, describes the use of home HD today, and discusses its advantages in comparison with PD.

What Is the History of Home Hemodialysis?

In 1963, home HD programs were started in Boston, London, and Seattle, primarily for financial reasons. At that time, no insurance or government sources provided funding for long-term dialysis other than research funds, so patients themselves or public donations paid for this expensive treatment. It soon became obvious that suitably trained and supported patients could safely perform HD themselves at home for a fraction of the cost of staff-assisted dialysis in a hospital or dialysis unit. Furthermore, these patients were better rehabilitated and had a better quality of life than those treated as outpatients in a dialysis center. For the next 10 years, until the introduction of the Medicare ESRD program in 1973, funds for dialysis in the United States remained in very short supply. As a consequence, in 1973, some 42% of the approximate 10,000 dialysis patients in the United States were on home dialysis, and almost all were on home HD for 6 to 8 hours, three times weekly.

What Was the Effect of the Medicare End-Stage Renal Disease Program on Home Dialysis?

The introduction of the Medicare ESRD program in 1973 provided almost universal entitlement to dialysis and transplantation for CKD patients; as a result, the picture changed radically. Funding was readily available for outpatient HD, resulting in the rapid proliferation of dialysis units across the United States. Many of these were for-profit units that were often reluctant to present home HD as a treatment option, and most were directed by nephrologists who lacked personal experience with a home HD program. At the same time, the treated patient population changed rapidly to include many more patients with diabetes, minorities, and older adult patients. As a result, the use of home HD decreased rapidly. By 1995, fewer than 1% of all dialysis patients in the United States were treated by home HD, although a few programs still persisted in providing this modality. In contrast, in 1995 in Australia, 14% of patients were undergoing home HD.

The next innovation in home dialysis occurred in the late 1970s with the development of CAPD by Moncrief and Popovich. This simple technique, which came at a time when access to home HD training programs was declining rapidly, gave more patients the opportunity to experience the benefits of self-care dialysis at home. Following the success of CAPD, other varieties of PD were developed. CCPD uses a cycler for treatment overnight with one or more exchanges during the day, and NIPD uses a cycler nightly for overnight PD.

What Is Daily Nocturnal Hemodialysis?

Daily nocturnal hemodialysis (DNHD) is an alternate home dialysis therapy in which the patient dialyzes at home at night while sleeping. The patient undergoing DNHD generally dialyzes for 7 to 10 hours, five or seven times a week.

DNHD allows patients to dialyze for longer periods and with greater frequency. As a result, blood flows are usually reduced to about 200 mL/min, and dialysate flows are reduced to 300 mL/min. Some patients are monitored by trained staff at a remote location via an internet connection. This live monitoring allows the dialysis staff to be alerted via the internet when a machine alarm occurs. If the patient does not respond to the alarm within the established protocol time frame, the staff monitoring the patient will call the patient's home. If no response is received from the home, the staff will call the emergency medical service. A benefit of monitoring by trained dialysis staff is that the patient and caregiver have a greater sense of comfort and confidence in performing the nocturnal dialysis treatment. Patients who dialyze daily reportedly have an increased sense of well-being, are hospitalized less often, and take fewer medications. Of all treatment options, nightly nocturnal dialysis is the best at removing large-molecular-weight particles. This is related to the long amount of time that it takes for large molecules to move from the intracellular space into the plasma (Curtis, 2004). Because there are fewer hours between dialysis treatments, removal of fluid and waste products more closely resembles normal kidney function.

What Is Short Daily Dialysis?

Short daily dialysis is performed over a 2-hour period in a highly efficient manner, six or seven times a week. This method of treatment resembles in-center HD in its intensity and rapid speed. Patients on this modality report using fewer medications and feeling better than in-center patients. Short daily dialysis allows patients to have fewer dietary and fluid restrictions and helps to reduce the number of medications they must take.

Why Is Frequent Dialysis Desirable?

The extent and rate of changes in the fluid and biochemical state of the body affect total body function. A large accumulation of wastes or fluid will make the patient ill. However, rapid reduction of this accumulation can also make the patient ill because of the shifts between the intracellular and extracellular compartments. Frequent HD reduces the interval during which metabolic wastes and fluid accumulate. Total accumulation and rate of reduction during dialysis are less.

Why Not Dialyze Every Day?

Dialysis is not performed every day because the equipment and supplies are expensive. The dialysis procedure also takes time that the patient would prefer to spend elsewhere. The duration and frequency of most dialysis prescriptions are a compromise between what is best for the patient's health and the practical limitations of money and time.

What Is Intermittent Nocturnal Dialysis?

Intermittent nocturnal dialysis is another option for the patients with ESRD. Nocturnal in-center dialysis allows the patient to dialyze at an in-center facility 3 nights a week. The patient is dialyzed at lower blood and dialysate flow rates for approximately 8 hours per treatment. Fewer hypotensive episodes and other dialysis complications are seen because the patient is dialyzed more gently. This is becoming a popular modality for some patients because they can sleep at night and continue normal daytime activities. Better clearances are observed, and these patients report a better sense of well-being because of the less intensive treatment.

What Is the Patient Selection Process for Home Hemodialysis?

Suitably trained and supported patients of all ages, including children and older adults, can perform HD at home. Careful consideration should be taken with serious cardiovascular or other problems during dialysis, lack of good blood access, documented noncompliance, lack of an assistant, lack of a suitable home, inability to learn, excessive anxiety on the part of the patient or family, and lack of patient motivation and willingness to undertake treatment at home. All other patients should be regarded as potential candidates for self-care and should be given information on the advantages of home dialysis, both home HD and PD, when they are selecting a treatment modality. A multidisciplinary team that works with the patient, family, and nephrologist should assess the patient's suitability for home HD while considering medical, psychosocial, and vocational factors that might affect the choice of treatment modality. It is always best to use the Match-D assessment tool to objectively evaluate patient suitability to a particular modality. There must be suitable plumbing, water, electricity, and space to store the equipment and supplies. Many homes and apartments require only minor modifications to allow for home HD, such as installation of a water softener or additional electrical outlets with ground fault circuit interrupters.

How Would You Train a Home Hemodialysis Patient?

Home HD training is best done in a separate area with specialized staff. Because of its specialized nature, consideration should be given to establishing regional training units. Training should begin as soon as possible once a patient has made the decision to be treated at home and is well enough to absorb information. The most difficult task for most patients is learning needle insertion, but this is something that patients do best for themselves. The buttonhole technique is commonly used for home HD and makes self-cannulation easier and less painful for the patient. See Chapter 12 for additional information on the buttonhole technique. From the beginning they must be reassured that home HD is a relatively simple and safe procedure and that when any problems occur at home, support and advice are always available from the training staff via telephone. In addition to the dialysis technique, patients must learn about diet, the disease and its complications, and the medical regimen. They should meet a social worker, a financial counselor, a nutritionist, an exercise coach, and when appropriate, a vocational counselor.

Training usually takes between 3 and 8 weeks after the patient becomes proficient with fistula puncture, and progress should be assessed at regular intervals. The training schedule should be arranged to maximize the patient's opportunities to continue working or to have access to vocational and other rehabilitation services as required.

WHAT ARE THE QUALIFICATIONS OF HOME HEMODIALYSIS TRAINING STAFF?

Selection of home HD training staff is most important. The staff should be experienced in dialysis, have good teaching skills, be committed to encouraging independence and self-care, and be willing to allow patients to learn by making mistakes. Written materials, videotapes, films, posters, models, and other educational aids can facilitate training. The CMS Conditions for Coverage require registered nurses responsible for home dialysis training to have at least 12 months of clinical experience plus 3 months of experience in the specific modality for which they will be training patients (HD, PD, or both).

WHAT PATIENT SUPPORT SERVICES ARE REQUIRED?

Provision of support services for home HD patients is very important. These services should include follow-up visits to the physician's office at least once a month; monthly routine laboratory testing; review of dialysis records; provision of supplies; equipment maintenance and repair; 24-hour availability of on-call advice from a training nurse; regular follow-up visits to the home by a training nurse; and access to social, nutritional, and other services as required. Patients can take their own blood samples for laboratory tests and mail them to the laboratory. The results of these tests are shared with the nephrologist, patient, and home dialysis training program.

Backup dialysis at a facility must be available when a patient develops medical, technical, or social problems that make dialysis at home difficult. Patients are able to take vacations either by arranging to dialyze at a center elsewhere or by using portable equipment. Backup dialysis should also be available to provide the opportunity for family members or other helpers to take vacations.

WHAT ARE THE ADVANTAGES OF HOME HEMODIALYSIS?

Although home dialysis was first introduced for financial reasons, its other advantages for patients soon became obvious. These include increased patient independence, a feeling of accomplishment, the opportunity to schedule dialysis into the patient's daily life, better quality of life, greater opportunity for rehabilitation, and a reduced risk of exposure to hepatitis and other infections. In contrast, patients treated in a dialysis unit have a fixed schedule and very easily become dependent on nursing and technical staff. Interestingly, very similar advantages have been reported with other treatment technologies that have been moved into the home. As Scribner pointed out many years ago, with any chronic disease, the more patients understand about the illness and the more responsibility and control they take for their own care, the greater will be the opportunity for adjustment and rehabilitation. A major aim in treating patients with ESRD should be to maximize the quality of life and encourage rehabilitation to the greatest extent possible. Studies have shown that the quality of life of home HD patients is better than that of CAPD patients, and, in turn, that the quality of life of CAPD patients is better than that of patients dialyzing at a center.

The recently revived interest in more frequent HD also has implications for home HD because it is much easier for patients to treat themselves six times per week at home than to have to travel to a center at such a frequency. Reports from Canada, Italy, and elsewhere have shown that much more dialysis can be provided with such a regimen. This results in remarkable improvements in blood chemistry, patient well-being, quality of life, and rehabilitation. As a result, knowledgeable patients are likely to demand home dialysis in the future.

CHAPTER 20

TRANSPLANTATION

Nephrology nurses who primarily care for patients undergoing dialysis treatment have several roles in the transplantation procedure. They educate and counsel patients regarding the option of transplantation and may assist patients undergoing pretransplant evaluation. They may also need to provide dialysis treatments to transplant recipients experiencing a temporary loss of kidney function from acute tubular necrosis (ATN) or a rejection episode and those with permanent loss of a transplanted kidney. Nephrology nurses and technicians may also provide dialysis to recipients of transplanted nonrenal organs, such as a liver or heart, who are experiencing acute kidney injury (AKI) or chronic kidney disease (CKD). Currently, there are approximately 102,718 patients waiting for a kidney transplant (United States Renal Data System [USRDS], 2017).

How Long Must a Patient Wait to Receive a Kidney Transplant?

The waiting list for a kidney transplant has decreased by 2.3% over the previous year for first time candidates (USRDS, 2017). In 2016, 20,161 kidney transplants were performed nationwide, and 19,301 were kidney-alone transplants (USRDS, 2017), making the active kidney transplant waiting list much larger than the supply of donor kidneys. The first step in organ allocation is to eliminate any transplant candidates on the waiting list for incompatibilities such as blood type, height, weight, and other medical factors. A computer application will then prioritize the order of candidates who may receive offers. Factors included in determining eligibility include:[a]

- Blood type (some are rarer than others)
- Tissue type
- Height and weight of the transplant candidate
- Size of the donated organ
- Medical urgency
- Time on the waiting list
- Pediatric status
- Distance between the donor's hospital and the recipient's hospital
- Number of donors in the local area over a period of time
- The transplant center's criteria for accepting organ offers

What Are the Advantages of Kidney Transplantation?

The most important advantage of kidney transplantation is an improved quality of life. Patients with successful kidney transplants report a better quality of life than patients receiving other forms of kidney replacement therapy. With no need for dialysis treatment and more complete resolution of uremic symptoms, successful transplant recipients can experience a more "normal" lifestyle that includes family, social, and vocational activities. Another benefit is cost. Although the initial year after transplantation is more costly than 1 year of dialysis treatment, the subsequent annual costs are significantly lower. Finally, although the long-term survival rate for patients undergoing dialysis therapies has considerably improved, transplantation may offer patients the opportunity for longer survival. Since the introduction of cyclosporine, survival rates of transplant recipients have been longer than those of dialysis patients. This difference is most pronounced in individuals with diabetes mellitus.

What Are the Disadvantages of Kidney Transplantation?

The disadvantages of transplantation stem from the need for lifelong immunosuppression to prevent the body from rejecting the transplanted organ. The necessity of daily medication compliance is a minor nuisance for some patients and an insurmountable hurdle for others. Family support can be crucial in ensuring adherence to what is often a daunting medication regimen, especially during the initial postoperative period.

The vast potential complications of immunosuppression probably represent a more important disadvantage of transplantation. The direct consequences of suppressing the immune system include an increased risk of infection and some malignancies. Immunosuppressive medications also carry the potential for some nonimmunologic complications (e.g., bone disease, cataracts, diabetes mellitus, hyperlipidemia, hypertension) and gastrointestinal complications (e.g., ulcers, hyperuricemia, and hyperkalemia). Obesity, as well as more cosmetic side effects such as hirsutism and gingival hyperplasia, may also occur.

Another major hurdle for many patients is the difficulty of paying for the costly immunosuppressive medications. Annual Medicare spending is approximately $91,000 per year for an individual on hemodialysis and $110,000 for a kidney transplant. However, after the first year of transplant, Medicare spends only about $35,000 for an individual with a

---

[a]US Department of Health and Human Services, Organ Procurement and Transplant Network: How organ allocation works. Retrieved from https://optn.transplant.hrsa.gov/learn/about-transplantation/how-organ-allocation-works.

functioning kidney transplant, making transplantation more cost effective than dialysis (USRDS, 2018). Although the Centers for Medicare & Medicaid Services (CMS) provides 80% coverage for the first 36 months after transplantation, many patients do not have other insurance coverage. Medicare did expand coverage of immunosuppressive medications from 3 years to lifetime for transplant recipients who are Medicare aged or Medicare disabled. Nondisabled transplant recipients younger than the age of 65 years continue to receive only 3 years of coverage after transplantation. Nephrology nurses practicing in transplantation, along with social workers, assist transplant recipients in finding solutions to this problem.

The process of transplantation, from evaluation and waiting for a donor organ to surgical hospitalization and threatened or actual rejection, places a great deal of stress on both the patient and family members. Again, strong social support is a crucial component of successfully coping with the stress of transplantation. Table 20.1 summarizes the risks and benefits of transplantation.

WHAT ARE THE RISKS AND BENEFITS OF COMBINED KIDNEY–PANCREAS TRANSPLANTATION?

A total of 835 combined kidney–pancreas transplants were performed in 2018 (Organ Procurement and Transplant Network [OPTN], 2018). Dialysis patients who also have diabetes mellitus may want to consider a combined kidney–pancreas transplant. For individuals with hypoglycemic unawareness, the combined procedure is a lifesaver. The major benefits of this procedure are as follows:

- Euglycemia, which may halt or slow the progression of diabetic sequelae
- Freedom from frequent insulin injections and finger sticks for glucose measurement. The combined kidney–pancreas transplant procedure is more complicated and carries more risks than kidney transplantation alone. These risks are associated with the following:
  - Longer surgery
  - Exocrine drainage of the pancreas. Many transplant surgeons choose to drain amylase, a digestive enzyme produced by the pancreas, to the urinary bladder using a piece of donor duodenum as a conduit. Although this procedure allows for monitoring of pancreatic function by measuring urinary amylase, amylase may cause acute or chronic cystitis or urethritis. In addition, patients lose a great deal of bicarbonate and fluid and thus have a tendency to develop acidosis and dehydration.
  - Increased immunosuppression-associated risks. A transplanted pancreas is much more prone to stimulate the body's immune system than a transplanted kidney; therefore, greater amounts of immunosuppression are required.

WHO SHOULD BE CONSIDERED AS A TRANSPLANT CANDIDATE?

In general, all patients should be offered the option of consultation with a transplant team to determine their eligibility. Variables such as advanced age, obesity, and other comorbid conditions are no longer viewed as absolute contraindications to kidney transplantation. Box 20.1 summarizes the absolute and relative contraindications to transplantation; however, exclusion and inclusion criteria may differ considerably among transplant centers and are individualized based on a close review of the patient's specific condition. For example, although active malignancy is a contraindication, a period of remission or cure may make the patient eligible for transplantation. A referral should be made as soon as possible because the patient can accrue valuable waiting time during the interim. Patients with a glomerular filtration rate of less than 30 mL/min should be referred to a transplant center for evaluation if deemed medically appropriate by the physician (OPTN, 2015.)

Table 20.1 Transplantation Trade-Offs	
BENEFITS	**RISKS**
• Improved quality of life	• Lifelong immunosuppression
• Freedom from dialysis	• Necessity for daily medication
• More normal lifestyle	• Increased risk of infection
• Longer survival rate	• Increased risk of malignancy
• Less costly than dialysis	• Difficulty paying for costly medications

• Increased ability to pursue normal activities: work, home, school
• More complete resolution of uremic symptoms
• Normal calcium–phosphorus product
• Improved cardiac function
• Improved appetite
• Less restrictive diet
• Improved sexual function
• Increased feeling of wellness
• Increased mental acuity
	• Steroid bone disease
	• Potential medication side effects:
	  • Hypertension
	  • Ulcers, dyspepsia, other gastrointestinal effects
	  • Hyperkalemia, hyperlipidemia, obesity
	• Body image changes (e.g., hirsutism, gingival hyperplasia)
	• Diabetes mellitus, gout, cataracts, tremor
	• Psychological stress

Box 20.1 Absolute and Relative Contraindications to Transplantation

Absolute Contraindications

- Active chronic infection or sepsis
- Active malignancy
- Active substance abuse
- Severe cardiovascular or pulmonary disease
- Inability to comply with the medication regimen

Relative Contraindications

- Age: very young or very old (biological vs chronological age)
- Severe comorbidities
- Lack of family support
- Mental or psychological problems
- Obesity: body mass index > 40 kg/m^2 (varies by transplant center)

Who Pays for a Kidney Transplant?

Medicare will help cover the cost of a kidney transplant provided the surgery takes place in a hospital approved by Medicare to perform transplants. Box 20.2 summarizes covered services for transplant recipients.

Can Patients Who Have a Viral Infection Receive a Kidney Transplant?

In the past, HIV was an absolute contraindication to transplantation because of concerns that the immunosuppressive therapy used in transplant recipients might exacerbate the HIV infection. Other reasons were the shortage of organs available for transplantation and the shortened life expectancy rates of those infected with HIV. Kidney transplants are no longer contraindicated for patients with well-controlled HIV, and more transplant centers across the United States now perform kidney transplants on carefully selected HIV-positive patients. HIV-positive patients must meet all of the standard criteria for kidney transplantation and undergo some additional screening. Patients with hepatitis B or C as well as those with well-controlled HIV would receive consideration for transplant by many transplant centers.

What Is the Immunologic Basis of Transplantation?

The immune system protects the body from foreign invasion by identifying invaders and then destroying them. Anything that produces this response is called an antigen. The basis of immunology in transplantation is to identify how the body recognizes foreign antigens. Transplant immunologists have identified two main antigen systems that affect the acceptance or rejection of a transplanted organ or tissue. These two systems are blood group and human leukocyte antigen (HLA). Blood group is the first determinant of compatibility for solid organ transplantation. In general, an organ must be ABO compatible with the transplant recipient. For this reason, transplant recipient waiting lists are arranged by the ABO group. The rhesus (Rh) factor is not applicable to solid organ transplantation. The four blood groups are O, A, B, and AB. Blood group O is the universal donor, and blood group AB is the universal recipient. Blood group O can receive organs only from blood group O donors; recipients with blood group A can receive a kidney from blood groups A and O; recipients with blood group B can receive a kidney from blood groups B and O; and recipients with blood group AB can receive a kidney from blood groups A, B, AB, and O.

The HLA system is composed of a group of genes found on the sixth chromosome. Three main sites or loci on this chromosome, A, B, and DR, have been identified as influencing the recognition of foreign tissue. Because each individual has two copies of each chromosome, one donated by each parent, six loci are identified in each person. When a tissue with different HLA genes is introduced in the body, the immune system is triggered, and the rejection process begins.

Box 20.2 Medicare Coverage for Transplant Services[a]

Part A Covers These Transplant Services	Part B Helps Pay for These Transplant Service
Inpatient services in approved hospital	Fee for physician services for transplant surgery
Kidney registry fee	Fee for physician services for kidney donor during hospital stay
Laboratory and other tests for donor and recipient evaluation	Immunosuppressive medications (for a limited time)
Finding proper kidney	Blood transfusion (if needed)
Full cost of care for kidney donor	
Blood transfusions if needed	

[a]If the patient has Medicare only because of permanent kidney failure, Medicare coverage will end 36 months after the month of a kidney transplant.
From Medicare: *Know Your Rights*, CMS product # 11360, July 2018.

The components of the immune system that are most important in transplantation are T lymphocytes and B lymphocytes. T lymphocytes recognize the foreign tissue and initiate the rejection process. B lymphocytes recognize foreign antigens and produce antibodies to destroy the invader. When primed, both T and B lymphocytes will remember a foreign antigen and attack it more quickly in subsequent presentations. Humans develop immunologic memory to HLA antigens through exposure via blood transfusions, pregnancy, and transplantation.

What Is Tissue Typing?

Tissue typing refers to blood tests designed to identify HLA genetic markers. Although HLA matching is used to distribute organs objectively, modern immunosuppressive medications have made HLA matching increasingly less important for successful outcomes. Many centers transplant organs with no HLA similarities (zero matched organs), as long as the cross-match is negative, with excellent results. When the body recognizes and acquires immunity to one HLA antigen, it often acquires immunity to other related antigens even though these antigens were not presented to the body. This crossover immunity has been recognized by the development of cross-reactive antigen group (CREG) tests. CREG matching may improve outcomes in minority groups. The HLA status is currently less critical with the availability of newer immunosuppressive medications; however, it is believed the better the HLA match, the more successful the transplant will be (National Kidney Foundation [NKF], 2017b).

What Is Cross-Matching?

Monthly serum samples from potential recipients are used to perform cross-matching tests. Cross-matching tests are blood tests that determine whether a recipient has acquired immunity to a given donor organ tissue. These tests are performed when a donor organ becomes available. Sera from all eligible recipients are tested against donor lymph cells. A positive cross-match means that the recipient has immunologic memory or acquired immunity to the donor and therefore cannot receive the organ because it would result in immediate rejection. The routine test is the Amos antiglobulin test, which takes about 6 hours to complete; however, more sophisticated and time-consuming tests, such as flow cytometric cross-matches, may sometimes be performed. In living donor transplantation, an additional test called a mixed leukocyte reaction may be ordered, although this test takes several days to complete and has not proven to be of great value. Sometimes a positive cross-match transplant may be performed with extreme caution at a transplant center with expertise in this area. Plasmapheresis or immunoglobulin therapy (or both) may be used to remove antibodies and minimize the chance of organ rejection.

What Are Percent Reactive Antibody Levels?

Another important cross-matching test is called percent reactive antibody (PRA). Antibodies form when the immune system is exposed to foreign antigens. The potential recipient's serum is tested against a panel of random donors. The number of positive reactions to the donor panel is expressed as a percentage. This percentage represents the risk of a positive cross-match and thus incompatibility with any random donor, along with an increased risk of acute or hyperacute rejection. Therefore, the higher a potential recipient's PRA level, the less likely it is that any given organ will be compatible and the more difficult it is to find a compatible kidney. For this reason, patients with high PRA levels are given preference in the distribution of organs from deceased donors. A patient with a PRA level greater than 80% is considered highly sensitized. Patients may be exposed to foreign HLAs through blood transfusions, viruses, pregnancy, or transplanted organs. In some cases, plasmapheresis, a procedure that separates blood plasma from the blood cells, can help to reduce the number of antibodies present in the blood. The percentage of preformed antibodies in your blood varies over time, which explains the frequency of testing.

What Is the Purpose of Monthly Serum Samples?

The number of sensitized lymphocytes that constitute preformed immunity to any particular antigen may wax and wane over time. Sometimes the number may be so low that the patient's PRA level may fall. Because of this phenomenon, a specific cross-match using current serum may be negative even though a cross-match using older or historic serum is positive. Because immunosuppression will be applied to block the memory response, a current negative cross-match may indicate a window of opportunity for a potential recipient. On the other hand, immunity provoked by blood transfusion after obtaining the most current serum sample could give a false-negative cross-match. The variability of the immune status necessitates monthly serum sampling for potential recipients.

What Does the Recipient Workup Entail?

The evaluation process for a kidney or other organ transplant begins with referral to the transplant center. The potential recipient and family members meet members of the transplant team. This team usually consists of transplant nurse coordinators, transplant surgeons, transplant nephrologists, and social workers. After the team has determined the initial eligibility of a candidate, the transplant nurse coordinator works with the patient, dialysis health care team, and primary health care provider to facilitate evaluation. Although the evaluation may find that transplantation is not a viable option for some potential recipients, the ultimate goal of the pretransplant workup is to find out as much about the patient as possible to perform a successful transplant.

The evaluation generally consists of blood, urine, and other diagnostic tests (e.g., chest radiography and electrocardiography), as well as a careful review of the patient's records. Special attention is given to the following areas:

- Cardiovascular assessment, which may include cardiac arteriography, echocardiography, and stress testing
- Infection surveillance, which usually includes dental examination
- Malignancy detection
- Genitourinary tract assessment
- Psychosocial evaluation, which may include screening for illicit drugs

WHAT ARE THE POSSIBLE SOURCES OF ORGANS?

The two main sources of kidneys for transplantation are living donors and deceased donors. Living donors can be related to the recipient by blood (parent, sibling) or otherwise emotionally connected (spouse, close friend, adopted child). The key requirements for living donation are voluntary informed consent and a completely healthy donor. Laboratory blood testing, immunologic testing, electrocardiogram studies, medical history and review, psychological evaluation, kidney function testing, and financial consultation are all investigated to determine whether someone can be a suitable donor.

Deceased donors are individuals who have died from irreversible brain death. Their bodies are kept functioning by artificial ventilation and medications. With the consent of the next of kin, organs and tissues are procured by the organ recovery team and distributed by the regional organ and tissue bank in accordance with national guidelines. There is no expense to the donor family, and usual funeral arrangements are not affected by organ and tissue donation. There is currently a shortage of organs from deceased donors in the United States.

WHO MANAGES THE SUPPLY AND ALLOCATION OF DONATED ORGANS IN THE UNITED STATES?

The United Network for Organ Sharing (UNOS) is a private, nonprofit organization under contract with the federal government. UNOS operates the OPTN. UNOS maintains the databases for all organ transplant information and manages the national transplant waiting list. UNOS develops policies to ensure fair organ allocation and coordinates the matching and distribution of donated organs.

WHAT ARE THE GUIDELINES FOR KIDNEY ALLOCATION?

Characteristics of both the donor and recipient are considered in the fair allocation of kidneys. A variety of factors are considered in the allocation process, including the following:

- Tenure on the waiting list
- Whether the organ recipient is a child
- Body size of the donor and recipient
- Tissue match between the donor and recipient
- Blood type
- Blood antibody levels

WHAT IS KIDNEY PAIRED DONATION?

Kidney paired donation (KPD) is an option for patients with an incompatible living donor. This procedure is considered when an individual who wishes to donate a kidney to a significant other or family member is unable to do so because her or his blood type does not match or some other incompatibility exists. In KPD, the incompatible donor and recipient are matched with another incompatible donor–recipient pair, and the kidneys are exchanged between the pairs. This procedure allows both donors to donate and both recipients to receive compatible kidneys (Fig. 20.1). The procedure usually involves two recipient–donor pairs, although the exchange may involve more than two pairs. The number of kidney paired donation transplants increased sharply since 2005, with 642 performed in 2016 (USRDS).

WHAT HAPPENS AFTER A PATIENT IS PLACED ON THE DECEASED DONOR WAITING LIST?

After a candidate is considered eligible for transplantation and no living donors are available, the transplant center places the candidate's name on the deceased donor waiting list. Kidneys are distributed according to a point system. Points are given for the length of time on the waiting, degree of HLA match, prior living donor, distance from donor hospital, survival benefit, and pediatric status for a kidney transplant. Because of the difficulty in finding suitable kidneys for these patients, additional points are given to patients with high PRA levels. In general, kidneys from deceased donors in one blood group are offered only to recipients in that same blood group; therefore, the waiting list is divided by blood group. In 2014, the OPTN revised the kidney allocation system (KAS) to more equitably allocate kidneys, decrease discard rates of kidneys, and provide access to transplants to those who have a more rigorous match requirement. The new system uses a metric called the Kidney Donor Profile Index (KDPI) for the donor and the Expected Post Transplant Survival (EPTS) score for the adult kidney transplant candidate. The KDPI combines a number of donor factors that determine the likelihood of graft failure after a deceased donor transplant. The lower the KDPI score, the longer the estimated length of time the transplanted kidney will function. The KDPI score is used in conjunction with the EPTS score. The EPTS scores the potential transplant recipient on four medical factors: age, time on dialysis, diabetic status, and previous history of a solid organ transplant. Lower EPTS scores are associated with longer estimated years of graft function from a transplanted kidney and range from 0% to 100%. Candidates with

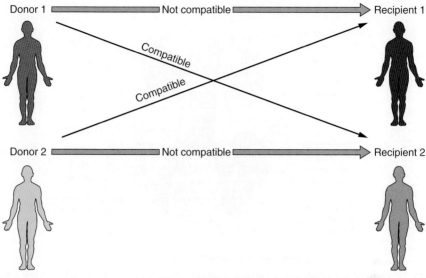

Fig. 20.1 Kidney paired donation.

lower EPTS scores (top 20%) will receive offers for kidneys from donors with KDPI score of 20% or less before others (US Department of Health & Human Services).

WHERE ARE TRANSPLANTED KIDNEYS PLACED, AND HOW LONG IS THE TRANSPLANTATION SURGERY?

The transplanted kidney and ureter are usually placed extraperitoneally in the right or left iliac fossa of the recipient. The incision extends from above the iliac crest to just above the symphysis pubis. Although the right iliac fossa is generally preferred for primary transplantation, either side may be used. If the recipient has had a previous transplant, the transplant surgeon will generally select the side not used previously. The donor renal artery is anastomosed end to end with the recipient internal iliac (hypogastric) artery or end to side with the external iliac artery. The venous anastomosis is generally end to side with the recipient's external iliac vein. The donor ureter is attached to the recipient's bladder or, rarely, the recipient's ureter (Fig. 20.2). If a pancreas is also being transplanted, it will be placed in the opposite iliac fossa (Fig. 20.3). The kidney transplantation procedure generally lasts 2.5 to 4 hours.

The iliac fossae are the preferred placement sites even when the patient has had two or more transplantations. Occasionally, adhesions and scarring from multiple transplantations or other surgical procedures or severe atherosclerotic disease preclude the use of these sites. In these extremely rare cases, the surgeon may place the kidney intraperitoneally and use other vasculature, including the abdominal aorta.

HOW LONG DO PATIENTS STAY IN THE HOSPITAL AFTER TRANSPLANTATION?

Transplant recipients are usually discharged 3 to 5 days after the transplantation procedure. Of course, surgical or medical complications may delay discharge, and the hospital stay may also be prolonged if the transplant team has concerns about the ability of the patient or the patient's family to provide adequate postoperative care.

WHY DO SOME TRANSPLANT RECIPIENTS REQUIRE DIALYSIS?

Like other individuals, organ transplant recipients may require dialysis treatment for fluid removal, electrolyte imbalance, uremia, or a combination of these reasons. Kidney, as well as other graft recipients (e.g., liver and heart), often need hemofiltration or ultrafiltration after surgery because of the vast amounts of fluids used to maintain cardiovascular stability during the procedure. The patient's new kidney may be slow to respond to this fluid load. Kidney transplant recipients with ATN or an acute rejection attempt may require temporary dialysis. Recipients of extrarenal organs often have concomitant kidney disease or acute kidney failure. Uremia or electrolyte imbalances may also occur in these patients. Fluid and solute removal via traditional hemodialysis, peritoneal dialysis, or methods such as slow continuous ultrafiltration or continuous venovenous hemofiltration may be used.

WHAT CAUSES DELAYED GRAFT FUNCTION?

Delayed graft function (DGF) is defined as failure of the kidney transplant to function immediately, necessitating dialysis in the first week after transplant. DGF affects up to 31% of deceased donor kidney transplantations but rarely affects living donor transplantations. DGF has been associated with poor short- and long-term outcomes as well as higher

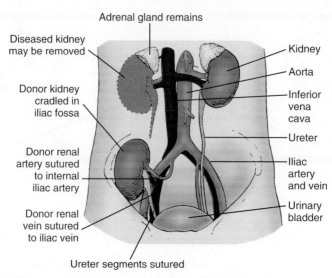

Adrenal gland remains

Diseased kidney may be removed

Donor kidney cradled in iliac fossa

Donor renal artery sutured to internal iliac artery

Donor renal vein sutured to iliac vein

Ureter segments sutured

Kidney

Aorta

Inferior vena cava

Ureter

Iliac artery and vein

Urinary bladder

Fig. 20.2 Transplanted kidney placement in the right iliac fossa. (Modified from Black JM, Hawks JH, Keene AM: *Medical-surgical nursing: clinical management for positive outcomes,* ed. 8, Philadelphia, 2009, Saunders.)

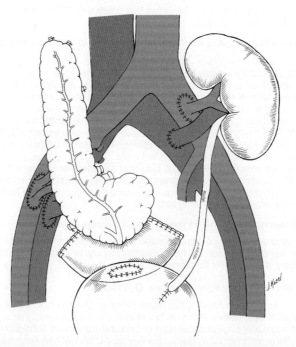

Fig. 20.3 Technique of combined kidney–pancreas transplantation with the duodenal segment bladder drainage technique. (From Sollinger HW, Stratta RJ, D'Alessandro AM, et al: Experience with simultaneous pancreas-kidney transplantation. *Annals of Surgery* 208(4):475–483, 1988.)

rejection rates (Mannon, 2018). DGF is characterized by oliguria (although high urine output DGF is occasionally seen) and failure of the serum creatinine to decrease after a technically successful transplantation procedure. Its cause is not well described, but it is probably caused by a combination of factors both donor and recipient mediated. Donor-related factors include advanced donor age or comorbidity, female gender, increased donor serum creatinine, body mass index (BMI), history of hypertension, preservation injury, prolonged cold storage time, vascular instability of the donor during the harvest or transplant procedure, and reperfusion injury. Recipient related factors include male gender, BMI, previous transplant, diabetes, duration and type of dialysis modality, and cardiac function (Nashan, Abbud-Filho, & Citterio, 2016). Calcineurin inhibitor (CNI) use may exacerbate or prolong DGF, and thus initiation of cyclosporine or tacrolimus therapy may be delayed in recipients with DGF. These individuals may require dialysis until the kidney begins to function, which generally occurs in several days to 2 weeks. DGF can last for several months with a good eventual outcome; however, oliguria and uremia that extend beyond 2 weeks may also be caused by rejection or drug-induced nephrotoxicity. Percutaneous biopsy of the kidney is usually performed to establish a diagnosis. Patients with DGF need reassurance and support from their caregivers. It is helpful to allow them to express their feelings about still requiring dialysis and to inform them that most transplanted kidneys with DGF will eventually function well.

WHAT SPECIAL PRECAUTIONS SHOULD BE TAKEN WHEN DIALYZING A TRANSPLANT RECIPIENT?

The following precautions are most notable when dialyzing a transplant recipient:

- During the initial 24 hours after surgery, internal bleeding is a concern, so hypotension should be carefully monitored and brought to the attention of the physician.
- Because of the susceptibility of the transplanted kidney to ischemia, avoid hypotension, even at the cost of decreased fluid removal.
- The integrity of the surgical incision must be maintained.
- Anticoagulation is also a concern in transplant recipients. Heparin-free or minimal anticoagulation is preferred, especially during the immediate postoperative period or if the recipient has undergone diagnostic percutaneous kidney biopsy.
- Electrolyte imbalances are common after transplantation. The most common is hyperkalemia. Hyperkalemia is common in patients with impaired graft function but is also caused by medications, such as cyclosporine and tacrolimus. Other electrolyte abnormalities are outlined in Table 20.2.

IS THERE AN INCREASED RISK OF INFECTION AFTER TRANSPLANTATION?

Increased risk of infection is an inevitable consequence of immunosuppression. During the immediate postoperative period, bacterial infections in sites such as the wound, urinary tract, and lungs are more common, whereas viral infections such as cytomegalovirus (CMV), herpes simplex, and herpes zoster are more prevalent after the first several weeks after transplantation. CMV is a major cause of morbidity and mortality in transplant recipients. Urinary tract infection was the most common cause of first-year infectious hospitalizations followed by septicemia and postoperative infection (USRDS, 2014).

Table 20.2 Electrolyte Abnormalities After Transplantation

ABNORMALITY	PREDISPOSING FACTORS	TREATMENT
Hyperkalemia	ATN Cyclosporine Tacrolimus Trimethoprim Sulfamethoxazole Blood transfusions	Dialysis IV 50% dextrose—insulin Kayexalate Diuretics Diet
Hypokalemia	Rapid posttreatment diuresis Diuretics	Potassium supplements Diet
Hypocalcemia (often with hyperphosphatemia)	Parathyroidectomy Hyperparathyroidism + ATN	Calcium supplements Increased calcium dialysate calcitriol (Rocaltrol) Phosphorus binders
Hypercalcemia (often with hypophosphatemia)	Hyperparathyroidism functioning kidney	Diet Phosphorus supplement calcitriol to suppress PTH (if calcium <11 mg/dL)
Hypomagnesemia	Diuresis Cyclosporine	Magnesium supplement
Acidosis	ATN Rejection Cyclosporine Pancreas transplant with bladder drainage	Sodium bicarbonate Dialysis Sodium citrate

ATN, Acute tubular necrosis; *IV*, intravenous; *PTH*, parathyroid hormone.

Many centers use prophylactic medications, such as ganciclovir or hyperimmune gamma globulin, to prevent CMV infection or reactivation. Strict adherence to Standard Precautions should reduce the number of infectious complications in these patients. Isolation is rarely required, and transplant recipients pose no special risk to other patients or staff.

DOES ANY ONE IMMUNOSUPPRESSIVE MEDICATION PLACE THE TRANSPLANT RECIPIENT AT HIGHER RISK FOR MALIGNANCY?

Cancer is the leading cause of death in kidney transplant patients with a functioning graft after the first year of transplantation. Transplant recipients have demonstrated a two- to threefold higher risk than the general population for certain malignancies such as colon, lung, liver, lymphoma, melanoma, and nonmelanoma skin cancer (Sprangers et al, 2017). No single immunosuppressant has been found to increase the risk; rather, the risk increases as the total amount of immunosuppression increases. Factors linked to an increased risk of malignancy after kidney transplant include age, sun exposure, previous cancer, concomitant viral infection, cumulative dose of immunosuppression, the type of immunosuppression, and the duration of pretransplant dialysis (Sprangers et al, 2017). When detected early, many of these cancers respond well to treatment. Transplant recipients should be made aware of their increased risk of malignancy and follow recommended screening guidelines. Transplant recipients should limit sun exposure to prevent skin cancer and should be discouraged from smoking. Recommendations for the cadence of screening vary based on the transplant center and patient risk for a specific cancer type. Most recommend intervals which are similar to those of the general population.

WHAT ARE THE MOST COMMONLY USED IMMUNOSUPPRESSIVE MEDICATIONS?

Maintenance immunosuppressive medications can be classified into four classes: corticosteroids, CNIs, antiproliferative agents, and mTOR (mammalian target of rapamycin) inhibitors. Most centers use triple-drug maintenance immunosuppressive therapies consisting of steroids, a CNI, and an antiproliferative. Antilymphocyte preparations are used for a short time as rejection prophylaxis or treatment. All immunosuppressive medications carry the risk of infection and malignancy.

Steroids

Oral prednisone and intravenous methylprednisolone sodium (Solu-Medrol) are the most commonly used steroids. Steroids are used to both prevent and treat acute rejection. Prednisone works by inhibiting interleukin-1 secretions, which result in decreased replication of cytotoxic T cells. Steroids, although easy to use and inexpensive, can potentially cause a vast number of side effects that can be minimized by using the lowest possible dose. Common side effects include acne, anxiety, depression, easy bruising, headache, insomnia, and a "moon face" appearance (UNOS, 2016).

Calcineurin Inhibitors

Cyclosporine (Sandimmune, Neoral) and tacrolimus (Prograf) are immunosuppressive drugs derived from fungi. These drugs block T lymphocyte action by blocking chemical signals via calcineurin. Cyclosporine and tacrolimus have similar side effect profiles. Nephrotoxicity is a major problem with both medications, complicating the diagnosis of rejection. Tacrolimus offers an advantage of not inducing the cyclosporine-related effects of hirsutism or gingival hyperplasia and may not have as deleterious an effect on serum lipids as cyclosporine, although it is more likely than cyclosporine to cause diabetes and gastrointestinal symptoms. Tacrolimus is a more powerful immunosuppressant than cyclosporine, so the doses used are much smaller. The doses of both medications are based on blood levels obtained 12 hours after the last dose of medication. In most cases, these drugs are used interchangeably rather than in combination. A change of medication is usually precipitated by a severe rejection episode or intolerable side effects while using one of these medications. Cyclosporine, either as Sandimmune or the more readily absorbed microemulsion form Neoral, is the primary drug used in kidney and heart transplantation. At many centers, tacrolimus is the primary agent used in patients undergoing pancreas, liver, and small bowel transplantation.

Antiproliferative

Azathioprine (Imuran) and mycophenolate mofetil (CellCept, Myfortic) are both antiproliferatives. Mycophenolate mofetil is rapidly replacing azathioprine in transplantation because it appears to have an improved immunosuppressive effect, including action against B lymphocytes. This makes mycophenolate mofetil the only immunosuppressant that may treat chronic rejection.

Antilymphocyte Preparations

Atgam and OKT3 (Orthoclone) are the primary antilymphocyte agents used as prophylaxis against, or to treat, rejection. These powerful immunosuppressants are made by immunizing an animal with human lymphocytes and using the resultant antibodies. These antibodies block the function of T lymphocytes in the recipient. Atgam is a polyclonal preparation, which means that it contains antibodies against a host of human blood cells, including platelets and red blood cells. It is administered in a manner similar to that used for other serum products using a central vein catheter. OKT3 is a product of genetic engineering; OKT3 targets only certain T lymphocytes known as CD3 cells. This monoclonal preparation is given as an intravenous push medication via a peripheral vein. The most serious side effects from OKT3 occur after the first or second dose (pulmonary edema and infection), and thus special precautions, including avoidance of fluid overload, are observed. KDIGO recommends the use of OKT3 for the treatment of acute rejection that does not respond to corticosteroids (Kasiske et al, 2010).

Monoclonal Antibodies

Several monoclonal antibodies have been developed for use in transplantation. Basiliximab (Simulect) and daclizumab (Zenapax) are similar drugs developed to prevent transplant rejection. These are either humanized or chimeric antibodies; in other words, the majority of the antibody molecule is from a partial human immunoglobulin, with only a small portion from a murine antibody molecule. This humanization means that the body is less likely to recognize the antibody as a foreign protein, thus minimizing the first-dose side effects and yielding a prolonged drug half-life. Both drugs prevent rejection by interfering with binding of interleukin-2 to lymphocytes. These drugs are administered intravenously after transplantation. Both drugs appear to be similar in efficacy and safety.

Mammalian Target of Rapamycin

In 2000, sirolimus (Rapamune) was approved for use by the US Food and Drug Administration for prevention of organ rejection in patients receiving a kidney transplant. Sirolimus inhibits T-lymphocyte activation and proliferation as well as antibody production, making it unique. This medication is initially taken in combination with cyclosporine and steroids. Cyclosporine can later be withdrawn from some patients at a low immunologic risk while the dose of sirolimus is increased. Side effects associated with this medication include increased serum cholesterol and triglycerides, hypertension, acne, fever, diarrhea, and rash. Increased creatinine levels may also be seen. This medication can be used for chronic rejection and is not nephrotoxic.

CAN A PATIENT RECEIVE VACCINATIONS AFTER A TRANSPLANT?

The immune system of a patient with a transplant does not function properly because of the required immunosuppressive medications taken to prevent rejection. Not all vaccines are safe for patients receiving these medications. Vaccines are either inactive or live. Inactive vaccinations are considered safe, but live vaccines should be avoided. The NKF (2017a) recommends that patients with a transplant avoid the following vaccinations:

- Influenza nasal (Flu Mist)
- Varicella (Varivax, Zostavax, "shingles vaccine," "chickenpox" vaccine)
- Measles, mumps, rubella (MMR)
- Yellow fever
- Smallpox
- Live oral typhoid
- Bacillus Calmette-Guérin (BCG)
  Vaccines that transplant recipients may regularly receive include the following:
- Influenza (flu) (the injectable form is inactive)
- Pneumonia vaccine (Pneumovax)

WHAT IS MEANT BY REJECTION?

When the body's immune system recognizes the transplanted organ as foreign, it will attempt to destroy it. This phenomenon is called rejection. Rejection occurs in two ways: cellular and humoral. Cellular rejection is initiated by T lymphocytes, and humoral rejection refers to destruction of the transplanted organ by specific antibodies.

WHAT ARE THE DIFFERENT KINDS OF TRANSPLANT REJECTIONS?

There are three basic types of rejection processes: hyperacute rejection, acute rejection, and chronic rejection. Rejection episodes place a great amount of stress on the recipient and his or her family.

Hyperacute Rejection

Hyperacute rejection is a humoral rejection process primarily caused by preformed antibodies against the transplanted tissue HLA or against ABO antigens. This type of rejection occurs within minutes to hours of the transplantation procedure. The onslaught of specific antibodies causes massive intravascular coagulation and cell death. There is no treatment for hyperacute rejection. It can be prevented by careful cross-matching.

Acute Rejection

When helper T lymphocytes recognize tissue cells as foreign, they initiate a cascade of events known as acute rejection. Acute rejection usually occurs weeks to months after transplantation. This form of cellular rejection generally occurs the first time the immune system is presented with a specific foreign tissue cell or antigen. The majority of immunosuppression is directed at preventing and treating acute rejection.

Chronic Rejection

In humoral rejection, beta cells are stimulated by nonself antigens and produce antibodies to destroy the transplanted organ. Chronic rejection, also known as chronic allograft nephropathy, is a slow humoral rejection process that occurs months to years after transplantation. The hallmark of chronic rejection is gradual loss of function caused by fibrosis in the organ's blood vessels. Chronic kidney rejection may be difficult to distinguish from chronic cyclosporine toxicity.

How Is Rejection Diagnosed and Treated?

In the absence of other causes, increased serum creatinine is most commonly used as a diagnostic indicator of rejection. Percutaneous biopsy may be used to confirm the diagnosis.

Hyperacute Rejection

Hyperacute rejection is often diagnosed as soon as the vascular anastomoses are completed and the clamps are released. The kidney will rapidly turn black and fail to produce urine, or the recipient may suffer have symptoms of oliguria, fever, and pain soon after the transplantation procedure. There is no treatment; the organ must be removed surgically.

Acute Rejection

Oliguria, fever, edema, weight gain, and graft tenderness are the cardinal physical symptoms of acute kidney transplant rejection. However, modern immunosuppressive therapy blocks these symptoms, causing transplant clinicians to rely on biochemical markers. A rapid rise in serum creatinine levels over several days with or without physical symptoms may indicate acute rejection. Nephrotoxicity is also a possible diagnosis, especially if drug levels are high.

Many rejection attempts can be treated with increased steroids. Steroids are delivered as intravenous boluses or "pulses" of methylprednisolone and/or increased oral prednisone that is rapidly tapered back to baseline doses over several days. If the rejection is severe or does not respond to steroids, antilymphocyte preparations (Atgam, OKT3) are used. Most acute cellular rejections are treated successfully.

Chronic Rejection

Patients with chronic rejection often do not experience symptoms until the rejection has progressed to serious kidney compromise. Serum creatinine slowly increases over months to years until the kidney ceases to function. A definitive diagnosis is made by biopsy. Traditionally there has been no treatment for chronic rejection; however, mycophenolate mofetil (CellCept), which acts against antibody-inducing beta cells, has demonstrated some success in treatment. Because it probably begins as very mild acute rejection, chronic rejection is best prevented by adequate immunosuppression and regular laboratory follow-up.

What Happens When the Transplanted Kidney Fails Irreversibly?

When the transplant team has determined that the transplanted kidney has failed irreversibly and that further treatment would be unsuccessful or detrimental, the patient returns to maintenance dialysis treatment. Except in cases of hyperacute rejection, early vascular catastrophe, or untreated acute rejection, the transplanted kidney usually slowly scars and shrinks as function ceases, so surgical removal is not necessary. Failed transplanted kidneys are removed in cases of severe hematuria, infection, or malignant hypertension. Immunosuppression is discontinued gradually to prevent superimposed acute rejection and to allow the adrenal glands to regain function.

These patients require special nursing care. In addition to the effects of immunosuppression, which may remain for several months, the failed transplant represents a crisis for the patient and family. Loss of the transplanted kidney may provoke depression and feelings of hopelessness, anger, and worthlessness. Individuals may experience a grieving process similar to the process described by those experiencing death. Emotional support is essential for these patients. If a patient has a failed transplant, retransplant is an option. The patient will need to undergo a pretransplant workup. An evaluation of how well the patient took care of his or her failed transplant as well as compliance with appointments and the medication regimen will also be assessed. The dialysis staff should encourage the patient to seek another transplant if appropriate.

CHAPTER 21

PEDIATRIC DIALYSIS

Children on long-term dialysis have a variety of social, cognitive, and nutritional needs in additional to their clinical issues. Treatment of children is complicated by the fact that they are still growing and developing, and chronic kidney disease (CKD) interferes with this normal growth and development. Therefore, pediatric nephrology nurses must have a comprehensive knowledge of pediatric nursing and childhood growth and development. Dialysis initiation should be considered for the pediatric patient when the glomerular filtration rate (GFR) is <15 mL/min/1.73 m^2 (National Kidney Foundation [NKF], 2006). End-stage renal disease (ESRD) is rare in children with approximately 1500 children developing the disease annually with a prevalence rate of 8500 children in the United States today (Deepa, 2017).

What Are the Causes of Chronic Kidney Disease in Children?

The causes of CKD in children are different from those in adults. The leading causes of ESRD in children and adolescents are glomerular disease (22.3%); CAKUT (congenital anomalies of the kidney and urinary tract; 21.9%); cystic, hereditary, or congenital disorders (11.7%); and secondary glomerular disease or vasculitis (10.7%). The most common individual diagnosis include focal glomerulosclerosis, renal hypoplasia or dysplasia, congenital obstructive uropathies, systemic lupus erythematosus, and unspecified kidney failure (United States Renal Data System [USRDS], 2017).

Unlike CKD in adults, diabetic nephropathy, chronic hypertension (HTN), autosomal dominant polycystic kidney disease, and membranous glomerulonephritis are rarely causes of CKD in childhood and adolescence.

What Are the Causes of Acute Kidney Injury in Children?

Acute kidney injury (AKI) in children usually results from hypoperfusion of the kidneys because of septic shock, hypotension, and severe dehydration from gastroenteritis or from acute blood loss because of surgery or an accident.

The pathology is that of acute tubular necrosis (ATN). ATN can also occur after treatment with nephrotoxic drugs, especially aminoglycoside antibiotics and amphotericin B. The most common cause of primary AKI in children in North America is hemolytic uremic syndrome. Acute poststreptococcal glomerulonephritis, although common in children, rarely leads to AKI severe enough to warrant dialysis.

Who Makes Up the Pediatric Interdisciplinary Team?

The pediatric interdisciplinary team (IDT) differs somewhat from the adult IDT and includes a nephrologist, dialysis registered nurse, social worker, dietitian, child life specialist, teacher, psychologist, urologist, surgeon, and vascular access surgeon. It is ideal when the team has experience in both the speciality and also in pediatric care. The family will play an integral part in the care-making decisions for the patient.

What Are the Staffing Considerations for a Pediatric Dialysis Population?

The hybrid services that a pediatric dialysis facility provides necessitate a good method of matching resources to patient workload activity. Staffing considerations should take into account factors such as developmental age versus chronological age along with the frequency and intensity of interventions required. Because of the many pediatric patient–dependency categories, staffing requirements for pediatric care comprise a complex matrix that is most easily implemented with a staffing and scheduling system that targets staffing by skill level. As a patient's dependency level increases, increased caregiver skills are usually required. The system must also recognize the potential for day-to-day variation in an individual child's care requirements and in the staff required to provide that care. Determining staffing by matching caregiver-to-patient ratios to patient ages or sizes can be a disadvantage because ratios presume that all patients of the same age or weight necessarily require the same level of care every day. Staffing ratios are mandated by various certifying organizations and agencies. Patient care technicians are prohibited from caring for pediatric dialysis patients weighing less than 35 kg. If the patient is less than 10 kg or in isolation, a one-to-one nurse-to-patient ratio is required. For patients 10 to 20 kg, a one-to-two ratio is acceptable, and a one-to-three ratio is allowed for children weighing more than 20 kg. Pediatric dialysis requires attentiveness and more frequent monitoring of hemodynamics. Children may not be able to verbalize or communicate their needs when a complication may arise during the dialysis treatment, so close visual monitoring as are vital sign monitoring are critical.

How Is a Modality Selected for Children Who Require Maintenance Dialysis?

The preferred modality of treatment for most pediatric patients who require maintenance dialysis is kidney transplantation. Modality selection is individualized to fit the lifestyle and health-related needs of both the patient and family. Patient size and additional comorbidities are also considered when selecting a modality for maintenance dialysis. Children initiate dialysis most often with hemodialysis (HD; 51%); however, peritoneal dialysis (PD; 25.7%) is used to a greater extent than in adults requiring maintenance dialysis. If a pediatric patient needs chronic dialysis, home PD is the usual choice but may not always be possible. Some family situations are unable to support chronic PD. Some patients may have lost peritoneal function from previous abdominal surgery or peritonitis. Currently, younger children, including infants and toddlers with CKD, who have failed PD and are not yet eligible for transplantation or who are waiting on the deceased donor transplantation list require chronic HD. USRDS found that in 2016, 72% of prevalent patients had a functioning kidney transplant followed by 17.2% receiving HD, and the remaining 10.6% on PD (USRDS, 2017). PD provides many benefits to infants, children, and adolescents such as preservation of residual kidney function, fewer dietary restrictions, avoidance of a vascular access, and less disruption to school and home activities. HD in a chronic setting is a good choice for those who lack the technical capacity to perform this modality at home and for those wanting a shorter treatment time (Warady, Neu, & Schaefer, 2014).

Technical advances in equipment and vascular access catheters have made chronic HD possible even in small children. Some adolescents may choose HD because of concerns about body image or their ability to comply with the discipline of chronic PD and the need for daily treatment.

WHAT IS THE SIGNIFICANCE OF BODY SURFACE AREA TO KIDNEY FUNCTION IN PEDIATRICS?

Normal serum creatinine level increases with age and body mass. The normal serum creatinine level in a 2-year-old child is 0.4 mg/dL, whereas that in an adult is about 1.0 mg/dL. A level of 1.0 mg/dL in a 2-year-old child would indicate kidney failure, with about 60% reduction in kidney function. To compare the parameters of kidney function in different-sized pediatric patients from infancy to adolescence, creatinine clearance and other measures of the glomerular filtration rate are usually normalized to the average adult BSA of 1.73 m^2. The normal range for creatinine clearance in a pediatric patient older than 2 years is 100 to 120 mL/min/1.73 m^2. When the creatinine clearance decreases to less than 10 mL/min/1.73 m^2, the pediatric patient has stage 5 CKD.

WHAT IS THE DIALYSIS PRESCRIPTION FOR HEMODIALYSIS AND PERITONEAL DIALYSIS?

Peritoneal Dialysis

The fill volume for PD is based on BSA, and the target volume is 1000 to 1200 mL/m^2 for patients 2 years of age or older and 600 to 800 mL/m^2 for children younger than 2 years of age. As children age up to adolescence, the fill volume can incrementally be raised up to 1200 to 1400 mL/m^2 for overnight dwell times, keeping in consideration patient tolerance and degree of intraperitoneal pressure. The standard automated peritoneal dialysis (APD) prescription is 5 to 10 cycles delivered over 9 to 12 hours overnight. The Kidney Disease Outcomes Quality Initiative (KDOQI) recommends the minimal "delivered" dose of small-solute clearance should be a peritoneal Kt/V$_{urea}$ of at least 1.8/wk.

Hemodialysis

The volume of the extracorporeal circuit is a consideration when dialyzing infants and children. The extracorporeal volume should be maintained at less than 10% of the patient's blood volume to maintain hemodynamic stability. Current KDOQI guidelines recommend a thrice weekly single-pool Kt/V of 1.2 for conventional dialysis (Warady, Neu, & Schaefer, 2014).

WHAT IS THE SAFE LIMIT FOR THE EXTRACORPOREAL VOLUME IN A CHILD?

The safe limit for the extracorporeal volume in a child is 10% or less of the child's blood volume (Table 21.1). This blood is returned to the patient at the end of the treatment unless it is needed for laboratory tests. In this case, no more than 3% to 5% of the child's blood volume should be removed on a given day. Many laboratories have microcontainers for sampling blood from small children or use minimal blood volumes for tests to help avoid excess blood loss in pediatric patients.

HOW DOES ONE CALCULATE THE EXTRACORPOREAL VOLUME?

Extracorporeal volume is the total volume of the dialyzer plus the bloodlines. Specific values are available from product manufacturers.

WHAT ARE THE VASCULAR ACCESS CONSIDERATIONS IN PEDIATRICS?

The smaller the pediatric patient, the more difficult it will be to establish adequate access for HD. In patients weighing less than 10 kg, placing an indwelling catheter of appropriate diameter in a major vessel is the only option. It is important to

Table 21.1 Approximate Blood Volume by Age

AGE	TOTAL BLOOD VOLUME (mL/K)
Premature infants	90–105g
Term newborns	78–86
>1 mo–1 yr	78
>1 yr–adult	74–82
Adult	68–78

ensure that the catheter does not approach or exceed the vessel size because this will lead to obstruction of normal venous flow. Double- and single-lumen cuffed catheters are now available for even very small children (5–10 kg in body weight). Blood vessel preservation is crucial, and the NKF KDOQI recommend using an arteriovenous (AV) fistula or graft for patients weighing 20 kg or more. An AV loop graft in the thigh may be possible for patients weighing more than 10 kg, and a primary AV fistula in the forearm may be possible for patients weighing more than 15 kg if a skilled pediatric access surgeon is involved. In general, permanent access is extremely difficult when the patient weighs less than 20 kg and should be placed only by a surgeon or pediatric nephrologist skilled in these procedures. Exceptions to placing a permanent vascular access would be if the patient weighs less than 20 kg, is scheduled to receive a kidney transplant within the next 2 years, or if HD is serving as a bridge to PD as a modality.

Do Children Require Special Dialyzers?

When choosing a dialyzer for a pediatric HD patient, the dialyzer surface area (available from the product manufacturer) often approximates the child's BSA. Dialyzers as small as 0.22 m² are available. The type chosen should be based on the blood volume of the dialyzer as well as the prescription for dialysis adequacy and ultrafiltration (UF) coefficient. Hollow-fiber dialyzers are preferred because of their low compliance and can have priming volumes of 28 ml to 100 ml, depending on the size.

Are There Special Pediatric Bloodlines?

Bloodlines for neonatal or pediatric patients are extremely limited in availability and selection. The bloodlines used for children offer a substantial decrease in the volume over adult lines. Neonatal bloodlines may have a volume as small as 29 ml and pediatric bloodlines about 73 ml compared to adult bloodlines which approximate 140 ml. Because these specialized bloodlines tend to be shorter, caution should be exercised to secure the lines so that there is no tension on the patient's access site to prevent an accidental disconnect.

Are There Hemodialysis Machines Specifically for Children?

Volumetric HD equipment used for adults can be safely used for children. Volumetric equipment decreases the margin of error for fluid removal. Note that all HD system manufacturers warn of the potential variance from the fluid removal target of 10%, which is especially important in small patients in whom 10% can be a substantial amount compared with the patient's total body water.

How Is Pain Associated with Hemodialysis Managed in Children?

For the discomfort of fistula needle insertion, pain management options include topical anesthetics or subcutaneous 1% lidocaine at the needle insertion site. Some children find topical anesthetics ineffective and consider subcutaneous 1% lidocaine "just another stick." For these patients, fistula needle insertion without an anesthetic may be the best-tolerated option. Additional pain management techniques include deep breathing, distraction (e.g., blowing bubbles or inverting a glitter wand), or visual imagery, such as focusing on a soft-colored light. Remember that crying is a normal response to pain or fear of a needle before there is pain. The key to pain management success is a consistent approach and good communication with the patient and family. The team should take every opportunity to soothe anxieties, offer an array of pain management options, and positively reinforce desired behaviors such as holding still.

If a child must be immobilized for needle insertion, minimize the number of personnel involved and focus on immobilizing the child's joints to prevent movement that will interfere with successful needle placement. Children who weigh less than 10 kg are best swaddled. Only rarely should a child require restraints and only for a short time period. When restraint is deemed necessary, a medical order should be written and refreshed with each HD treatment for which restraint is used.

Is Sequential Ultrafiltration Used in Children?

Ultrafiltration is appropriate only in older children and adolescents. Small infants requiring 5% albuminized saline or reconstituted whole blood prime should not undergo sequential UF. Prolonged UF in a small child can lead to hypothermia because the blood compartment will not be warmed by the dialysis fluid.

How Does One Determine the Target Weight for a Child Undergoing Hemodialysis?

If the patient is growing, his or her weight should gradually increase. The target weight is the weight at which a patient with an adequate dialysis clearance is normotensive and euvolemic. Noninvasive in-line monitoring devices, such as Crit-Line, can help to refine target weight determinations during dialysis treatment. In growing children, the target weight should be reassessed at least monthly or more often when indicated by HTN. Fluctuations in weight can occur frequently in children because of changes in dietary intake, compliance with fluid restrictions, or vomiting and diarrhea. Chronic fluid overload in children may masquerade as false weight gain and mislead even experienced dialysis nurses.

What Is the Optimal Blood Flow Rate for a Pediatric Hemodialysis Patient?

The optimal blood flow rate (Qb) is a function of what the access will allow as well as the body size of the patient. Care must be taken to maintain a blood flow rate that will not compromise cardiac stability. An optimal blood flow is usually not higher than 10% of blood volume in milliliters per minute (Skorecki et al, 2016).

How Does Intradialytic Monitoring Differ in Children?

The advent of volumetric HD equipment has made the procedure much safer in children. Blood pressure (BP) monitoring intervals should match the individual patient's care requirements. BP should always be measured immediately after initiating HD and every 30 minutes thereafter. When a patient is perceived to be unstable, monitoring should be increased. Resist the urge to take BP measurements every 15 minutes just because the patient is a child. The child may become agitated and uncooperative, creating technical difficulty in obtaining reliable readings. Monitors designed to noninvasively and automatically measure systolic and diastolic pressure, mean arterial pressure, and pulse rate for neonatal or pediatric patients are effective and versatile. These continue to monitor during most clinical crises when other indirect measurement methods may fail. Acute HD treatments in unstable patients nearly always require continuous arterial pressure monitoring for safety.

In addition to BP measurement in patients weighing less than 20 kg, continuous monitoring of heart rate (electrocardiography) and oxygenation (pulse oximeter) is required to detect deterioration in the patient's condition, which is most often related to acute fluid removal. Continuous nursing assessment is also needed to detect subtle changes of impending hypotension, such as irritability, yawning, or fidgety movements. Because these subtle signs vary from patient to patient, their inclusion in an individual patient's plan of care will facilitate communication of a particular patient's care to the entire team.

Do Children Ever Require Isolation?

Communicable diseases, such as varicella (chickenpox), are common in childhood. In addition to isolation for blood-borne pathogens, children may need to be isolated during periods when they are at a risk of manifesting communicable diseases after recent exposure. Each facility should develop general recommendations for isolating children exposed to communicable diseases such as varicella to avoid exposure of susceptible adults and patients in the dialysis unit.

What Is High Blood Pressure in Children?

Kidney parenchymal disease and structural abnormalities account for nearly 34% to 76% of secondary HTN in children, and 12% to 13% are caused by vascular diseases of the kidney. The subcommittee on the Screening and Management of High Blood Pressure in Children recommend the following guidelines for children and adolescents with Chronic Kidney Disease:[a]

- Children and adolescents with CKD should be evaluated for HTN at each medical encounter.
- Children or adolescents with both CKD and HTN should be treated to lower 24-hour mean arterial pressure by less than the 50th percentile by ambulatory blood pressure monitoring (APBM).
- Children and adolescents with CKD and a history of HTN should have BP assessed by ABPM at least annually to screen for masked HTN, even with apparent control with office visits.

The committee defines elevated BP as a BP above the 90th percentile in children 1 to 18 years of age (Table 21.2). BP differs by gender and increases with age and size, so the parameters for HTN differ from those for adults. Girls and shorter children have slightly lower BPs than boys and taller children at a given age. BP must be taken with an appropriately sized cuff, the air-filled bladder of which should have a width equal to approximately 40% of the circumference of the arm, measured at a point midway between the olecranon and acromion, and a length sufficient to extend around the arm, covering at least 80% of the circumference. Cuff size is not standardized by industry, so the label "infant," "child," or "small adult" on the cuff should be disregarded, and the above parameters should be followed for proper sizing. If the

Table 21.2 Updated Definitions of Blood Pressure Categories and Stages

FOR CHILDREN AGED 1–13 YEARS	FOR CHILDREN AGED 13 YEARS AND OLDER
Normal BP: <90th percentile	Normal BP: <120/<80 mm Hg
Elevated BP: ≥90th percentile to <95th percentile or 120/80 mm Hg to <95th percentile (whichever is lower)	Elevated BP: 120/<80–129/<80 mm Hg
Stage 1 HTN: ≥95th percentile to <95th percentile + 12 mm Hg or 130/80–139/89 mm Hg (whichever is lower)	Stage 1 HTN: 130/80–139/89 mm Hg
Stage 2 HTN: 95th percentile + 12 mm Hg or ≥140/90 mm Hg (whichever is lower)	Stage 2 HTN: ≥140/90 mm Hg

BP, Blood pressure; *HTN*, hypertension.
Reprinted with permission from Flynn JT, Kaelber DC, Baker-Smith CM, et al: Clinical practice guideline for screening and management of high blood pressure in children and adolescents [published correction appears in *Pediatrics* 140(6):e20173035, 2017]. *Pediatrics* 140(3): e20171904, 2017.

---

[a]Key Action Statement 23: *Chronic Kidney Disease, Clinical Practice Guidelines for screening and management of high blood pressure in children and adolescents*, 2017.

cuff is too small, the BP measurement will be falsely high. An oversized adult cuff or large thigh cuff is needed for obese adolescents.

What Is the Significance of Latex in the Pediatric Hemodialysis Setting?

Certain groups of children are at a high risk of developing latex allergy. Children with spina bifida or urologic disorders and those who have frequent medical procedures are at risk. Other children who require clean intermittent urinary catheterization are also at a high risk. Repeated exposure to latex products is purported to be a significant risk factor that can trigger a reaction, which can begin as contact urticaria or can be as dramatic as an anaphylactic reaction. There are two basic exposure routes: direct mucosal contact and airborne latex particles. Treatment of latex allergy is best directed toward preventing exposure to the numerous items that contain latex, such as gloves and catheters. In addition to identifying pediatric patients at risk, each facility should develop protocols for latex precautions.

How Does Anemia Management Differ in Children?

Two multicenter trials have shown that pediatric patients younger than 5 years frequently require initial recombinant human erythropoietin at higher doses than those required by older pediatric patients and adults. Achieving target iron levels to support erythropoiesis requires administration of either oral or intravenous (IV) supplemental iron. KDOQI recommends oral iron (or IV iron in CKD HD patients) administration when the transferrin saturation (TSAT) is 20% or less and ferritin is 100 ng/mL or less for pediatric patients with anemia and not on erythropoietin-stimulating agent (ESA) therapy. For pediatric patients on ESA therapy, the recommendation is oral iron (or IV iron in CKD HD patients) to maintain the TSAT above 20% and ferritin above 100 ng/mL (Kliger et al, 2013). When administering IV iron dextran, heed the differences in pediatric test doses, for patients weighing less than 10 kg and for those weighing 10 to 20 kg, and pediatric dosing by body weight. The 2006 NFK KDOQI clinical practice guidelines note the differences in anemia management in children and are a good guideline to follow for pediatric care. The dose of ESA will vary depending on the patient's treatment modality, route of administration, and age. The NKF guidelines recommend that evaluation for anemia should begin when hemoglobin levels fall below the fifth percentile for age and sex, recognizing that hemoglobin differentiation between boys and girls is minimal between gender before girls reach menarche (NFK, 2013). The hemoglobin goal for children is the same as that for adults (11–12 g/dL) and should not exceed 13.0 g/dL. (See Appendix A for additional information on NKF KDOQI.)

Why Are Children with Chronic Kidney Disease Short in Stature?

Growth retardation is a significant consequence of CKD in children; therefore, frequent monitoring of nutritional status is necessary to ensure the patient is reaching developmental goals. KDOQI suggests monitoring of children with CKD be performed twice as frequently as they would be performed in a healthy child of the same age. Infants and children experiencing polyuria, growth delay, those with a body mass index above or below safe levels, having comorbidities influencing growth or intake, and recent acute changes in medical status require more frequent monitoring (NKF, 2009). The age of onset is an important variable affecting growth: the younger the patient at the onset of CKD, the greater is the potential for growth retardation. Many factors contribute to poor growth, including chronic metabolic acidosis, sodium wasting and chronic dehydration, chronic fluid overload, poorly controlled osteodystrophy, anorexia and malnutrition from poor caloric intake, steroid therapy for underlying kidney disease control, and disturbances of normal growth hormone regulation. To best achieve normal or catch-up growth, efforts should be made to correct as many of these abnormalities as possible before the patient needs chronic dialysis.

How Can Growth Be Maximized in a Pediatric Dialysis Patient?

To maximize growth potential during chronic HD, efforts should continue to include correcting acidosis, minimizing fluid overload, controlling osteodystrophy of kidney failure, and promoting optimum nutrition and should include optimizing dialysis adequacy. Each patient's height and target weight should be monitored closely (at least every 3 months) until the bone growth plates close. Head circumference as well as the length and target weight should be measured in children younger than 3 years of age. Gender-specific growth charts should be maintained and plotted quarterly or more frequently if the patient is falling off his or her percentile on the growth chart. When height falls below the fifth percentile for age in a child more than 1 to 2 years old, initiation of recombinant human growth hormone therapy should be considered. Children with CKD are relatively resistant to normal levels of growth hormone, so supplementation can help to normalize their growth and improve muscle mass. The NKF KDOQI guidelines provide recommendations for the nutritional needs of children with CKD to include the dietary intake of sodium, potassium, calcium, phosphorous, and fat. Other topics include nutritional assessment, acid–base balance management, use of kinetic modeling, energy and protein intake, and vitamin and mineral requirements (NKF, 2008). It is important to monitor dietary intake, and parents and caretakers should be counseled on how to keep a food diary to include a 3-day diet record or three 24-hour dietary recall. Recombinant human growth hormone therapy should be considered in children with CKD stages 2 to 5 and those on dialysis, who are short in stature, with a potential for linear growth if growth failure persists beyond 3 months despite treatment of nutritional deficiencies and metabolic abnormalities (NKF, 2009).

Can Children Receiving Hemodialysis Treatments Attend School Regularly?

Most school-age children on HD are able to attend school regularly with their peers. Missing school is often related to hospitalizations or the HD treatment schedule. When scheduling HD, every attempt should be made to facilitate school attendance. School constitutes a framework for daily behavior that imposes discipline and regularities, skills that are essential to achieving adult independence and ultimately entering the job market.

WHAT ARE THE OPTIONS FOR MEASURING FUNCTIONAL STATUS IN CHILDREN?

Denver II developmental screening tests are easy to perform and are recommended for the assessment of children younger than 6 years of age. Developmental delays are common in this chronically ill population. Another functional status tool for older children is the Children's Health Questionnaire, which is the pediatric version of the Short Form 36.

HOW IS QUALITY OF LIFE ASSESSED IN PEDIATRIC PATIENTS WITH END-STAGE RENAL DISEASE?

The social worker is critical to help assess the pediatric patient's quality of life (QoL) as well as to work with family members to assure the special needs of the pediatric dialysis patient are being met. QoL assessment is required every 6 months after initiation of dialysis and then annually. Two tools used in this population are the Pediatric Quality of Life inventory and PedsQL 3.0 ESRD Module. There are different versions of the model based on the child's age (toddlers to young adults) to measure ESRD-specific health-related QoL.

WHEN DO CHILDREN TRANSITION TO ADULT CARE?

Optimally, early preparation should begin during the stage of late adolescence (ages 17–21 years), which is characterized by a teenager's ability to define future goals, make close and intimate friendships, and begin rapprochement with parents and other authoritative adults. During the stage of mid-adolescence (ages 14–17 years), a teenager is at the height of risk-taking behavior, peer conformity, poor future orientation, and parental conflict; this is a very difficult time to implement the transition to adult responsibilities. Some patients who are developmentally delayed may not be ready for transition at age 17 years. Transition preparation includes teaching self-care skills, such as taking responsibility for adhering to a medication schedule, arranging clinic visits, and arriving for treatments on time. Ideally, late preparation should also incorporate a visit to the adult dialysis center while accompanied by a trusted nurse or social worker. Actual transfer to adult care should occur between 18 and 21 years of age, depending on patient readiness, disease management, and availability of service. Being in an integrated pediatric and adult care facility should not preclude having the adolescent participate in a defined transition preparation program to ensure that the patient is ready for the demands of adult-oriented care.

CHRONIC KIDNEY DISEASE IN THE ELDERLY

Patients older than 65 years of age have the highest adjusted prevalence of end-stage renal disease (ESRD) in the United States. The incident rate is highest in the oldest group ($\geq$75 years); however, ESRD prevalence is a little lower in this group because of a higher mortality rate among the oldest patients (Fig. 22.1). Regardless of the treatment modality selected, some changes are required to adapt the therapy to the special needs of older adult patients. As will become clear during the course of this chapter, besides presenting some limitations, older adult patients bring certain assets to their treatment regimens. All maintenance dialysis treatment modalities are available to older adult patients, subject to the usual considerations such as an adequate vascular access or an intact peritoneal membrane.

ARE THE CAUSES OF CHRONIC KIDNEY DISEASE DIFFERENT IN OLDER ADULT PATIENTS?

Not really. The most common cause is nephrosclerosis secondary to either diabetes or hypertension. Causes such as chronic glomerulonephritis and pyelonephritis are as common in older adult patients as in younger patients, although there may be a slightly higher number of older adult patients with an "unknown" kidney diagnosis. (Biopsies are rarely performed in older adult patients with kidney failure of undetermined cause.)

HOW DO OLDER ADULT PATIENTS DIFFER FROM YOUNGER CHRONIC KIDNEY DISEASE PATIENTS?

Comorbid conditions are much more common in older adult patients and can complicate the treatment of chronic kidney disease (CKD). Examples of significant comorbidities include an impaired cardiovascular system, osteoporosis, type 2 diabetes, delayed protein synthesis, reduced protein intake, impaired pulmonary function, impaired cognitive function, poor vision, poor mobility, and poor coordination.

Although these are not physical factors, adverse psychosocial and socioeconomic factors complicate the treatment regimens for a larger proportion of older adult patients than younger patients.

CAN OLDER ADULT PATIENTS BENEFIT FROM KIDNEY REPLACEMENT THERAPY?

Many, perhaps most, older adult patients can benefit from kidney replacement therapy and often return to a level of physical functioning and quality of life (QoL) that is either equivalent to that of people their age without CKD or at least acceptable to the patient. Some older adult patients do not achieve an improvement in their QoL and may experience significant distress or disability with dialysis therapy. Treatment selection should take into account the patient's functional status, cognition, QoL, and social support. Some patients, usually but not necessarily older adults, may not benefit from treatment. Examples include those with irreversible dementia or extremely debilitating or imminently terminal comorbid conditions, such as cancer or advanced congestive heart failure. However, there are few firm medical or community standards with respect to withholding treatment, and decisions regarding initiating therapy vary among individual physicians or family members. Older adult patients and their significant others are often not informed of the high morbidity and mortality rates accompanying dialytic therapy. Additionally, physicians and social workers do not always discuss end-of-life issues with newly diagnosed ESRD patients.

CAN OLDER ADULT PATIENTS BE SUCCESSFULLY TRANSPLANTED?

Transplantation remains the treatment of choice for older adult CKD patients requiring maintenance dialysis. Transplantation provides increased survival and improved QoL in older adults compared with those on dialysis (Scherer & Bitzer, 2015). Although the proportion of older adult CKD patients who qualify for transplantation is not as high as that of younger patients, graft survival in those who do receive transplants is about the same. Kidneys are becoming more available to older adult recipients because some transplant surgeons believe that organs donated by an older person should go to another older person using the Kidney Donor Profile Index (see Chapter 20). Physical frailty, cardiovascular disease, infection risk, and malignancy are associate with less positive outcomes and require additional consideration. Older adult patients often require less intensive immunosuppressive therapy because their immune systems may already be compromised by age.

Although the survival of older adult patients is not as good as that of younger patients because of an increased number and severity of complications, data show satisfactory results for transplantation in older adult patients. By the same principle, dialysis is also safer than ever for older adult patients, so making a decision between modes of therapy is not simple.

WHAT ARE THE ADVANTAGES OF PERITONEAL DIALYSIS FOR OLDER ADULT PATIENTS?

Older adult patients benefit from being at home in a number of ways. First, they are spared the considerable time, effort, and expense of being transported to and from a dialysis center. The transportation effort is in itself very debilitating for some

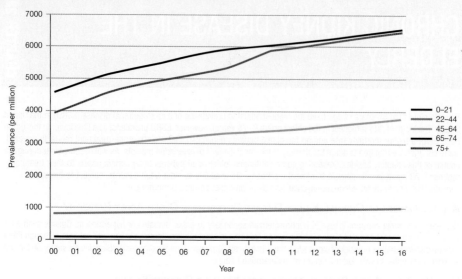

Fig. 22.1 Trends in the standardized prevalence of end-stage renal disease age group in the US population, 2000 to 2016. (United States Renal Data System. 2018 USRDS annual data report: Epidemiology of kidney disease in the United States. National Institutes of Health, National Institute of Diabetes and Digestive and Kidney Diseases, Bethesda, MD, 2018. Publications based on USRDS data reported in the Annual Data Report or on the USRDS web site or supplied upon request must include the above citation and the following notice: The data reported here have been supplied by the United States Renal Data System (USRDS). The interpretation and reporting of these data are the responsibility of the author(s) and in no way should be seen as an official policy or interpretation of the U.S. government.)

older adult patients. Second, home dialysis patients are in full charge of administering their own therapy. This not only fosters independence but also preserves their usual lifestyle, allowing patients to perform exchanges at their convenience, within reason, rather than requiring them to conform to a rigid in-center schedule.

PD patients do not need a vascular access with its attendant problems (although they must have a peritoneal access catheter with its attendant problems), and many older adult patients have inadequate peripheral vessels. Because PD is a continuous—or at least daily—therapy, blood chemistries and fluid statuses approach a steady state; thus PD patients do not suffer the effects of the rapid biochemical and fluid changes common in HD. This can be a significant advantage, because older adult patients are more prone to adverse reactions to these changes. For example, PD patients with diminished cardiac reserves experience less orthostatic hypotension or other cardiac symptoms in response to fluid removal. Slow, continuous therapy allows better correction of brain electrophysiological and cognitive function abnormalities, which incurs less risk of destabilizing the fragile mental equilibrium of some older adult patients.

Another advantage of daily therapy is that dietary and fluid restrictions are less rigid, which can be important for those with diminished appetites or impatience with restrictions. Despite the advantages of PD, only 6.0% of all prevalent patients older than 65 years use this modality (US Renal Data System [USRDS], 2016).

CAN OLDER ADULT PATIENTS LEARN HOW TO PERFORM PERITONEAL DIALYSIS?

Many older adult patients can perform PD very well by themselves, and others can perform PD with assistance from family members. PD is often underused in the older adult population because of the inability of the patient to perform the required PD exchanges due to functional or cognitive impairments. In addition, several assistive devices are available that allow all patients who are blind or who have limited dexterity to perform their own fluid exchanges. Automated overnight dialysis systems eliminate all but a single connection and disconnection procedure.

WHAT ARE THE DISADVANTAGES OF PERITONEAL DIALYSIS FOR OLDER ADULT PATIENTS?

The incidence of certain complications (dementia, hernia, *Staphylococcus epidermidis* peritonitis, abdominal and catheter leaks) is higher in older adult PD patients compared with younger PD patients and compared with older adult HD patients.

If the patient frequently requires significant ultrafiltration (UF), the resulting increased dialysate glucose concentration can significantly suppress the appetite, resulting in substantial malnutrition. This can be difficult to diagnose at least initially because the dry weight may be stable or even increase (dextrose provides many calories but little nutrition). This can be a special problem with older adult patients who are already at a higher risk of malnutrition. Kidney failure exacerbates malnutrition in older adult patients, and PD may cause significant protein losses in the dialysate. Along with the decreased appetite seen in older adult patients and the protein losses, the potential for malnutrition needs to be closely monitored.

Older adult patients experience some age-related changes in the peritoneal membrane, placing them at an increased risk of problems such as diverticulosis, bowel perforation, and constipation. Older adult patients may have also experienced other abdominal surgeries, increasing their risk of adhesions and abdominal wall leaks (Sakacı et al, 2015).

Loss of the opportunity to socialize during in-center therapy may also be a drawback to PD because many older adults are socially isolated.

What Are the Advantages of Hemodialysis for Treating Older Adult Patients with Chronic Kidney Disease?

Most HD in the United States is provided as an in-center therapy. There may be psychosocial advantages for older adult patients provided by human interactions during dialysis center treatment, as mentioned earlier.

Another advantage is frequent observation by trained personnel. Older adult patients are more prone to complications of both CKD and dialysis. When they develop such complications, these patients often exhibit less obvious symptoms. Earlier recognition and intervention (with resulting reductions in patient discomfort and health care costs) are more likely in a dialysis center setting.

Modern HD equipment, with its sophisticated monitoring and UF control systems, is better able to provide controlled rates of biochemical and fluid removal and thus safe and comfortable treatments for a larger range of older adult patients than was possible in the past. Some patients prefer short, thrice-weekly treatments rather than continuous dialysis, as with PD. Treatment "burnout" is less common in the HD population. Also, many older adult patients grew up in an era when physicians and nurses, rather than patients, were expected to provide health care. Self-treatment, whether in a dialysis center or at home, is not acceptable to every older adult person. Most older adult dialysis patients in the United States are undergoing HD.

Is Hemodialysis More Complicated for Older Adult Patients?

Some practitioners claim that older adult patients are easier to dialyze. They tend to have lower fluid gains, lower creatinine levels, and lower urea generation rates; thus, they do not necessarily require extremely aggressive treatment with its higher risk of intradialytic complications. Also, older adult patients are generally more compliant with all facets of the treatment regimen and express higher life satisfaction than younger patients.

With one exception, the nature and frequency of intradialytic complications are similar to those in younger HD patients. The exception is hemodynamic instability, which is more common in older adult people; thus, intradialytic cardiac arrhythmias and hypotensive episodes are likely in this group. In most cases, the episodes of hemodynamic instability can be minimized and often prevented if staff members are properly trained in the methods to achieve this.

Measures to prevent hypotensive episodes include using an extracorporeal circuit with the smallest possible priming volume; equipment with a volumetric UF control system; and a bicarbonate dialysate with sufficiently high sodium, calcium, and dextrose levels to help maintain blood pressure during UF. No patient, especially older adults, should be allowed to eat during dialysis because blood is diverted from the peripheral circulation (where it maintains blood pressure) to the digestive organs immediately after a meal. As a result, hypotension is usually inevitable. There is now ample evidence that a brief episode of simple exercise, especially if performed during the last hour of dialysis, is an effective way to support blood pressure and minimize muscle cramping. Dietary sodium, protein, and fluid intake and antihypertensive medication regimens should be reevaluated on a regular basis.

Arrhythmias are common in older adult HD patients and may not be associated with any detectable symptom. They arise in conjunction with anemia, hypokalemia, hyperkalemia, acidosis, hypoxia, hypotension, hypertension, digoxin use, or cardiac abnormalities caused, for example, by metastatic calcifications, amyloid deposition, or cardiac hypertrophy. Arrhythmias that are associated with symptoms such as weakness or hypoxia should be reported to the physician, who may elect to adjust the patient's diet, dialysate composition, or medication prescriptions. Nasal oxygen may provide symptomatic relief for hypoxia. Transfer to PD may be necessary, if feasible, for patients who do not respond to the aforementioned measures.

What Are the Disadvantages of Hemodialysis for Older Adult Patients?

As mentioned, patients with significant cardiovascular disease do not tolerate the rapid biochemical and hemodynamic changes that accompany HD procedures and are at a higher risk of intradialytic complications. As also mentioned, debilitated older adult patients undergo considerable physical and emotional stress in relation to the thrice-weekly transportation to and from the dialysis center. Patients in either group would probably do better with a daily home dialysis regimen, such as PD or daily home HD, if feasible. Older adult patients may also experience more vascular access problems.

It is important to realize that older adult patients whose comorbidities are no more severe than those seen in younger patients do as well as younger patients.

What Special Precautions Should Be Taken with Respect to Monitoring the Nutrition of Older Adult Patients?

All patients lose nutrients during dialysis, whether HD or PD. Compared with the general dialysis population, older adult patients are at a higher risk of malnutrition, in addition to being less likely to replace the nutrients lost during treatment. For this reason, staff must be able to recognize and regularly probe for factors that signal poor nutrition.

In addition to the usual impediments to good nutrition, older adults experience a number of losses that interfere with their ability to achieve good nutrition. There are physical losses such as loss of teeth and loss of senses of taste and smell that make eating difficult or uninteresting or loss of mobility that makes it difficult to get to the grocery store or prepare meals.

Mealtimes, often occasions for social interaction, can remind older adult patients of their social losses, such as the loss of a spouse, companions, or access to community support. Some patients have psychological conditions, such as dementia, depression, or simply mental inertia, which can impede their will to eat. Financial constraints can be a factor because many older adult people live on fixed incomes and may have to make choices between paying for heat or food, for example. Medical factors, such as anorexia, constipation, and medication effects, can interfere with eating. Even with adequate meals, there can still be nutritional losses because of vomiting, diarrhea, or loss of protein through persistent exudates from wounds or sores. Some of the factors that impede good nutrition can be corrected if they are recognized.

You should suspect malnutrition if the patient has an increase in the episodes of intradialytic hypotension or symptomatic congestive heart failure, develops depression or dementia, reports episodes suggestive of hypoglycemia (when not on hypoglycemic agents), experiences a steady decline in dry weight, or shows symptoms of adult failure-to-thrive syndrome.

A low predialysis blood urea nitrogen level is always caused by poor nutrition, not great dialysis. Resist the temptation to decrease dialysis; such patients usually need more dialysis, not less. By the same principle, patients who are unstable during dialysis should not be taken off treatment early. This leads to underdialysis, which decreases appetite, leading to lower plasma protein levels and, shortly, to even greater intradialytic instability.

The physician or dietitian should be contacted if any of the situations discussed in this section are identified.

What Are the Problems with Medications in Older Adult Patients with Chronic Kidney Disease?

Dialysis patients, especially older adults, are likely to take a great many drugs, also known as polypharmacy. Older adult patients are much more susceptible to drug reactions and interactions. Thus, the dose of each drug must be carefully calibrated by the physician, taking into consideration many factors common in older adult patients, such as poor intestinal absorption, impaired hepatic clearance, and alterations in distribution space. Various elements can alter a patient's response to the prescribed dosage or combination of drugs; therefore, any unexplained change in the physical or mental condition should be reported to the physician.

However, the main issue for staff is to check with the patient on a regular basis if he or she is having problems taking all of the prescribed medications and to be alert to the possibility of polypharmacy, which is the tendency of some older adults to see several physicians and, unknown to the physicians, acquire multiple prescriptions from each.

What Are the Outcomes of Various Chronic Kidney Disease Treatment Modalities in Older Adult Patients?

In terms of treatment selection, the most recent information available (USRDS, 2018) offered the following statistics as of the end of 2011: 73% of US patients aged 65 years or older were receiving in-center HD, fewer than 1% were undergoing home HD, 6% were undergoing PD, and 20% had a functioning transplant.

The mortality rates for prevalent dialysis patients aged 65 years and older are almost seven times higher than those for the general population. The rates have been decreasing over the past 5 years. Among dialysis patients aged 65 years and older, the mortality rate is twice as high as that for patients in the general population with diabetes, cancer, congestive heart failure, cerebrovascular accident or transient ischemic attack, or acute myocardial infarction. Mortality rates among ESRD patients increase with age, as expected. Dialysis patients 80 years old or younger are expected to live less than one third as long as their counterparts without ESRD, and dialysis patients 85 years and older are expected to live around half as long as their counterparts without ESRD. Male dialysis patients older than the age of 75 years experienced mortality rates 3.7 times higher than their peers, and the mortality rate for female dialysis patients was 3.8 times higher (USRDS, 2018). There is an overall improvement in the mortality rates of patients aged 65 years and older, and this may reflect improvements in maintenance dialysis therapies and experience with treating older adult CKD patients.

CHAPTER 23

CASE MANAGEMENT OF THE CHRONIC KIDNEY DISEASE PATIENT

The diagnosis of chronic kidney disease (CKD) provides numerous challenges for patients and families who must navigate the complexities associated with this chronic illness. CKD and its requisite treatment can be very costly and time consuming, placing a burden on the patient, family, and health plan. Patients on maintenance dialysis typically have multiple morbidities such as diabetes, hypertension, bone disease, anemia, cardiovascular disease, and malnutrition. Both end-stage renal disease (ESRD) and advanced CKD patients are cared for by a myriad of physicians and other health care providers. Many times little to no coordination takes place between the patient and her or his care providers. This fragments the care received by the patient, causing confusion, increasing the potential for duplication of services, and adding to overall health care expenditures. Another untoward effect is the potential for adverse medication events caused by several health care providers ordering different dosages of the same medications. The care team at a dialysis center commonly spends approximately 15 hours per week with each ESRD patient as they receive their dialysis treatments. This can provide a good opportunity to activate patients in their care and to address dialysis and non–dialysis-related issues and needs, including mental health and social determinants of health. Although dialysis and kidney-related issues cannot be overlooked, so too must mental and social factors be addressed in the plan of care because they impact the patient's overall health and well-being.

Patients receiving Medicare assistance for their dialysis and kidney related services comprise fewer than 1% of the Medicare population and accounted for at least 7.2% of total Medicare spending, accounting for more than $35.4 billion Medicare (United States Renal Data System [USRDS], 2017). A kidney disease management program takes a patient-centric approach and provides a plan of care with targeted interventions and self-management activities along with an emphasis on coordination of care and communication with other health care providers. Care coordination has many benefits, including improved quality of care and clinical outcomes, increased patient satisfaction, decreased emergency department (ED) utilization, and fewer hospitalizations and readmissions, all of which significantly decrease overall medical costs and increase patient health care–related quality of life (QoL).

Most kidney disease management programs focus on the mid to late stage CKD or on patients already undergoing kidney replacement therapy. This chapter looks at the goals of kidney disease management for both patients on maintenance dialysis and patients not yet on dialysis therapy.

WHAT IS CASE MANAGEMENT?

Case management is a collaborative process that assesses, plans, implements, coordinates, monitors, and evaluates the options and services required to meet the client's health and human service needs. It is characterized by advocacy, communication, and resource management and promotes quality and cost-effective interventions and outcomes. Retrieved from https://ccmcertification.org/about-ccmc/about-case-management/definition-and-philosophy-case-management.

Patient advocacy is promoted through communication and the use of other resources to promote quality and cost-effective outcomes (Case Management Society of America, 2016, p. 8). Successful case management involves collaboration between the patient and health care providers, patient involvement in the management of their self-care, and health coaching and patient empowerment. Case management is holistic because it addresses the patient's medical, psychosocial, behavioral and spiritual needs while motivating the patient to engage in self-care activities and decision making whenever possible. Case management seeks to defragment care by involving and collaborating with the entire interdisciplinary team. An emphasis is placed on transitions of care as well as the promotion of medication and plan of care adherence to move the patient to an optimal level of health and improved QoL.

WHAT IS THE ROLE OF THE RENAL CASE MANAGER?

Case management of patients with CKD is practiced across a variety of settings with various degrees of complexity and intensity. Most disease management programs risk stratify eligible members as high, medium, low, or rising risk by using health care claims and laboratory studies information. The number and types of comorbid conditions, psychosocial difficulties, and lifestyle risk factors such as smoking and obesity may be factored into some models. After a patient is stratified, the appropriate level of care can be provided with interventions and resources customized based on level of intensity and patient risk. CKD case managers practice in an ambulatory or outpatient care setting, or remotely, with the use of telecommunication technologies. Other CKD case managers visit the patient in her or his home if part of the contract of the particular health plan. Kidney disease case managers manage patients through all stages of CKD and when on kidney replacement therapy. After being enrolled in a kidney disease management program, the patient is assigned a nurse manager specific to the kidney disease stage. The CKD case manager will work with enrolled members and initiate a plan of care after a thorough patient assessment.

A thorough needs assessment of the patient is made from the following target areas:

- **Activities of daily living (ADLs).** The patient is assessed to determine if he or she can perform activities necessary for independent living at home. The Katz Index of Independence in Activities of Daily Living is one tool that can be used to assess the patient's functional status (Wallace & Shelkey, 2008). Categories assessed include personal hygiene, dressing, eating, continence, and transferring or mobility. Patients may require family or caregiver assistance. The results of an ADL screening are reflective of a patient's cognitive, motor, and perceptual skills and abilities. The CKD case manager can make referrals as necessary for home health assistance if indicated.

- **Access management.** The goal for all patients is to have a permanent vascular access after maintenance dialysis is initiated. This requires coaching patients predialysis to select a suitable modality, whether it is hemodialysis or peritoneal dialysis, and after it has been selected, having the appropriate permanent access placed. This helps the patient have a smooth transition from CKD to the need for maintenance dialysis.

- **Advance care planning.** Advance care planning is the process of thinking about and determining preferences for future health care decisions and life-prolonging treatment preferences if the need arises. Identification of a health care proxy or medical power of attorney is a part of the process of advance care planning. Patients sometimes require guidance on selecting a suitable agent who will ensure the patient's wishes are respected when she or he can no longer speak for her- or himself. Advance care planning should be included throughout all stages of CKD because patients with kidney disease have a shortened life expectancy and a high burden of symptoms (Moran, 2018). Living wills should be revisited when the patient has a change in health status and at transitions of care at a minimum. Case managers are in a prime position to engage patients in conversation involving their thoughts about future medical care and their wishes when the time comes when they are unable to make medical decisions for themselves. The positive relationship between the patient and the CKD case manager facilitates the partnership necessary to introduce and discuss advance care planning. It is important to be familiar with the specific documents required by the state where the patient resides because differences exist in the documentation and process of living wills and advance care planning.

- **Caregiver support.** Many patients with CKD rely on family and friends to help manage and support their medical care. Often family dynamics change when a friend or family member has a chronic illness. The physiological, psychological, and functional changes imposed by CKD may result in strain, isolation, and sometimes anger in the caregiver. *Caregiver burden* is a general term describing the emotional, physical, and stress experienced by caregivers as a result of providing care (Mashayekhi, 2015). A caregiver burden questionnaire can be administered to those in that supportive role to identify caregiver strengths or areas of stress. The CKD case manager can assist in finding resources where gaps in caregiver skills or abilities may exist. A variety of caregiver assessment tools and measures may be used to target specific areas of burden the caregiver may experience. Some states have specific measurement tools that can be used for caregiver assessment.

- **Cognitive function.** Cognitive function is commonly impaired in patients with CKD and increases in prevalence with severity of the disease. Cognitive impairment can impact patient adherence with treatment plans and can decrease overall QoL (Weiner & Seliger, 2014). Cognitive impairment may be manifested by diminished memory, concentration, and attention span, confusion, and disorientation. Early screening helps to establish a baseline so that deviations may be promptly identified and interventions initiated to minimize the impact on the patient's ADLs and QoL.

- **Comorbid management.** Patients with CKD develop other diseases that either cause CKD or contribute to their overall health-related QoL. The prevalence and severity of comorbidities increase as CKD progresses. An increased number of morbidities is associated with greater medication burden and poorer survival (Fraser, 2015). Treatment of comorbidities can help to delay the progression of CKD and decrease cardiovascular events of all patients. Malnutrition, diabetes, hypertension, anemia, cardiovascular disease, depression, and osteoporosis are just a few comorbidities associated with CKD. Early identification and collaborative care with primary or other specialized health care providers can help to improve kidney and cardiovascular outcomes.

- **Depression and behavioral health.** Depression and other behavioral health conditions are associated with a poorer QoL and can accelerate mortality among the CKD population. Depression is highly prevalent and can be attributed to the psychosocial and biological changes that accompany the disease process and kidney replacement therapy. Two commonly used depression screening tools used for patients with CKD or ESRD are the Patient Health Questionnaire (PHQ-9) and the Beck Depression Inventory (BDI). More information on the psychosocial aspects of living with CKD can be found in Chapter 24.

- **Diabetes management.** Almost half of all CKD patients have diabetes (National Institutes of Health, 2016). The CKD case manager assists patients to self-manage their diabetes to prevent complications such as heart attack, stroke, blindness, and limb amputations. Key self-care behaviors include daily blood sugar monitoring and HbA_{1c} monitoring, blood pressure monitoring, foot and eye examinations, medication compliance, and physical activity.

- **Environment, home safety, and fall risk.** Falls are a concern for older adults as well as those with a chronic disease. One of every four older Americans reported a fall in 2014, making falls the leading cause of injuries among those 65 years of age and older (Centers for Disease Control and Prevention, 2016). Falls place a major social, psychological, and financial burden on the patient as well as their caregivers (Paliwal, 2017), and an even greater concern is the risk of a hospital admission. Risk factors for falls include age-related changes, cognitive and sensory deficits, gait or strength deficits, certain medications such as psychoactive medications, use of assistive devices, and environmental factors in the home.

It is important to assess home safety to ensure the patient has well-lit hallways and walkways, clutter-free living areas, handrails on stairwells, and grab bars near the toilet and bathtub and that the patient wears firm shoes. Other important areas of assessment include stairs into and in the home, the presence of fire and smoke detectors, accessible phone and emergency phone numbers, and functional and safe durable medical equipment such as wheelchairs and walkers. Medication storage can be part of a safety assessment because medications stored under improper conditions such as heat, light, air, or moisture can impact the potency of the drugs. Patients should be advised to notify their health care practitioners after a fall even if they do not have an obvious injury. A variety of fall risk assessment tools are available to use, but regardless of the tool used, it is important to involve the patent, family, and interdisciplinary team.

- **Fluid management.** Fluid-related admissions represent a significant driver of cardiovascular-related hospitalization rates in those on dialysis, with an estimated annual cost of $250 million (Assimon, 2016). Fluid management is a critical part of the case manager's assessment to identify patients whose fluid status indicates the need for intervention to avoid a fluid-related hospitalization. The case manager can assist the member with fluid management strategies and engage the patient in self-management to help control fluid intake and treatment adherence. Coaching the patient on completing full hemodialysis sessions or peritoneal dialysis treatments is essential to avoid preventable fluid-related admissions.

- **Medication management.** Medication problems are common in patients with CKD. Patients with CKD have a high incidence of nonadherence and a lack of knowledge of reasons for taking medications, dosing, and monitoring (Galura & Pai, 2017). Risk factors for medication mismanagement include age, multiple comorbidities, polypharmacy, and frequency of dosing. CKD case managers conduct regularly scheduled comprehensive medication interviews with patients. Medication interviews should also take place when the patient's medical condition changes or after a hospitalization.

After the patient needs assessment is complete, the case manager will help the patient identify pertinent goals and create a plan of care that will result in maintaining or optimizing the patient's health and QoL. Care plans include interventions or actions that can reasonably be accomplished by the patient or responsible care team member.

WHAT ARE SOME INTERVENTIONS THE CHRONIC KIDNEY DISEASE CASE MANAGER CAN TAKE TO SLOW THE PROGRESSION OF CHRONIC KIDNEY DISEASE?

Case managers will implement plans of care to help delay the progression of CKD and prevent other complications such as cardiovascular disease. These may include nutritional and lifestyle modifications as well as interventions to control blood pressure, blood glucose, and albuminuria. The CKD case manager works with the health care team to monitor for other comorbidities such as dyslipidemias, anemia, malnutrition, and mineral and bone disorders. Patients may need education on dietary modifications such as limiting sodium use to help control blood pressure. Some patients are placed on a lower protein diet to help reduce proteinuria, which may help to slow the progression of CKD. It is especially important to monitor for malnutrition when placed on a protein restriction and when the GFR declines. The CKD case manager should monitor the patient's GFR and assist the patient with limiting phosphorus-containing foods as well as foods higher in potassium content when ordered by the physician.

Lifestyle modifications to help delay the progression of CKD include assisting the patient with smoking cessation and encouraging physical activity as tolerated to support blood pressure control. The case manager coaches the patient to monitor blood glucose and promotes glycemic control through diet and medication adherence. And finally, the case manager works with and coordinates with other providers to ensure the patient receives CKD education well in advance of the need for maintenance therapy to avoid crashing into dialysis.

The term "crash into dialysis" is used when a patient begins dialysis without prior planning or education. This may include not having any formal or informal education on CKD, modality, or access education and not having an assigned nephrologist involved in his care. These patients typically have their first dialysis treatment in an acute care setting with a temporary central venous catheter as opposed to a permanent access such as an arteriovenous fistula or graft. Patients who "crash" into dialysis often have poor outcomes and higher mortality rates (Molnar et al, 2016). Requisite guidance to prevent this includes providing treatment and access education once a modality is selected or referral for a transplant workup if applicable. Patients are positioned best if they are fully prepared for their treatment modality when the glomerular filtration rate falls and uremic symptoms indicate the need to initiate dialysis.

WHAT IS A SPECIAL NEEDS PLAN?

A Special Needs Plan (SNP) is a Medicare Advantage Plan that limits members to those with a specific disease type or chronic conditions such as ESRD, HIV, cancer, dementia, diabetes mellitus, drug dependencies, and others. Participants must have Medicare Parts A and B, live in the plan's service area, and meet other eligibility requirements. There are three types of SNPs:

1. Chronic Condition SNP (C-SNP): The patient must have one or more severe or disabling conditions.
2. Institutional SNP (I-SNP). The patient must live in an institution or require nursing care at home.
3. Dual Eligible SNP (D-SNP). The patient must have both Medicare and Medicaid.

Special Needs Plans modify benefits, providers, and drug formularies specific to the needs of the groups served in that model. An ESRD SNP uses special tools that address the clinical needs of the kidney patient such as fluid management, access management, comorbid management, infection prevention, foot care, and other services. Patient education is provided to enhance treatment and medication adherence, to help manage complex and multiple comorbidities, and to reduce or avoid hospitalizations.

Medicare SNPs are available through private insurance companies and can include care-coordination services to help patients better manage their comorbid conditions.

A comprehensive care team can provide patient management and integrated care and may include a case management registered nurse, dietitian, social worker, nephrologist, pharmacist, and dialysis center staff. Risk stratification is used to determine at risk patients for hospitalizations so that through collaboration with the health care team, these may be avoided. The SNP is an opt-in program, meaning the patient determines whether she or he wants to participate in the program.

What Is an ESCO?

An End-Stage Kidney Disease Seamless Care Organization (ESCO) is a Comprehensive ESRD Care (CEC) model introduced by the Centers for Medicare & Medicaid Services in 2015. The purposes of this model are to improve outcomes, increase patient QOL, and reduce costs associated with the treatment for patients with ESRD by integrating care for Medicare's ESRD population. ESCOs are accountable for clinical quality outcomes and financial outcomes, including all spending on dialysis services for those ESRD beneficiaries. Financial incentives are extended to dialysis facilities, nephrologists, and other Medicare-enrolled health care providers for coordinating care and reducing the cost of care for all providers. Each ESCO must include at least one dialysis facility and one nephrologist or nephrology practice to be eligible to participate. The ESCO model can improve ESRD care by addressing the complex care needs of its members. CKD case managers supplement the care received by dialysis patients by coordinating the care a patient receives with the dialysis clinic and by supporting the patient needs outside of the clinic. This integrated model of care helps to meet the patient's medical, social, and behavioral needs in collaboration with the dialysis clinic, nephrologist, and other health care providers. The ESCO model differs from the SNP model in that it is not an opt-in program. Any patient who is dialyzing at an ESCO-approved facility must be part of the program.

What Are the Keys to Effective Case Management?

Effective case management requires a proactive approach in assessing and identifying actual and potential health problems before a major event occurs placing the patient at risk for hospitalization. The CKD case manager will need to intervene early and frequently to address key issues. Patients on dialysis are likely to experience ongoing problems with access, fluid, and diabetes management as well as challenges with other comorbidities. The goals of assessment and monitoring are to improve clinical outcomes and increase the overall QoL for this population of patients.

What Is Transition of Care?

Transition of care is the movement of a patient from one health care practitioner or setting to another. This occurs when the patient's status or care needs change. Examples of transition of care include home to hospital, acute care setting to a skilled nursing facility or rehabilitation, ED to intensive care unit, or discharge to home from any setting. Estimates from the USRDS (2017) suggest 35% of patients with ESRD are readmitted within 30 days of discharge. Telephonic or in-person follow-up with a patient after transitioning can help to reduce avoidable readmissions and identify and prevent complications by addressing patient concerns, reinforcing medication and treatment adherence, and ensuring the patient is following discharge instructions.

What Are Some Transitions of Care Considerations?

The potential for information gaps is quite common when a patient transitions across sites of care. Transitions of care can become critical when pertinent health information, such as medication management, laboratory test follow-up, device maintenance, home health services, durable medical equipment needs, medication management, or follow-up appointments, is not communicated. Transitions of care, if not managed appropriately, can lead to a hospital readmission. The goal of transition of care planning is that the patient has an optimal transition and avoids complications and hospital readmission.

Important details to communicate when a patient with CKD transitions include:
- Dry weight review
- Medication reconciliation
- Heparinization changes
- Antibiotic orders
- Laboratory studies
- Primary care physician appointments
- Cardiologist, pulmonologist, endocrinologist, and other specialist referrals
- Durable medical equipment orders
- Home health referrals
- Advance directive updates

What Is the Impact of Successful Case Management of the Chronic Kidney Disease Patient?

The overarching goal of case management of the patient with CKD is to improve the patient's QoL. Through successful case management implementation and motivational interviewing (see Chapter 25), patients may benefit from reduced hospitalizations, readmissions, and ED visits; decreased medical complications through management and treatment of comorbid conditions; and patient engagement, empowerment, and education. This can be accomplished through complex care coordination and patient advocacy. Early identification of CKD provides the time needed to educate patients on ways to prevent the progression of the disease process and prolong the need for kidney replacement therapy.

Patients on maintenance dialysis benefit from coaching on fluid management and medication and treatment adherence. Diabetes surveillance and blood glucose monitoring help to reduce complications associated with nerve and blood vessel damage, infection, and amputations. Through close monitoring of the patient's comorbidities, psychosocial status, and medication regimen, hospital and ED utilization will be reduced. It is necessary for the CKD case manager to activate the member in his or her own care. It is well known that patients who are active in their own care are more successful in other self-management areas such as medication adherence, demonstrate better QoL, and have fewer hospital admissions than patients who are less involved (Schober et al, 2017).

CHAPTER 24

PSYCHOSOCIAL ASPECTS OF DIALYSIS THERAPY

Dialysis, as a means of prolonging life for an indefinite period, took on new psychosocial implications on July 1, 1973, when the Medicare End-Stage Renal Disease (ESRD) Program (Public Law 92-603, Section 2991) became effective in the United States. The Medicare Act made major financial coverage available to 90% of patients with kidney failure irrespective of age or complicating disease processes.

Medical and mental health professionals recognized psychosocial issues as impediments to adjustment and a satisfactory quality of life (QoL) for patients with chronic kidney disease (CKD) long before Medicare entered the dialysis picture. This became even more apparent when federally supported dialysis treatment was determined to be a right of all people with kidney failure. Some of the psychosocial factors involved in dialysis therapy are changes in an individual's work and family situation, financial concerns, and the stress of living with a life-challenging illness. The rate of depression is up to four times higher in patients with CKD and ESRD than in those with other chronic conditions (Shirazian, 2016).

WHAT ARE THE PSYCHOLOGICAL CONSEQUENCES OF LONG-TERM DIALYSIS?

Dialysis may have a major impact on a patient's psychosocial status. Some patients have a gradual decline in their QoL, particularly as medical complications become more severe. This can lead to depression and an increased risk of suicide. Other patients experience an excellent QoL and are highly rehabilitated and productive. What distinguishes these two patient groups remains uncertain. Close attention to psychosocial adaptation, with psychiatric intervention and counseling when needed, can help patients optimize the quality of their lives while undergoing dialysis.

HOW DOES DEPRESSION AFFECT THE PATIENT WITH CHRONIC KIDNEY DISEASE?

Depression often goes unnoticed or undiagnosed in the CKD patient as the symptoms such as fatigue, lack of appetite, sleeping difficulties, and lack of concentration are misinterpreted as being caused by uremia rather than depression. Depression is a prevalent and undertreated problem in patients with CKD and is associated with increased morbidity and mortality, functional impairment, and decreased QoL (Hedayati et al, 2012). The burden of the demands of the disease and treatment both contribute to the higher rates of depression seen in this population. Factors such as frequency of dialysis treatments, health care provider appointments, pill burden, hospitalizations, and self-monitoring of health can be overwhelming and contribute to the development of depression (Shirazian, 2016). After a diagnosis of depression is made, treatment including medication and cognitive behavioral therapy should be initiated.

IS IT POSSIBLE TO PREDICT HOW A PATIENT WILL REACT TO MAINTENANCE HEMODIALYSIS?

Little work has been done to help health care professionals predict how patients will react to the multiple changes and stresses associated with life on dialysis. Most studies have involved small numbers of patients and showed little agreement regarding predictive parameters. An individual's method of coping with past life stresses remains the single best indicator of his or her adaptability to daily life with dialysis. Frustration tolerance, aggression, denial of sickness, and obsessive-compulsive characteristics are personality traits that can be evaluated and used to help predict a patient's potential adjustment to dialysis.

Partial evaluation of the patient's coping methods is conducted by a mental health professional (usually a clinical social worker) in the dialysis treatment team. In-depth psychosocial evaluation that includes interviews with both the patient and the family is conducted by the social worker at the initiation of chronic dialysis treatment. Based on this evaluation, a treatment plan is formulated to include psychosocial counseling and community resource referrals that can enhance the patient's ability to cope. Often the social worker can provide support and reassurance to the patient and family as well as help to alleviate pressing resource needs by assisting with social, financial, and insurance problems.

WHAT STAGES OF ADJUSTMENT TO DIALYSIS MIGHT A CHRONIC KIDNEY DISEASE PATIENT EXPERIENCE?

When the onset of CKD is gradual, the patient has time to adjust to the idea of dialysis and to make well-informed treatment choices. The initial response to dialysis itself can be one of relief, especially if the patient has been feeling ill for a period of time. Unfortunately, some patients delay beginning dialysis until they are quite ill and then may require the initiation of dialysis on an emergency hospitalized basis.

When the onset of CKD is sudden, there can be an acute crisis phase of adjustment, often marked by feelings of shock, disbelief, desperation, and depression. In such cases, a crisis intervention approach by a trained mental health professional is indicated. Three stages of patient adjustment to dialysis have been identified:

- The "*honeymoon*" *period* is defined as a patient's initial response to dialysis, which can last from a few weeks to 6 months or more. Usually this phase is one of physical and psychological improvement and is accompanied by renewed feelings of hope and confidence. During the honeymoon period, patients may respond to staff in a positive and grateful manner. This does not mean that patients do not also experience periods of anxiety and depression but rather that they may view dialysis in a more positive way overall because they feel better than they did before initiation of dialysis.

- The *period of disenchantment and discouragement* is marked by reduced feelings of confidence and hope and can last from 3 to 12 months. This phase is usually triggered when an individual returns to some previous routine or employment and is forced to confront the limitations that dialysis places on these activities. During this time, feelings of sadness and helplessness may arise.
- The *period of long-term adaptation* is characterized by the patient's arrival at some degree of acceptance of the limitations, shortcomings, and complications that dialysis brings into his or her life. Patients can experience long periods of contentment alternating with episodes of depression. Adaptation can often be facilitated by return to some form of meaningful work or by settling down to doing little or no work at all. Incorporation of diet and activity restrictions and the dialysis procedure into the daily lifestyle is part of long-term adaptation.

These periods of adjustment are presented as general guidelines only. Not all researchers and practitioners agree about this sequence of phases. There is not always a linear progression from one stage to another, and for individual patients, the various stages may be much briefer or much longer than indicated earlier. Furthermore, patients may shift back and forth from stage to stage for a variety of reasons, including medical complications.

How Can the Quality of Life of a Dialysis Patient Be Evaluated?

Quality of life is a phrase that is sometimes used interchangeably with such terms as *life satisfaction, well-being,* and *morale.* Usually, *quality of life* is defined as encompassing major areas of functioning in the physical, psychological, and social realms. Furthermore, feelings about this issue are relative perceptions of each individual, and any attempt to evaluate the QoL must take into account the significance of these highly subjective perceptions. An intolerable situation for one patient may not be intolerable for another.

Several instruments that measure the QoL for research purposes may be used for clinical assessment as well. In addition to using formal measures, dialysis personnel should provide patients with opportunities to talk about their own feelings and perceptions regarding their QoL.

What Are the Common Sources of Stress for Dialysis Patients?

Maintenance dialysis patients are confronted with severe limitations and demands on themselves and their families. They must contend with changes in family relationships, such as role reversal and deteriorating sexual responsiveness, as well as accompanying feelings of guilt, depression, and loss. It has been suggested that 20% of all patients with CKD have significant depressive symptoms (Shirazian et al, 2017). Depression has been found to have profound effects on the overall health and well-being of patients with chronic diseases. The threat of reduced job responsibility or unemployment can contribute to feelings of worthlessness and a loss of self-esteem. Many patients experience conflict between the need to be dependent on a machine and on other people and the desire to remain independent. They may feel that they have relinquished control of their lives to the dialysis team. Underlying many of these feelings is the basic fear of dying. Dependence on the dialysis machine can be a constant reminder for the patient that he or she has been rescued from death.

How Can the Dialysis Team Assist Patients and Families in Coping When Dialysis Becomes Necessary?

Dialysis patients and family members who regard kidney failure and the need for dialysis as a loss may grieve over that loss. Dialysis personnel should be familiar with the issues of grief and the grieving process and be prepared to provide appropriate intervention or call on a resource person, such as a psychiatric nurse, social worker, psychologist, or psychiatrist, as needed. If members of the dialysis team are able to recognize periods of exceptional stress and use appropriate crisis intervention approaches, they can help patients cope with such periods and prevent major adjustment problems.

Patients who are unable to accept the restrictions imposed on them by dialysis may become depressed and unable or unwilling to adhere to their dialysis regimens. When this occurs, the diminished QoL and increased potential for death should be addressed by prompt recognition and social work or psychotherapeutic intervention.

What Are Some Psychological Reactions and Common Coping Mechanisms of Maintenance Dialysis Patients?

Anxiety is the initial reaction of most patients and families when faced with the prospect of life on dialysis. Such anxiety is entirely normal, and the dialysis staff needs to reassure patients that this is the case.

Depression may occur early in the treatment process. Again, this is a rational reaction to the prospect of a limited and risky life that will require totally different objectives than would have been planned otherwise.

Hostility and anger are frequent reactions of dialysis patients. Hostility toward dialysis personnel and the medical regimen is actually a reaction to the limitations imposed by the disease, but this anger is directed to the treatment staff and procedure.

A difference of opinion exists regarding the role that the denial mechanism plays in patients who have become stabilized on dialysis. To the staff involved in the primary care of these patients, denial seems to be a common defense that allows patients to cope with the realities of the situation while regarding it as not a part of their real selves. Denial used in this way can be very useful for the patient because it shuts out negative aspects of the illness. However, denial can be carried to extremes, subverting medical management, and the result can be disastrous.

In What Ways Does Nonadherent Behavior Affect Patients' Physical Condition?

Nonadherent behavior can manifest in a number of ways, including the following:
- Nonadherence to the prescribed diet is a manifestation of the denial mechanism gone astray. This can contribute to increased morbidity and even mortality.
- Ingestion of excess fluid represents denial of kidney failure, with potentially harmful results.
- Inadequate care of the vascular or peritoneal access is sometimes a problem. A clotted or infected vascular access may not be discovered until it is time for dialysis treatment. With peritoneal dialysis, use of an improper technique may lead to infection.
- Manipulation of treatment time can be another manifestation of nonadherent behavior. Skipping treatments and shortening treatment times are examples of this behavior.

    Such behaviors can contribute to malnutrition, neuropathy, bone disease, cardiac failure, and the like. If these behaviors persist, they result in physical deterioration and, in extreme cases, death—a form of passive suicide.

How Can Such Adverse Behaviors Be Countered?

Patients sometimes resent consultation with a psychiatrist. In such cases, patients may be defensive and unwilling to admit that a problem exists or that problems may have an emotional basis. Even if the psychiatrist is recognized as a member of the treatment team, there is a tendency to avoid such counsel. Group sessions that involve patients as well as family members and are guided by a skilled and accepted social worker or psychiatric nurse (using the psychiatrist as a resource person) may be a more readily accepted form of help. Within such a group setting, ventilation, sharing of problems, and discussions with peers can help resolve many problems. The psychiatrist, psychiatric nurse, or social worker can also help medical and other personnel deal with a patient's resistant behaviors. These professionals can offer reassurance and suggest approaches to help other members of the dialysis team assist patients in handling the challenges of dialysis.

What Emotional Problems Are Commonly Seen in Family Members?

Anxiety is a common and normal response in family members, particularly when the patient first begins dialysis. With the passage of time, other stresses may bring added reactions. The continued drain on financial resources and the need for role changes within the family may create additional problems and resentment. Often a dialysis patient may become increasingly dependent, demanding, and irascible. Resenting the loss of a positive self-image and self-esteem, either real or imagined, the patient may become antagonistic toward the rest of the family. Family members, in turn, may become hostile toward the patient and then experience guilt for having these feelings.

    Nurses and other dialysis personnel can provide opportunities for family members to express hostility and anxiety through the use of active listening techniques. Staff can offer reassurance that these are normal reactions. Furthermore, other team members may act as liaisons with the psychiatrist or social worker for developing a realistic plan to help the patient and family resolve any problems that arise.

What Are Some of the Physical Problems That Can Adversely Affect the Psychosocial Adjustment of Dialysis Patients?

Insomnia, chronic pruritus, neuropathy symptoms, muscle cramps, and bone and joint pain are some of the most commonly identified physical problems that contribute to a diminished QoL in dialysis patients. Ongoing assessment of the physiological response to CKD and dialysis therapy is essential. In many cases, medical management can alleviate physical problems, enhancing patients' psychological adjustment and improving their QoL. Some patients need to be encouraged to report physical symptoms because they may otherwise assume that nothing can be done about them.

How Does the Dialysis Procedure Itself Affect the Psychosocial Adjustment of Dialysis Patients?

The time commitment involved is probably the single aspect of the dialysis regimen that exercises the largest influence on a patient's adjustment to treatment. The time demand may interfere with the patient's ability to perform activities of daily living, resulting in loss of independence and, ultimately, lowered self-esteem and depression. Dialysis personnel need to work with the patient to design the least restrictive regimen possible. Encouraging the patient to perform self-care activities and to maintain some degree of independence will sustain a more positive psychosocial adjustment.

What Types of Self-Care Skills Can Patients Learn?

Patients who participate in and are accountable for their care are empowered and have greater control over their life and health. Patients can be trained to perform both hemodialysis as well as peritoneal dialysis in the home setting. An alternative form of self-care in which the patient assumes responsibility of certain aspects of the treatment can take place in the dialysis clinic. Some dialysis centers offer in-center self-care programs in which the patient shares responsibility with the clinic staff for performing the dialysis treatment. Some activities that the patient can learn to perform include the following:
- Determination of pretreatment and posttreatment weights
- Preparation of the vascular access

- Measurement of vital signs
- Administration of some medications
- Setting up and programming the dialysis machine
- Retrieval of laboratory specimens
- Cannulation of the vascular access

Patients performing in-center self-care may encourage other patients to take part in their own treatment as they see the benefits firsthand. This modality provides a potential bridge for patients to transition their treatment fully to home as they become more confident in their skills and abilities.

WHAT TYPE OF RELATIONSHIP SHOULD EXIST BETWEEN THE DIALYSIS PATIENT AND THE NURSE OR TECHNICIAN?

It is common for dependence to develop between dialysis personnel and patients. This type of relationship may be very satisfying to the nurse or technician and may fulfill a desire to be needed. However, an excessively close relationship may cause the health care professional to exercise faulty judgment, which can be detrimental to the patient. Patients need to be encouraged to do things for themselves whenever possible to preserve and promote a sense of independence.

It is best if one staff member can be responsible for working with a given patient and his or her family. This helps to prevent problems that can be created by inconsistent responses to questions. Because of anxiety, patients and family members tend to ask everyone slightly different versions of questions, which can result in ambiguity and chaos. Questions should be answered consistently, accurately, and honestly, and this is best accomplished if one team member serves as the primary source of information for each patient and his or her family.

WHAT ARE PROFESSIONAL BOUNDARIES?

Professional boundaries are the limitations that health care providers impose on themselves to maintain a safe and comfortable therapeutic relationship with their patients. The National Council of State Boards of Nursing (2018) defines *professional boundaries* as "the spaces between the nurse's power and the client's vulnerability." The nurse or dialysis technician is in a position of power because he or she has the ability to perform life-sustaining treatments that patients require for survival. The dialysis staff is typically involved with the care of the patient 3 days a week over a duration of many years. This situation lends itself to the potential development of personal relationships between patients and nurses or patients and technicians. Although most relationships are therapeutic, health care personnel sometimes become overly involved with the patient's needs. An employer or state board of nursing may interpret these boundary crossings or violations as inappropriate.

It is never appropriate to have anything other than a professional relationship with a patient. Neither a business relationship nor a personal relationship should be established between a patient and staff member. Health care professionals should not spend time with patients outside the workplace or socialize with them. Intimate relationships with a patient are never appropriate; any type of sexual relationship with a patient is misconduct and a serious violation of the Nurse Practice Acts of most states. It is the responsibility of the nurse or technician to ensure that professional boundaries are maintained. The patient is always considered vulnerable if litigation occurs as a result of an inappropriate relationship. Gifts, monetary or otherwise, should never be accepted from a patient or a patient's family member.

Health care professionals are responsible for maintaining professional boundaries. A good rule to determine the appropriateness of a relationship is to ask if you would establish the same relationship or engage in the same activities or behaviors with every patient in the clinic. If the answer is no, the chances are that the relationship, activities, or behaviors constitute a boundary violation.

DO PATIENTS HAVE UNREALISTIC EXPECTATIONS OF DIALYSIS THERAPY?

It is common for patients to expect a greater degree of curative capability than dialysis can actually provide. Dialysis provides a lifesaving therapy, but it does not cure the disease. The patient and his or her family must still live and cope with a chronic illness.

WHAT IS THE PURPOSE OF PREDIALYSIS EDUCATION FOR CHRONIC KIDNEY DISEASE PATIENTS?

Education programs are necessary and can help to ease the transition of patients with CKD through all phases of the disease. Predialysis education is known to lower stress for both the patient and the family, improve mortality and morbidity, enhance self-care and decision making, play a role in continuation of employment, and allow for more informed decision making when replacement therapy must finally be initiated. The 2006 Kidney Disease Outcomes Quality Initiative Clinical Practice Guidelines for Hemodialysis Adequacy recommend planning for kidney failure when the patient reaches stage 4 CKD. Education about kidney failure and options for its treatment should be provided to patients at that time. Early education allows the patient and family to weigh their treatment options and begin to make decisions before an imminent situation in which dialysis is needed urgently. Some education programs are offered to patients as early as stage 3 CKD.

The American Association of Kidney Patients provides a CKD patient resource library with easy to read patient-centric learning materials on its website. DaVita, Inc. offers "Kidney Smart," a comprehensive education program for patients with CKD. This program offers instructor-led classes in the community or online learning from home. Fresenius Medical Care North America offers KidneyCare:365, a free class led by an expert on CKD. Topics include symptoms and stages of CKD, treatment options and modality review, nutrition and CKD, coping, and other resources.

Kidney School, an online and self-management learning program, is also available to patients with stage 3 to 5 CKD. Its materials were developed at the seventh- through ninth-grade reading levels and contain graphics and animations to keep the learner engaged.

Centers for Medicare & Medicaid Services (CMS) guidelines state that patients have the right to be informed about and, if desired, participate in all aspects of their care. They must also be informed about all treatment modalities and all aspects of their care, such as diet, blood tests, access options, medications, rights, responsibilities, and rehabilitation. Most education programs help to address these required topics and provide patients with additional written materials and resources.

Is the Sexual Dysfunction Experienced by Many Dialysis Patients Emotional?

Sexual dysfunction in dialysis patients involves both emotional and organic factors. Organic elements that contribute to decreased sexual functioning can include severe anemia, impaired testosterone and other hormone levels, and an increased parathyroid hormone level. These conditions can lead to reduced fertility and libido. Medications, particularly some antihypertensive agents, may also contribute to sexual dysfunction. In addition to these organic causes, depression also seems to be an important element in the sexual dysfunction of dialysis patients. Even after correction of anemia with erythropoietin, sexual dysfunction remains a major problem.

Both the patient and his or her partner need to be aware of the potential for sexual dysfunction and be provided with a framework for discussion about sexuality. In many cases, the nephrologist or mental health professional will need to initiate the discussion about sex rather than expect patients to bring up the topic on their own. Together, the physician and social worker can provide a forum for discussion. Counseling may be helpful in some cases, and it should be possible for a couple to work out acceptable alternatives.

What Is an Advance Directive?

An advance directive (AD), also known as a living will, is a written document that specifies in advance what kind of medical treatments an individual wants or does not want in the event of an incapacitating condition. In 1991, the Patient Self-Determination Act (Danforth Bill: Public Law 101-508) came into effect. The law applies to most health care organizations and providers in the United States. It requires that patients be given information concerning their legal right to make decisions about the medical care and treatment they are about to receive. An AD can include a durable power of attorney for health care, a living will, or both. The durable power of attorney for health care is also known as the health care proxy or agent and will make health care decisions for the patient in the event she or he is not able to make decisions for her- or himself. The AD or living will provides the specific instructions or wishes about medical treatments the patient wishes to receive should he or she not be able to speak for him- or herself. The laws and required forms for ADs vary state to state. Some states require the forms to be notarized, but others do not. The National Hospice and Palliative Care Organization can be found online and provides a link to access the specific forms for all 50 states. Educational materials on hospice and palliative care for both patients and health care providers can also be accessed on this site. ADs are for anyone older than the age of 18 years and allow for health care decisions to be made based on the person's values and preferences. Having an AD in place can remove the burden of decision making about end-of-life care for family members and can improve end-of-life care for both patients and families when the time comes.

After it has been prepared, it is important to share an AD with physicians, family, clergy, and dialysis centers. It is also important to review ADs periodically, especially when there is a change in health status. This is a difficult subject to discuss with anyone, but it can be particularly difficult to explore with someone who is confronting a life-threatening illness. Often it is the role of the social worker to provide information about ADs to patients and their families, but all staff should be familiar with the laws and issues surrounding ADs.

What About Patients Who Decide to Discontinue Dialysis?

In planning the treatment regimen, the staff should include a comprehensive and open discussion about the options available to patients. The right not to begin dialysis and the right to withdraw from dialysis are among these options. Such decisions are based on the specific needs and desires of the individual patient, with consideration of his or her medical condition. A decision to discontinue or not initiate dialysis is usually made in conjunction with family members, the physician, and other members of the dialysis team, including the chaplain and the psychiatrist. In general, older adults who have complications because of underlying illnesses are more likely to discontinue dialysis than are younger individuals. When a patient has elected to discontinue dialysis, members of the professional team need to provide supportive care with an emphasis on physical and emotional comfort. The patient must be informed of the consequences of refusing medical treatment.

What Is The Difference Between Hospice and Palliative Care?

There is confusion at times between the services provided and intentions of hospice and palliative care. Although the two resources share similarities, they are also different in some ways. Palliative care is for anyone with an illness, serious or otherwise, and can be delivered at any stage of the illness. Palliative care is meant to help improve the patient's QoL while providing symptom management. Palliative care is provided along with curative treatment and does not rest on the patient's diagnosis and includes medical, social, and emotional support during the course of illness. Palliative care is a bridge of hospice care that treats the patient earlier in the course of the illness or disease process. Patients' needs are assessed throughout the course of the illness, and changes are made on the basis of these needs, with a transition to hospice care when indicated. A core belief of hospice and palliative care is that the patient deserves to die pain free and with dignity. When it is determined that palliative care is no longer helping, the decision can be made to transition to hospice care. Those enrolled in Medicare can receive hospice care if their physicians believe they have 6 months or less to live. Hospice care can be extended beyond the 6 months if the patient lives longer than the initial 6 months when determined and certified by the physician. Bereavement support is provided to the family for a period after the death of the patient (National Institute of Aging, 2019).

Hospice care should be discussed with any CKD patient who requires maintenance dialysis but opts to decline dialysis or transplantation, as well as with any patient who wishes to discontinue the current dialysis therapy. For referral to the CMS for benefits, the patient must have a life expectancy of less than 6 months. The ESRD benefits will be covered when a patient withdraws from dialytic therapy or when a terminal disease will result in death in less than 6 months. The patient can continue to undergo dialysis in the form of ultrafiltration to ease the symptoms of fluid overload if dialysis is discontinued.

In What Ways Can Chronic Kidney Disease Patients Achieve More Control Over Their Own Situations?

Patients who previously led independent lives may be at increased risk for psychosocial difficulties with the onset of dialysis treatment. It is especially important that these individuals be given opportunities to participate in their treatment regimens as much as possible. Patients may feel a greater sense of control over their situations if they are encouraged to perform self-care dialysis in the hemodialysis unit or during home hemodialysis. Peritoneal dialysis can be a positive choice for patients with a need or desire for freedom from dialysis schedules. Self-care is a good option for most patients who are suffering from a lack of control and is becoming a more popular treatment option. Patients can become involved in various levels of care, including setting up the machine and dialyzer, cannulating their own access, and monitoring their own treatment and alarms.

What Is the Health Insurance Portability and Accountability Act, and How Does It Affect the Dialysis Community?

The Health Insurance Portability and Accountability Act (HIPAA) was enacted in 1996. New privacy regulations, which came into effect on April 14, 2003, protect patients' medical records and other health information that might be provided to insurance groups, doctors, hospitals, and other health care providers. The new privacy regulations developed by the Department of Health and Human Services ensure patient privacy by limiting the ways in which health plans, hospitals, and other health care providers can use a patient's personal medical information. Any identifiable health information that is on paper, in computers, or communicated orally is protected under this law.

CHAPTER 25

PATIENT EDUCATION GUIDELINES

Patients with chronic kidney disease (CKD) require a considerable amount of education to manage and understand the manifestations of their disease and treatment requirements. New-onset CKD and maintenance dialysis require the patient to acquire knowledge about new medications, procedures, dietary changes, and treatment plans. Patient education is an essential role of the nurse in the dialysis setting and is an important component of patient care. Dialysis technicians play a key role in reinforcing the education initially provided to the patient by the registered nurse. Patients are often encouraged to learn all they can about their disease in order to become informed and develop a positive approach to manage their condition. Ineffective or incomplete patient education results in failure of the patient to understand the treatment regimen, leading to lack of compliance, poor health outcomes, and increased health care costs. Effective patient education helps improve compliance with the treatment plan and patient outcomes.

WHAT IS HEALTH LITERACY?

Health literacy is the extent to which a patient is capable of obtaining, processing, and understanding basic health information. The degree of health literacy directly impacts a patient's ability to understand health information so that appropriate health decisions can be made. A patient is considered "health literate" when he or she possesses skills to understand the information needed to make appropriate decisions about health. The following areas are commonly associated with health literacy (US Department of Health and Human Services [USDHHS], 2010):

- Patient–physician communication
- Drug labeling
- Medical instructions
- Health information materials
- Informed consent
- Response to medical and insurance forms
- Health history

  Limited health literacy is not exclusive to those with limited reading abilities or for whom English is a second language. Limited health literacy affects people of all ages, races, incomes, and educational levels; however, people belonging to lower socioeconomic and minority groups, adults older than the age of 65 years, recent refugees and immigrants, and those without a high school degree or GED are more significantly impacted. USDHHS has a program to address these issues under the name "Healthy People 2020 Initiative" (USDHHS, 2019).

WHAT ARE THE BARRIERS TO EFFECTIVE PATIENT EDUCATION?

Many factors serve as barriers to providing effective patient education. Those specific to health care providers include the following:

- Lack of time to spend with the patient
- Lack of educational materials
- Lack of training and skills regarding how to educate patients
- Failure to assess patient learning styles and preferences
- Failure to determine patients' readiness to learn
  Patient-specific barriers include the following:
- Physical obstacles such as vision and hearing deficits
- Cultural variables such as language differences
- Lack of understanding or health illiteracy
- Anxiety
- Complexity of information
- Anxiety, depression, or fear
- Pain
  Environmental barriers include the following:
- Temperature (too hot or cold)
- Lighting
- Noise level
- Privacy

WHAT ADULT LEARNING PRINCIPLES SHOULD BE CONSIDERED WHEN TEACHING PATIENTS?

Andragogy is the art and science of teaching adults. Adult learning theories emphasize that adults want information that is relevant to their lives and that they can put to use immediately.

Malcolm Knowles, a pioneer in the science of adult learning theories, asserted five assumptions about how adults learn:

1. Adults are independent and self-directing.
2. Adults have accumulated a great deal of experience, which is a rich resource for further learning.
3. Adults value learning and knowledge that integrates with the demands of their everyday life.
4. Adults are more interested in immediate, problem-centered approaches rather than in subject-centered approaches.
5. Adults are more motivated to learn by their personal internal drives rather than by external drives.

Knowles also suggested the following principles on how to teach adult learners:

1. Establish a learning environment where the learner feels safe and comfortable to speak freely.
2. Involve the learner in lesson planning.
3. Include the learner when establishing her or his learning needs.
4. Allow the learner to have control when formulating his or her learning objectives.
5. Support the learner in carrying out her or his learning plan.
6. Involve the learner when evaluating his or her learning.

WHAT IS LEARNING STYLE ASSESSMENT?

Learners have different preferred methods of learning and processing new information. For example, some prefer to learn by looking at pictures or diagrams (visual), listening (auditory), reading information displayed as words (reading and writing), or through practice (kinesthetic or tactile). The majority of learners are characterized as visual learners. By assessing learning styles, you are more likely to promote patient engagement and improve learning. The characteristics of each learning style and recommended strategies to use when teaching each can be found in Table 25.1.

WHAT SHOULD I ASSESS IN MY PATIENTS BEFORE I BEGIN AN EDUCATION SESSION?

It is of critical importance to assess a patient's readiness to learn before planning a teaching session. This is a commonly missed opportunity. Evaluation of the patient's health literacy is another important and often overlooked component. Avoid making assumptions about the skill and knowledge level of the learner. Cultural beliefs regarding health, illness, and medical treatment will influence a patient's responsiveness to the teaching session and willingness to learn.

Finally, learning style preferences must be assessed in order to personalize the delivery of health information. Assessing how the patient learns best—by reading, listening, or hands-on techniques—is fairly clear-cut, but a variety of formal assessment tools are available. Fleming and Mills have developed a learning style assessment tool known as VARK that can be adapted to assessing a patient's learning style preferences. The acronym "VARK" represents the sensory modalities of visual, aural, reading and writing, and kinesthetic. The questionnaire provides users with a profile of their learning style preferences. It is important to keep in mind that learners' preferences often cross learning styles, and they may rely on multiple modalities. A variety of tools and methods of instruction should be used when teaching patients to ensure that learning is successful.

Table 25.1 Characteristics of Learning Styles and Recommended Strategies	
LEARNER PREFERENCES	**TEACHING STRATEGIES**
Auditory Learns best by listening to spoken words	• Provide verbal instructions. • Read instructions to patients while they demonstrate a procedure. • Engage in discussions. • Listen to audiotapes or videotapes. • Have patients read aloud or verbalize written instructions.
Visual Learns best by reading words on paper or seeing the information	• Use handouts with lots of images and pictures. • Use charts, videos, and flashcards.
Kinesthetic or Tactile Learns best by doing or being physically involved	• Have learners trace or highlight words as you say them. • Give patients paper to take notes. • Give patients a colored pen to emphasize important points. • Have patients hold the materials rather than placing them on the table for them to read. • Have patients provide return demonstrations. • Use models as examples whenever possible and let patients touch or hold them.

After you have assessed your patient, you can formulate your education plan with clearly identified goals and objectives. The goals of your plan are the desired outcomes upon completion of education and the learning objectives are the actions that will be performed to achieve the goals (Redman, 2007).

How Do I Assess My Patient's Readiness to Learn?

A sign of readiness and motivation to learn is when patients begin to ask questions about their treatment regimen or procedures specific to their care. Redman (2007) recommends screening the patient as part of the general nursing assessment. Patients should be asked about what they know, how they perceive their problems, what skills they currently possess, and what is their confidence level to perform the skill or task. Patients who have greater knowledge about their health are more likely to engage in self-care activities. Often this information can be gathered during a simple conversation with the patient and family. This is especially appropriate for patients who will be performing self-care in the dialysis unit or using a home dialysis modality.

What Are Some Effective Ways to Communicate with My Patient?

Begin by determining the most important concepts you want to teach, present no more than three or four concepts at a time, and limit the session to no longer than 15 minutes. Begin your teaching sessions with simple concepts and later move on to more complex concepts. Patients will be more confident to learn new information after they have accomplished and mastered simple concepts. Make your instructions clear and specific and try to avoid "nice to know" information. For example, telling the patient the percentage of patients undergoing peritoneal versus hemodialysis, although nice to know, would not be necessary to achieve the desired learning outcomes. Focus on desired behaviors and avoid technical or medical jargon. Summarize what the patient needs to do at the end of the teaching session. Check for patient understanding by asking them to repeat the intended information back in their own words. Always ask, "What questions do you have?" as opposed to "Do you have any questions?" Praise them when they achieve success to reinforce the expected behaviors. It is best to always use open-ended questions rather than "yes" or "no" questions. Finally, it is very important to evaluate whether the learning objectives have been met. Reinforcement or reteaching may be needed if the patient did not achieve the objectives. It is important to document any patient education completed as well as the outcome. As with any patient with a chronic disease, reinforcement of information will be required as needed to help maintain their health.

How Effective Are Print Materials for Reinforcing Patient Education?

Written materials are an excellent source for reinforcing any verbal education that has been presented to the patient, provided they are designed with the patient in mind. The more senses that are engaged in a learning episode, the greater the likelihood of patient understanding.

Poorly designed patient education materials can overwhelm and confuse the patient, thus preventing learning from taking place. The National Assessment of Adult Literacy found that 30 million adults struggle with basic reading, and only 12% of consumers have proficient health literacy skills. Patient education materials should be created for individuals with a wide range of literacy abilities. Written materials should be written at no greater than the fifth or sixth grade level. There are a number of tools to determine the reading level of written materials. The Flesch-Kincaid Readability Test, Fry Readability Graph, and Gunning "FOG" Readability Test are tools that can assess the readability of your written materials.

It is always best to tell your patient what to do versus what not to do. Sentences should be no longer than 8 to 10 words, and paragraphs should be limited to 3 to 5 sentences per paragraph.

Scientific language should be kept at a minimum, if used at all, and abbreviations and acronyms should be avoided.

Text formatting affects the readability of educational materials. Font size should be between 12 and 14 points, and headings should be at least 2 points larger than the main text size. Avoid using fancy or script lettering and never use all uppercase letters. Important words should be bold-faced instead of underlined or italicized to emphasize their importance. The USDHHS Agency for Healthcare Research and Quality (2017) advocate that patient educational materials are understandable when consumers of diverse backgrounds and varying levels of health literacy can process the information. This can be assessed using the Patient Education Materials Assessment Tool (PEMAT) found on the USDHHS website. Educational materials should be actionable in that consumers of diverse backgrounds and varying levels of health literacy can determine what they need to do based on the information presented. Two versions of PEMAT are available to evaluate print materials (brochures, pamphlets, PDFs) and audiovisual materials (videos, multimedia materials).

How Can I Recognize a Patient with Low Health Literacy?

It is not very easy to identify a patient with low health literacy because people of all ages, races, education levels, and socioeconomic statuses are affected. Low health literacy is not confined to those who cannot read or are not highly educated. Patients will go to great lengths to conceal their lack of understanding. Illiteracy can be masked by making excuses such as not having the time to read patient education literature or having left their eyeglasses at home, not filling out medical forms completely or correctly, or recognizing pills by their appearance rather than by reading the medication vials. Redman (2007) provides some strategies to use when teaching patients with limited literacy (Box 25.1).

Box 25.1 Teaching Techniques and Strategies

- Eliminate anything that is extraneous.
- Move from simple to complex concepts.
- Break contents into components or chunks.
- Build on information with review, feedback, and questions.
- Allow patients to demonstrate what they have learned.
- Reward patients who lack confidence in their abilities.
- Deliver oral instructions in a conversational style using short words and sentences.
- Visual aids should contain only one idea for each image, and captions should be no longer than 10 words.
- Organize material in the order in which the patient will use it.
- Use words familiar to the patient.

Modified from Redman BK: *The practice of patient education,* ed. 10, St. Louis, 2007, Mosby.

CAN MOTIVATIONAL INTERVIEWING BE USED TO HELP FACILITATE CHANGE IN A PATIENT?

Motivational interviewing (MI) is an approach that can be used to help promote behavior change by strengthening a person's own motivation and commitment to change. MI was first introduced in the early 1980s by William R. Miller for use in the treatment of patients with alcohol disorders. MI can be defined as "a collaborative conversation style for strengthening a person's own motivation and commitment to change"(Miller, 2013). This process has since evolved to be useful in individuals with substance abuse disorders and other medical conditions such as diabetes, heart disease, and asthma. MI interventions can also be used successfully in a clinical setting to assist with smoking cessation, medication adherence, and weight loss. MI uses a series of techniques in a collaborative spirit to guide and strengthen a patient's motivation to change while assessing patient understanding, motivation, and confidence. The spirit of MI includes the three key elements, the first of which is collaboration between the health care provider and the patient. MI is done for and in partnership with a patient, not "to" or "on" a patient. The patient is seen as an expert in her or his own health, and the goal is to activate the patient's motivation to make healthy behavior changes. Evocation and autonomy are two additional elements encompassing the spirit of MI. Evocation is an approach in which the health care provider draws out the patient's own thoughts and ideas rather than imposing her or his own opinions on why and how the patient needs to change. Finally, autonomy is practiced and allows the patient to take the lead in deciding what goals to commit to and how to achieve the desired change. You can say that MI is a conversational approach in helping patients consider making a positive lifestyle change while helping them work through any ambivalence or knowledge gaps they may have around making the change.

WHAT ARE THE GUIDING PRINCIPLES OF MOTIVATIONAL INTERVIEWING?

Miller and Rollnick (2013) developed a set of four guiding principles when practicing MI that are represented by the acronym RULE:

Resist the Righting Reflex

As nurses and health care providers, we have a tendency to provide advice to patients because we believe we know what is best for them. We have an innate sense of responsibility to make things right for the patient and have them engage in positive health behaviors. This may be interpreted as arguing or pushing for change with the patient who may not be ready or have the desire or confidence to change. This may be seen as pushing back on the patient and may cause them to become more resistant to change. In the spirit of MI, the nurse or health care provider needs to resist the righting reflex and focus on eliciting change talk by asking open-ended questions, being empathetic and nonjudgmental, and helping the patient to identify barriers to positive health behaviors.

Understand

It is incumbent on the HCP to identify and understand the patient's reason or motivation for change. This requires attentiveness and active listening and giving the patient cues that you understand why the change is important to him or her.

Listen

Listening can take place at many levels, but a health care professional hoping to help a patient become actively involved in her or his health requires active and intentional listening. It is listening not just to hear the words but also to understand the patient's concerns, fears, and readiness to make a change in health behaviors while identifying barriers.

Empower

Nurses, case managers, and all health care professionals need to empower the patient and respect that she or he is in control of her or his health and health-related behaviors. It is only then that the patient will begin to take control of her or his actions and make steps toward positive change.

What Are Some Skills Used with Motivational Interviewing?

Motivational interviewing involves the skillful use of a communication technique represented by the acronym OARS (Table 25.2), which helps to build rapport with the patient and generate information. Using OARS helps to establish a therapeutic relationship while eliciting change talk. Change talk is when the patient begins to consider motivation or commitment to change. Statements such as "I want to change," "I need to change," and "I am taking steps to change" are all examples of change talk. When the patient is talking about change, he or she is more likely to commit to the behavior change.

The Change Ruler is another tool that can facilitate change talk by assessing for importance and confidence. The Change Ruler is used to explore and rate a patient's readiness and confidence to change by asking the patient to identify on a scale of 1 to 10 her or his readiness and confidence to change. If the patient answers a "6" as an example, the nurse can follow up by asking "Why did you not choose a lower number such as a 3 or 4?" This encourages the patient to engage in positive change talk and serves as an impetus to commit to positive behavior changes.

Another skill is to present information using an "elicit, provide, elicit" framework. The nurse first assesses a patient's understanding of a problem and need for additional information. This is followed by the nurse providing correct or additional information to the patient with her or his permission. The nurse can then ask the patient what the new information means to her or him while assessing the patient's sense making of the new information (Resnicow & McMaster, 2012).

The process of MI and the use of specific skills requires practice with an understanding that MI is not a one for all and linear process. Whatever skills are used to assist patients in making positive health behavior changes, the most important thing is to fully listen to and seek to understand where your patient is in the change process while assessing his or her level of understanding and sense making. By being empathetic, understanding, and empowering, we can better support change in the manner that works best for the patient.

Table 25.2 OARS for Client-Centered Communication

SKILL	DESCRIPTION	EXAMPLE	FUNCTION
Open questions	Asking questions that can't be answered with a "yes" or "no"	"Can you tell me how you have been feeling?"	• Invites patient to elaborate • Allows for reflection and gathering of more meaningful information • Opens the door for exploration
Affirmations	Noticing and acknowledging something positive the patient has done	"You really worked hard on managing your fluids this week!"	• Demonstrates support of the patient • Provides encouragement • Builds rapport
Reflections	Repeating back to patients in the exact words or paraphrases the essence of what they just shared with you	"So at this time, you are not concerned about your fluid gains."	• Clarifies that you understood what the patient said and meant • Conveys respect • Strengthens the empathic relationship
Summaries	Pulling together what has been discussed with a patient during a contact and offering it back to the patient	"So to summarize what we have talked about, you have not yet decided on a modality for when your GFR indicates you will need dialysis. You have been feeling pretty well and do not see a need to make this decision at this time. You are going to ask your PCP to draw another GFR. We will discuss on our next call. Did I miss anything?"	• Pulls together content and results of session • Highlights important aspects of the discussion • Useful to transition to new topic or to end contact

GFR, Glomerular filtration rate; *PCP*, primary care physician.
Modified from Miller WR, Rollnick S: *Motivational interviewing: helping people change*, New York, 2013, Guilford Press.

MANAGEMENT OF QUALITY IN DIALYSIS CARE

Like all health care providers, dialysis programs are undergoing a revolution in accountability. The government, accrediting and regulatory agencies, payers, and patients are holding health care organizations accountable for the delivery of high-quality, low-cost health care. Health care providers are being asked to explain the rationales behind their decisions and plans of care. Increased competition in the managed care environment also demands that providers be responsive to quality and cost issues. Continuous quality improvement (CQI) is a method used to address these concerns. CQI must be supported by a leadership style of total quality management (TQM), in which all members of the organization are motivated to go beyond meeting minimum standards by continually evaluating their performance with the goal of improving care and outcomes and surpassing the minimum regulatory requirements.

What Is the Medicare Improvements for Patients and Providers Act?

The Medicare Improvements for Patients and Providers Act (MIPPA) was approved and passed by Congress in July 2008. This act has significant implications for the nephrology community. The core of this act is development of a case-mix–adjusted bundled payment rate, a pay-for-performance quality incentive, and an educational condition to help patients with chronic kidney disease (CKD) manage their disease process. This is the only modification in the payment rate since the composite rate was introduced in 1983.

The new composite rate is a fixed rate that Medicare pays for each dialysis treatment; the rate was introduced through a transition period, with full implementation as of January 1, 2014. This fixed or composite rate covers all services rendered, including supplies, equipment, and medications associated with dialysis treatment. Since the composite rate was established, many new treatment-related pharmaceuticals have become part of the standard dialysis treatment. These additional drugs, such as erythropoiesis-stimulating agents, vitamin D, and iron, were not included in the original composite rate and were billed separately over and above the composite rate. Additionally, many new laboratory studies and supplies did not exist when the composite rate came into effect, so these too were billed separately. With the increase in Medicare use for end-stage renal disease (ESRD) services, MIPPA charged the Centers for Medicare & Medicaid Services (CMS) to develop a new bundled payment that will include the additional drugs and laboratory services. This rule aligns dialysis facility payments on the basis of quality performance measures. The new payment system was phased in over a period of 3 years beginning in January 2011.

What Is Continuous Quality Improvement?

Continuous quality improvement is the ongoing process of identifying opportunities to improve quality. It involves collecting data on the current situation, identifying ways to improve performance, introducing new and better approaches and methods to achieve desired outcomes, and then evaluating the interventions. When CQI is operating as intended, important aspects of care in need of improvement are identified and prioritized, and action steps are initiated before problems occur. All personnel contribute to CQI by being vigilant in recognizing care practices in need of improvement. A patient-centered perspective and questioning (e.g., "What about my work interferes with my ability to do what needs to be done to achieve the best possible outcome for patients?") are effective ways to identify practices in need of improvement. The goal of CQI is to use data to make objective decisions without assigning blame or finding fault.

What Is the Origin of Continuous Quality Improvement?

Quality management efforts began in manufacturing, where the focus was on product inspection. Quality management experts such as W. Edwards Deming recognized that it was not enough to simply evaluate the end product. He introduced the principles of CQI to improve and manage the production processes used to achieve a quality product.

What Is Quality Assessment and Performance Improvement?

Quality Assessment and Performance Improvement (QAPI) is the name given by the CMS to an internal program that ESRD facilities must develop to promote continuous improvement and outcomes (Box 26.1). The program is data driven with input from the entire interdisciplinary team (IDT).

Quality of care issues to address include, but are not limited to, dialysis adequacy, dialyzer reuse program, nutritional status, anemia management, vascular access, bone disease management, infection control, medical injuries and errors, patient education, patient survival, vaccinations, and physical and mental functioning. Facilities are expected to prioritize areas affecting patient safety. The Measures Assessment Tool is a reference list of acceptable standards and values for clinical and quality outcomes (Table 26.1). CMS requires that all facilities have a written plan describing their QAPI program. Facilities are also required to constantly monitor their performance using quality indicators or performance measures and to make performance improvements as needed. Action plans must be prioritized, and actions that result in performance improvement must be taken.

> **Box 26.1** V626 Quality Assessment and Performance Improvement Condition Statement
>
> The dialysis facility must develop, implement, maintain, and evaluate an effective, data-driven quality assessment and performance improvement program with participation of professional members of an interdisciplinary team. The program must reflect the complexity of the dialysis facility's organization and services (including services provided under arrangement) and must focus on indicators related to improved health outcomes and prevention and reduction of medical errors. The dialysis facility must maintain and demonstrate evidence of its quality improvement and performance improvement program for review by the CMS.

From the Centers for Medicare & Medicaid Services (CMS): Interpretive guidance. April 2008.

How Does CMS Link Quality Measures to Payment?

The End-Stage Renal Disease Quality Incentive Program (ESRD QIP) is a value-based program established by CMS. It links the quality of care provided to dialysis patients to the payment received by the facility delivering that care when meeting established performance standards. When the quality of care provided is not met to established standards, CMS can lower facility payments by up to 2% for an entire payment year. Quality is based on eight clinical performance measures and four reporting measures (Box 26.2). Holding facilities accountable to their quality outcomes financially incentivizes them to improve patient care. Facilities receive a Total Performance Score (TPS) indicating how they performed overall, which becomes publicly reported. ESRD QIP measures are updated every 2 years.

What is the Consumer Assessment of Healthcare Providers and Systems Survey?

The Consumer Assessment of Healthcare Providers and Systems (CAHPS) survey is a patient experience survey administered to eligible patients who have been treating for more than 90 days, are older than 18 years of age, and do not reside in an institution or in hospice care. The CAHPS survey is a government mandated survey through CMS and is administered to in-center hemodialysis patients. CAHPS is a QIP measure and contributes to a facility's overall score. Facilities must have a minimum of 30 patients and receive 30 or more total survey responses in a combined biannual survey period. The surveys are conducted by third-party vendors by mail only, telephone only, or mail with telephone follow-up. The survey itself contains 44 core questions and demographic identifiers. Questions involving patient care, staff, communication, and treatment options are asked. Results are provided to the facility after analysis so that quality improvements can be made as necessary (CMS, 2019).

What Are the Basic Tenets of Quality Management?

Efforts to manage quality in health care continue to be influenced in particular by three sets of guides: Deming's 14 points; Donabedian's structure-process-outcome framework; and The Joint Commission's (TJC; formerly the Joint Commission on Accreditation of Healthcare Organizations) 10 steps. The basic tenets of CQI and TQM are focus on customers, broadly defined to include personnel and patients. A commitment to gather and use data to identify opportunities to improve quality outcomes by modifying processes that result in higher quality care at a lower cost is another tenet of the process. Efforts to achieve quality are dynamic and continuous, and everyone in the organization is involved and responsible. Failures in quality are more often caused by flaws in processes rather than failures of people doing the work.

Why Is Continuous Quality Improvement Relevant for Health Care and Dialysis Programs?

The health care industry is one of the largest and most costly industries in the United States. CQI was introduced in the health care industry in part as an effort to slow the ever-increasing percentage of the country's gross domestic product being devoted to health care. Total Medicare costs for patients with ESRD increased 4.6% between 2015 and 2016 from \$33.8 billion to \$35.4 billion, accounting for 7.2% of the overall Medicare paid claim costs. Total Medicare expenditures for peritoneal dialysis increased 5.7% in 2016 compared with increases of 3.6% for transplantation. Spending for hemodialysis care increased to \$28 billion in 2016. Costs reached \$1.5 billion for peritoneal dialysis and \$3.4 billion for transplantation (US Renal Data System, 2018).

What Is the Connection Between Quality and Cost?

Health care personnel are committed to providing high-quality care to patients. Consideration of the costs of this care has not always been addressed, and providers may not realize that poor care is costly. For example, if optimal dialysis is not achieved for any number of process- or system-related reasons, the patient may have outcomes that require hospitalization for emergency treatment and additional dialysis. The end result is an increased cost and poor financial performance.

How Does Continuous Quality Improvement Differ From Quality Assurance?

Quality assurance (QA) was an early effort to address quality care issues in health care. QA, initiated in response to the requirements of accrediting organizations, tended to use retrospective data collection in which audits of medical records identified problems. These audits evaluated documented, existing problems but did not necessarily result in improved

Table 26.1 Measures Assessment Tool (MAT)

TAG	CONDITION OR STANDARD	MEASURE	VALUES	REFERENCE	SOURCE
494.40 Water and dialysate quality					
V196	Water quality	Max. chloramine (must determine)	≤0.1 mg/L daily/shift	AAMI RD52	Records
V196	Use max. chloramine value if only one test is performed	Max. total chlorine (may determine)	≤0.5 mg/L daily/shift		
V178		Action / Max. bacteria - product water / dialysate	50 CFU/mL / <200 CFU/mL		
V180		Action / Max. endotoxin - product water / dialysate	1 EU/mL / <2 EU/mL (endotoxin units)		
494.50 Reuse of hemodialyzers and blood lines (only applies to facilities that reuse dialyzers &/or bloodlines)					
V336	Dialyzer effectiveness	Total cell volume (hollow fiber dialyzers)	Measure original volume Discard if after reuse <80% of original	KDOQI HD Adequacy 2006; AAMI RD47	Records Interview
494.80 Patient assessment: The interdisciplinary team (IDT), patient/designee, RN, MSW, RD, physician must provide each patient with an individualized & comprehensive assessment of needs					
V502	• Health status/comorbidities	• Medical/nursing history, physical exam findings	Refer to Plan of care & QAPI sections (below) for values	Conditions for Coverage	Chart
V503	• Dialysis prescription	• Evaluate: HD every mo; PD first mo & q 4 mo		KDOQI Guidelines	
V504	• BP & fluid management	• Interdialytic BP & wt gain, target wt, symptoms		(see POC)	
V505	• Lab profile	• Monitor labs monthly & as needed			
V506	• Immunization & meds history	• Pneumococcal, hepatitis, influenza; med allergies			
V507	• Anemia (Hgb, Hct, iron stores, ESA need)	• Volume, bleeding, infection, ESA hypo-response			
V508	• Renal bone disease	• Calcium, phosphorus, PTH & medications			
V509	• Nutritional status	• Multiple elements listed			
V510	• Psychosocial needs	• Multiple elements listed			
V511	• Dialysis access type & maintenance	• Access efficacy, fistula candidacy			
V512	• Abilities, interests, preferences, goals, desired participation in care, preferred modality & setting, expectations for outcomes	• Reason why patient does not participate in care, reason why patient is not a home dialysis candidate			
V513	• Suitability for transplant referral	• Reason why patient is not a transplant candidate			
V514	• Family & other support systems	• Composition, history, availability, level of support			
V515	• Current physical activity level & referral to vocational & physical rehabilitation	• Abilities & barriers to independent living; achieving physical activity, education & work goals			
494.90 Plan of care The IDT must develop & implement a written, individualized comprehensive plan of care that specifies the services necessary to address the patient's needs as identified by the comprehensive assessment & changes in the patient's condition, & must include measurable & expected outcomes & estimated timetables to achieve outcomes. Outcome goals must be consistent with current professionally accepted clinical practice standards.					

Continued on following page

Table 26.1 Measures Assessment Tool (MAT) (Continued)

TAG	CONDITION OR STANDARD	MEASURE	VALUES	REFERENCE	SOURCE
V543	(1) Dose of dialysis/volume status Monitor each treatment	Management of volume status	Euvolemic & BP 130/80 (adult); lower of 90% of normal for age/ht/wt or 130/80 (pediatric)	KDOQI HD Adequacy 2006 KDOQI Hypertension 2004	Chart
V544	(1) Dose of dialysis (HD adequacy) Monitor adequacy monthly	Adult HD <5 hours 3x/week, minimum spKt/V Adult HD 2x/week, RKF <2 mL/min. HD 2, 4-6x/week, minimum stdKt/V	≥1.2; Min. 3 hours/tx if RKF <2ml/min Inadequate treatment frequency ≥2.0/week	KDOQI HD Adequacy 2006	DFR
V544	(1) Dose of dialysis (PD adequacy - adult) Monitor 1st month & every 4 months	Minimum delivered Kt/V_{urea}	≥1.7/wk	KDOQI PD Adequacy 2006	Chart
V544	(1) Dose of dialysis (PD adequacy - pediatric) Monitor 1st month & every 6 months	Minimum delivered Kt/V_{urea}	≥1.8/wk	KDOQI PD Adequacy 2006	Chart
V545	(2) Nutritional status - Monitor albumin & body weight monthly; other parameters at V509, monitor as needed for impact on nutrition	Albumin Body weight & other parameters listed at V509	≥4.0 g/dL BCG preferred; if BCP: lab normal % usual wt, % standard wt, BMI, est. % body fat	KDOQI Nutrition 2000 KDOQI CKD 2002	Chart
V546	(2) Nutritional status (pediatric) monitor monthly	Length/ht-for-age % or SD, dry wt & wt-for-age % or SD, BMI-for-ht/age % or SD, head circ/age % (age ≤3), nPCR	nPCR normalized-HD teen (nPCR and albumin are not predictive of wt loss/nutritional status in younger children)	KDOQI Pediatric Nutrition 2008	Chart
V546	(3) Mineral metabolism & renal bone disease Monitor calcium & phosphorus monthly Monitor intact PTH every 3 months	Calcium corrected for albumin (BCG) Phosphorus Intact PTH (consider with other MBD labs, not in isolation)	Normal for lab; preferred upper level <10/ mg/dL All: 3.5-5.5 mg/dL Adult: 150-300 pg/mL (under review); Peds: 200-300 pg/mL	KDOQI Bone Metabolism & Disease 2003	Chart
V547	(4) Anemia - Hgb non-ESA - monitor monthly	Hemoglobin (Adult & pediatric)	>10.0 g/dL	KDOQI Anemia 2006	DFR

V547	(4) Anemia - Hgb on ESA - monitor monthly	Hemoglobin (Adult & pediatric) Hemoglobin (Adult & pediatric) Hemoglobin (Adult & pediatric)	<12.0 g/dL[1] 10-12.0 g/dL[2] 11-12.0 g/dL, ≤13.0 g/dL[3]	[1]FDA "box" warning [2]Medicare reimbursement [3]KDOQI Anemia CKD 2007	DFR
V548					
V549	(4) Anemia - Monitor iron stores routinely	Adult & pediatric: transferrin saturation Adult & pediatric: serum ferritin	>20% (HD, PD), or CHr >29 pg/cell HD: >200 ng/mL; PD: >100 ng/mL HD/PD: <500 ng/mL or evaluate if indicated	KDOQI Anemia 2006	DFR
V550	(5) Vascular access	Fistula Graft Central Venous Catheter	Preferred[4,5] Acceptable if fistula not possible[4,5] Avoid, unless bridge to fistula/graft or to PD, if transplant soon, or in small adult/peds pt[4]	[4]KDOQI Vascular Access 2006 [5]Fistula First	DFR Interview CW
V551					
V552	(6) Psychosocial status	Survey physical & mental functioning annually KDQOL-36 survey annually or more often as needed	Achieve & sustain (case-mix adjusted) scores of average or above, with no declines of ≥10 points.	Conditions for Coverage CMS CPM 4/1/08; DOPPS	Chart Interview
V553	(7) Modality	Home dialysis referral Transplantation referral	Candidacy or reason for non-referral	Conditions for Coverage	Chart Interview
V554					
V555	(8) Rehabilitation status	Productive activity desired by patient Pediatric: formal education needs met Vocational & physical rehab referrals as indicated	Achieve & sustain appropriate level, unspecified	Conditions for Coverage	Chart Interview
V562	(d) Patient education & training	Dialysis experience, treatment options, self-care, QOL, infection prevention, rehabilitation	Documentation of education in record	Conditions for Coverage CMS CPM 4/1/2008	Records Interview

494.110 Quality assessment and performance improvement (QAPI): The dialysis facility must develop, implement, maintain, & evaluate an effective, data-driven QAPI program with participation by the professional members of the IDT. The program must reflect the complexity of the organization & services (including those under arrangement), & must focus on indicators related to improved health outcomes & the prevention & reduction of medical errors. The dialysis facility must maintain & demonstrate evidence of its QAPI program including continuous monitoring for CMS review. Refer to your ESKD Network's goals for targets for aggregate patient outcomes.

Continued on following page

Table 26.1 Measures Assessment Tool (MAT) (Continued)

TAG	CONDITION OR STANDARD	MEASURE	VALUES	REFERENCE	SOURCE
V627	Health outcomes: Physical & mental functioning	Survey adult/pediatric patients KDQOL-36 survey annually or more often as needed	Achieve & sustain appropriate status ↑ % completing survey	Conditions for Coverage CMS CPM 4/1/2008	Records
V627	Health outcomes: Patient hospitalization	Standardized hospitalization ratio (1.0 is average, >1.0 is worse than average, <1.0 is better than average)	↓ hospitalizations	Conditions for Coverage	DFR
V627	Health outcomes: Patient survival	Standardized mortality ratio (1.0 is average, >1.0 is worse than average, <1.0 is better than average)	↓ mortality	Conditions for Coverage CMS CPM 4/1/08	DFR
V629	(i) HD adequacy (monthly)	HD: Adult (patient with ESKD ≥3 mo)	↑ % with spKt/V ≥1.2 or URR ≥65% if 3 times/week dialysis; stdKt/V ≥2.0/week if 2 or 4–6 times/week dialysis	Conditions for Coverage CMS CPM 4/1/2008, MIPPA	DFR Records
V629	(i) PD adequacy (rolling average, each patient tested ≤4 months)	PD: Adult	↑ % with weekly Kt/V$_{urea}$ ≥1.7 (dialysis + RKF)	Conditions for Coverage CMS CPM 4/1/2008	DFR Records
V630	(ii) Nutritional status	Facility set goals; refer to parameters listed in V509	↑ % of patients within target range on albumin and other nutritional parameters set by the facility	Conditions for Coverage	Records
V631	(iii) Mineral metabolism/renal bone disease	Calcium, phosphorus, & PTH	↑ % in target range on all measures monthly	Conditions for Coverage CMS CPM 4/1/2008	Records
V632	(iv) Anemia management Patients taking ESAs &/or patients not taking ESAs	Mean hemoglobin (patient with ESKD ≥3 mo) Mean hematocrit Serum ferritin & transferrin saturation or CHr	↑ % with mean 10–12 g/dL ↑ % with mean 30–36% Evaluate if indicated	Conditions for Coverage CMS CPM 4/1/2008, MIPPA	DFR Records

Code	Topic	Measures	Target / Change	Standard	Data Source
V633	(v) Vascular access (VA) Evaluation of VA problems, causes, solutions	Cuffed catheters > 90 days AV fistulas for dialysis using 2 needles Thrombosis episodes Infections per use-life of access VA patency	↓ to <10%[6] ↑ to ≥65%[6] or ≥66%[7] ↓ to <0.25/pt-yr at risk for fistulas; 0.50/pt-yr at risk for (grafts ↓ to <1% (fistula); <10% (graft) ↑ % with fistula >3 yrs & graft >2 yrs	[6]KDOQI 2006 [7]Fistula First CMS CPM 4/1/2008	DFR Records CW 2/09
V634	(vi) Medical injuries & medical errors identification	Medical injuries & medical errors reporting	↓ frequency through prevention, early identification & root cause analysis	Conditions for Coverage	Records
V635	(vii) Reuse	Evaluation of reuse program including evaluation & reporting of adverse outcomes	↓ adverse outcomes	Conditions for Coverage	DFR Records
V636	(viii) Patient satisfaction & grievances	Report & analyze grievances for trends CAHPS In-Center Hemodialysis Survey or any patient satisfaction survey	Prompt resolution of patient grievances ↑ % of patients satisfied with care	Conditions for Coverage CMS CPM 4/1/2008	Records Interview
V637	(ix) Infection control	Analyze & document incidence for baselines & trends	Minimize infections & transmission of same Promote immunizations	Conditions for Coverage	DFR Records
V637	Vaccinations	Hepatitis B, influenza, & pneumococcal vaccines Influenza vaccination by facility or other provider	Documentation of education in record ↑ % of patients vaccinated on schedule ↑ % of patients receiving flu shots 10/1-3/31	Conditions for Coverage CMS CPM 4/1/2008	Records

Sources: *Chart,* patient chart; *CW,* CROWNWeb; *DFR,* dialysis facility reports; *Interview,* patient/staff interview; *Records,* facility records.

BCG/BCP, Bromcresol green/purple; *BMI,* body mass index; *CAHPS,* Consumer Assessment of Healthcare Providers & Systems; *CFU,* colony forming units; *CHr,* reticulocyte hemoglobin; *CMS CPM,* Centers for Medicare and Medicaid Services Clinical Performance Measures; *DOPPS,* Dialysis Outcomes & Practice Patterns Study; *ESA,* erythropoiesis stimulating agent; *KDIGO,* Kidney Disease Improving Global Outcomes; *KDOQI,* Kidney Disease Outcomes Quality Initiative. *nPCR,* normalized protein catabolic rate; *NQF,* National Quality Forum; *RKF,* residual kidney function; *spKt/V,* single pool Kt/V. *SD,* standard deviation; *spKt/V,* single pool Kt/V.

From Centers for Medicare & Medicaid Services: Interim Version 1.8. Retrieved from https://www.qirn3.org/Files/Conditions-for-Coverage/2017/03-MAT-2-5-White-508.aspx.

Box 26.2 Centers for Medicare & Medicaid Services Clinical Performance and Reporting Measures

Clinical Performance Measures	Reporting Measures
In-Center Hemodialysis Consumer Assessment of Healthcare Providers and Systems Survey	National Healthcare Safety Network Dialysis Event
Standardized Readmission Ratio	Clinical Depression Screening and Follow Up
Standardized Transfusion Ratio	Ultrafiltration 13ml
Kt/V Dialysis Adequacy	
Vascular Access Type	
Hypercalcemia	
National Healthcare Safety Network Bloodstream Infection in Hemodialysis Patients	

From Dialysis Facilities and the End-Stage Renal Disease Quality Incentive Program (ESRD QIP): Linking quality to payment. Retrieved from https://www.medicare.gov/dialysisfacilitycompare/#qip/quality-incentive-program.

---

quality of care. CQI is a more proactive method that focuses on seeking every opportunity to improve processes and systems to achieve quality outcomes. Concurrent data collection for analysis is a vital aspect of CQI. The focus of CQI is evaluation of interventions to improve quality rather than documentation of problems.

Is Continuous Quality Improvement Essential in Dialysis Facilities?

As a high-volume, high-risk, problem-prone, high-cost health care program, dialysis is a model for CQI. Dialysis facilities can use CQI techniques to identify processes in need of improvement; implement interventions or corrective actions; and evaluate costs, measurable improvements, and quality outcomes.

What Are Some Tools Used in Continuous Quality Improvement?

Quality improvement efforts use the scientific method to search for, find, and fix the root cause of a problem. FOCUS is a CQI tool used to examine and analyze a specific process.

The first step is to *find* a process to improve by analyzing data. Statistical control is used to distinguish between common and special causes of variation in processes. Data are displayed in control charts to track performance. Variations outside the control limits are special cause variances and require investigation. For more detailed instructions on the use of statistical control and other tools, such as flowcharts, Pareto charts, cause-and-effect (fishbone) diagrams, and run charts, refer to a CQI reference text.

The next step is to *organize* a team to work together to improve the situation.

Clarify the problem by collecting and analyzing data specific to the process being targeted for improvement. A cause-and-effect diagram might be useful in this step.

To truly *understand,* health care providers examine data for the causes of variation and the changes over time.

The final FOCUS step is to *select* a method for improving outcomes and initiate the plan–do–check–act (PDCA) cycle of CQI.

What Is the Plan–Do–Check–Act Cycle?

The PDCA cycle is a framework for implementing the methods to improve the outcomes selected during the FOCUS process.

Plan, the first step in instituting a change for improvement, requires investment of time because a hastily determined solution may not produce the desired result. Use of brainstorming techniques encourages all members of the team to contribute ideas to the plan. Reviewing relevant literature is a critical element of planning. One outcome of planning by the multidisciplinary team may be a decision to develop a clinical care pathway or to adopt a clinical practice guideline as a way to improve the quality and cost outcomes of an important aspect of care.

After the plan is agreed upon, the second phase of PDCA—*do*—is applied. Typically, *do* means implementing an intervention or series of steps to reach the desired outcome.

During the *check* phase, the results of the intervention are checked for measurable improvements against the goals of the plan. The interventions may be modified as needed to continue with the improvements.

The final phase of the PDCA cycle is *act,* in which the implementation phase is conducted. Ongoing monitoring is necessary to ensure that the improvement persists over time.

What Is the Role of the ESRD Networks?

Congress established the ESRD Networks in 1977 to provide support to Medicare through administration of the ESRD program. The nonprofit ESRD Networks function as an intermediary between the payer (CMS) and the provider (dialysis facility). The Networks service assigned geographical areas according to the number and concentration of patients. They operate under contract with the CMS, with renewals awarded every 3 years. Currently, 18 ESRD Networks function to promote and improve the quality of care provided to CKD patients through education and management of quality improvement. The program ensures that patients get the right care at the right time. Some responsibilities of the program include the following (ESRD Network Organizations, CMS, 2013):

- Assuring effective and efficient administration of benefits
- Improving quality of care for ESRD patients
- Collecting data to measure the quality of care
- Providing assistance to ESRD patients and providers
- Evaluating and resolving patient grievances

Greater focus is currently being placed on quality improvement through use of patient- and family-centered care and reducing the costs of ESRD through improved care.

DOES THE NATIONAL KIDNEY FOUNDATION HAVE A QUALITY IMPROVEMENT INITIATIVE?

In March 1995, the National Kidney Foundation established the Kidney Disease Outcomes Quality Initiative (KDOQI) to develop evidence-based clinical practice guidelines to improve the care of patients with ESRD. The guidelines were completed in 1997 and have been translated into practice through professional education programs. The Clinical Practice Guidelines have been evaluated for their effect on patient outcomes.

ARE THERE OTHER NETWORKS THAT MONITOR FOR PATIENT SAFETY AND QUALITY?

The National Healthcare Safety Network promotes CQI education and tools to help reduce infection rates in dialysis facilities. They allow facilities to track blood safety errors, vaccination status of employees, and infection control adherence. The Centers for Disease Control and Prevention offers educational webinars, quality improvement tools, and other resources to reduce or prevent hepatitis, pneumonia, flu, and other bloodstream-related infections.

CHAPTER 27

ON BEING A PRECEPTOR

Many employers elect to use preceptorship as a model for clinical education of their newly hired employees. This model is based on the assumption that a stable and consistent relationship optimizes socialization into clinical practice and bridges the gap between theory and practice (Billings & Halstead, 2012). In most instances, the preceptor and preceptee have a one-to-one relationship. Some states require a student-to-preceptor ratio of one to one. The terms *preceptee* and *student* are used interchangeably throughout this chapter.

Preceptors help to enhance student learning, assist in the development of clinical skills, and facilitate the transition of recently hired dialysis employees to their new role by providing guidance and support and serving as a role model. Both the preceptor and the student benefit from the learning relationship. A preceptor is normally selected because of his or her clinical strengths, knowledge, and skills. Many preceptors find the role of teaching and mentoring to be the most fulfilling aspect of their professional practice. Preceptors will most often maintain their normal clinical workload, so the ability to prioritize and multitask is essential.

Often a preceptor has increased opportunities to move up the clinical ladder as well as to receive increased financial compensation. Box 27.1 outlines some of the functions and roles of a clinical preceptor.

What Qualities Should a Preceptor Possess?

Preceptors should first and foremost exhibit clinical expertise in the modality in which they practice and be able to communicate their knowledge to students. Preceptors should demonstrate consistent use of written policies and procedures and exhibit good problem-solving skills. Preceptors must naturally assist and guide others because of an inherent desire to do so. Good communication skills, both oral and written, are necessary to provide feedback and evaluation. Preceptors are expected to serve as role models for those they precept as well as for the entire clinical team. Motacki and Burke (2011) relate that to be effective in the role of a clinical educator, one must be knowledgeable and able to convey concepts to students in effective ways, be clinically competent, have interpersonal skills that positively influence students' learning, and have the ability to establish collegial relationships that last once the clinical obligation is complete.

What Are the Initial Steps in Establishing a Preceptor–Student Relationship?

The initial steps should include meeting the student and evaluating his or her learning style preferences. Teachers tend to teach how they learn best, which may be in conflict with how the student learns best. It is important for preceptors to have a clear understanding of their own philosophy of teaching and learning before understanding that of the student.

The second step in establishing a strong preceptor–student relationship is to identify the learning goals and clinical needs of the student. This would include becoming aware of the strengths and weaknesses of the student to plan the best clinical experiences while building on the strengths and working on the weaknesses. It is difficult to provide good clinical experiences if you are not aware of the learning needs of the student. Individualized learning is crucial and should help link classroom knowledge to the clinical setting. Finally, developing a positive relationship with the student is critical in the initial meeting to foster trust and encourage open communication.

How Do I Prepare Students for Their Clinical Experience?

Make sure that students have directions to the clinic location or training site. It is helpful if they have a point person to contact as well as a telephone number in case they have difficulties finding the clinic on their first day. Information about parking and whether they should bring lunch will make their first day transition smoother. Students should also be notified of any items that they should bring with them, such as a lab coats, goggles, scrubs, stethoscopes, pens, and nametags. Ask students to come prepared to address their strengths and weaknesses, describe what they hope to accomplish during this preceptor experience, and define any areas in which they need additional experience and practice. A tour of the clinic and an introduction to staff after they arrive is beneficial.

What Are Some Characteristics of an Effective Learning Environment?

The preceptor needs to maintain his or her role as an instructor and thus maintain the boundaries of the preceptor–student relationship. This can sometimes be a challenge for the preceptor as he or she attempts to establish trust and provide a nurturing environment in which to learn. Care must be taken to maintain this relationship as such to avoid role conflict and confusion.

Forming a strong interpersonal relationship is critical to the success of the preceptor–student experience. A strong interpersonal relationship will give both parties permission to openly verbalize their thoughts and feelings; however, the preceptor must be able to provide honest ongoing feedback throughout the experience.

Box 27.1 Preceptor Functions

- Assist a new nurse or technician to acquire knowledge and skills
- Tailor the program specifically to needs
- Orient to the unit
- Socialize within the group
- Orient to unit functions
- Teach unfamiliar procedures
- Assist in development of skills
- Act as a resource person
- Familiarize with policies and procedures
- Act as a counselor
- Act as a role model
- Assist in time management
- Delegate tasks
- Assist with priority setting

From Motacki K, Burke K: *Nursing delegation and management of patient care*, St. Louis, 2011, Mosby.

WHAT IS THE ROLE OF EVALUATION IN THE TEACHING–LEARNING ENVIRONMENT?

Evaluation of both clinical performance and learning outcomes is an important task of the clinical preceptor. The student must always be evaluated against the established criteria and learning outcomes of the specific training program. This judgment of the student's performance involves pointing out her or his strengths and weaknesses compared with established criteria. The overall purpose of evaluation is to determine whether learning has occurred and objectives are met.

Evaluation is both formative and summative. Formative evaluation is one that occurs at the time of the learning activity or shortly thereafter and is carried out throughout the preceptor experience. The advantage of this type of evaluation is that the areas of weakness can be addressed early, allowing the instructor to shape the learning environment and help the student to be successful. Formative evaluation also allows the student to make early adjustments to his or her performance to accomplish the established program and clinical objectives. Formative assessments tend to be less formal and are often done on a daily basis, thus providing a good picture of student achievement.

Summative evaluation is one that occurs at the end of the preceptor experience (e.g., 2, 4, or 8 weeks, depending on the timeline of your program). Summative evaluation looks at the entire learning experience and judges whether the course or program objectives have been met. Summative evaluation is formal in nature and focuses on the program or training outcomes. A disadvantage of summative evaluation is that students are not given the opportunity to change behaviors or improve performance if they are not meeting the program objectives.

Most programs use a combination of both formative and summative evaluation to assess learning and achievement of program objectives.

HOW DO I EVALUATE MY STUDENT?

Evaluation and providing feedback are the most difficult parts of the preceptor experience for some. It is necessary to know what knowledge, behaviors, and skills the student is expected to assimilate and apply in his or her clinical role to provide fair evaluation. The personal learning goals of the student should also be assessed at this time. Evaluation should be ongoing and the student should have knowledge of how well he or she is meeting the objectives at all times.

Self-assessment by the student is a helpful tool to use when completing evaluation. Self-assessment helps the student to identify his or her areas of strengths and weaknesses. Reviewing self-assessment before the final evaluation will give the preceptor time to prepare a response if the thoughts are disparate.

At the time of evaluation, the outcomes should be explained with specific examples of where the student excelled and underperformed. It is very important to cite specific examples to validate the results of evaluation. It is helpful to keep anecdotal notes throughout the preceptor experience so that your evaluation is reflective of the entire clinical experience and not just the most recent few days or weeks. Anecdotal notes are helpful to recall specific examples of performance.

Feedback should be given in a friendly and nonthreatening manner, and you should relate your feedback to specific observations. Avoid "whitewashing" in which you comment only on the student's strengths and omit any areas in which she or he was deficient. Billings and Halstead (2012) provide some guidelines to consider at the start of the evaluation process (Box 27.2).

WHAT ARE SOME EFFECTIVE COMMUNICATION STRATEGIES I CAN USE WHILE ACTING AS A PRECEPTOR?

Feedback, whether positive or negative, is necessary to reinforce good behaviors or to discourage undesired behaviors. Feedback is best delivered as soon as possible. This "point-in-time" feedback is necessary to have the desired effect and greatest impact on the student. Negative or constructive feedback should always be delivered privately and in person. It is important when providing negative feedback that you focus on the problem and not the student. Table 27.1 provides some communication strategies to use in the clinical setting to foster positive behaviors.

Box 27.2 Quick Tips for Clinical Evaluation

- Clearly define both knowledge and skills that the preceptee will need to demonstrate.
- Use multiple sources of data for evaluation: anecdotal notes, observations by other staff members, case study reviews, student self-assessments.
- Be reasonable and consistent in evaluation of all preceptees.
- Use formative mini evaluations and suggest minor, easy corrections at the time they are needed.
- Present feedback and evaluation in nonjudgmental language, confining comments to a preceptee's behavior.
- Provide evaluation "sandwiches" by commenting first on a strength, then a weakness, and then a strength of the preceptee's behavior.
- Carry an anecdotal record and maintain privacy of the information.
- Make specific notes focusing on the specific details of a preceptee's behavior.
- Document patterns of the preceptee's behavior over time through compilation of records.
- Invite preceptees to complete self-assessments and summarize what they have learned.
- Help preceptees prioritize learning needs and turn feedback into constructive challenges with specific goals for each day.

Modified from Billings DM, Halstead JA: *Teaching in nursing,* ed. 4, St. Louis, 2012, Elsevier, p. 486.

Table 27.1 Communication Strategies

Setting goals	• Set goals for the entire experience and for each clinical session. • Establish the instructor's expectations for student performance. • Address goals for both patient care and student learning.
Communicating values	• Identify and articulate the impact of preceptor's values on patient care. • Demonstrate how to operationalize values.
Motivating performance	• Review the rationale for each activity performed and how it contributes to safe patient care.
Praising	• Recognize successful performance by focusing on the observed behavior and how it positively influenced patient care.
Providing corrective feedback	• Focus on the behavior and how it impacted patient care. • Describe what was wrong, why it was wrong, and how to correct the behavior.

Modified from O'Connor A: *Clinical instruction and evaluation: a teaching resource,* Sudbury, MA, 2001, Jones and Bartlett.

WHAT ARE SOME ISSUES I MIGHT FACE AS A PRECEPTOR?

Occasionally, a problem may arise when a student faces some performance difficulties or may be dissatisfied with his or her clinical learning experience. Other problems include an inability to transfer didactic knowledge to the clinical setting; poor communication with patients, clinical staff, or the preceptor; failure to improve; or regression of clinical skills. Although these situations are rare, they should be resolved sooner than later. The student may be overwhelmed, frustrated, or distracted. The preceptor should not hesitate to have a conversation with the student to explore the reasons for underperformance or any other issues that may have a negative impact on the clinical experience. Any serious issues should be addressed immediately, and the faculty or manager should be informed of the situation. A poor preceptor–preceptee match should also be considered. It is important to keep meticulous documentation of any performance behaviors that may be "red flags." Box 27.3 lists quick tips to identify whether your student is learning or struggling in the clinical setting.

HOW CAN I MOTIVATE MY STUDENT?

A little bit of praise can go a long way to help motivate your student. Setting small and achievable goals initially will help to instill confidence. Be prepared to allow your student to begin working on the skills that he or she has learned early in the clinical experience. Providing an opportunity for hands-on practice quickly engages the student and will increase motivation. Bridging the gap between classroom didactics and clinical learning experiences can be accomplished by giving the student ample hands-on learning opportunities. Be aware of any teaching and learning moments and include the student in any uncommon occurrences that may take place in the clinical setting. Strengthen learning and retention by frequently providing rationales for procedures and actions performed. Giving your student a variety of learning opportunities will increase his or her interest and motivation. Remember: the better prepared your student is to perform the duties and clinical skills required of the position, the greater an asset he or she will be to you and your colleagues.

Box 27.3 Red Flags

"Red Flag" Behaviors

- Hesitant or anxious when performing patient care procedures
- Defensive attitude or hostile behavior toward the preceptor, clinic staff, or patients
- Difficulty in establishing therapeutic rapport with patients
- Unable to explain rationale for procedures or tasks
- Fails to recognize treatment complications or patient problems
- Unsure of steps in common dialysis procedures
- Inconsistent clinical performance

"Learning" Behaviors

- Performs patient care procedures with confidence and acknowledges when assistance is needed
- Shows positive attitude in assignments and interactions with staff and patients
- Uses therapeutic communication and establishes rapport with patients
- Articulates rationale for completed procedures and tasks
- Responds appropriately to treatment complications or patient complaints
- Executes treatment procedures according to written policy
- Consistently performs procedures with confidence

Modified from Burns C, Beauchesne M, Ryan-Krause P, Sawin K: Mastering the preceptor role: challenges of clinical teaching. *Journal of Pediatric Health Care* 20(3):172–183, 2006.

CHAPTER 28

BASIC MATH CALCULATIONS

This chapter covers basic math calculations that dialysis personnel may need to use while providing care to patients in a chronic or acute dialysis setting. Working with numbers and calculations can sometimes induce anxiety in even the most seasoned student or practitioner. Being able to convert numbers and perform math calculations is critical to safely administering the correct dosage of medication or determining a patient's dialysis treatment prescription. It is imperative that you are able to correctly calculate medication dosages to ensure that your patients are appropriately treated. In this chapter, you will have the opportunity to review basic math skills and practice some problems to strengthen your skills and increase your comfort level in working with numbers and calculations.

THE METRIC SYSTEM

The metric system is the most widely used system of measurement in the world. In health care, it is the most commonly used system to measure medications. It is well suited for this purpose because it can be used to name very large numbers and, more important, very small numbers. The three base units used in the metric system are the meter (m), liter (L), and gram (g). The gram is used to measure weight, the liter is used to measure volume, and the meter is used to measure length. You will most often use grams and liters to calculate medication dosages and meters to measure height or size (Boxes 28.1 and 28.2).

You will use the metric system to calculate not only medication dosages but also your patients' treatment parameters. For example, a patient's weight is always converted into kilograms when determining how much fluid the patient gained interdialytically, how much over "dry" weight the patient is, and how much fluid was removed intradialytically.

How Do you Convert Units Within the Metric System?

It is easy to convert units within the metric system when you reference the metric line, which is illustrated in Table 28.1. Make note of the base units in the center of the metric line: meter, gram, and liter. Everything to the left of the base units gets larger and is represented by a whole number. Everything to the right of the base units gets smaller and is represented by fractions of whole numbers. Prefixes are used with the base units to determine whether the units are larger or smaller than the base unit. The prefixes indicate the size of the unit in multiples of 10. The size of a base unit can be changed by multiplying or dividing by 10. When converting larger units to smaller units, multiply by 10 or move the decimal point to the right for each unit changed; when converting smaller units to larger units, divide by 10 or move the decimal point to the left for each unit changed. The prefixes in the metric line are based on powers of 10. When you make a conversion within the metric system, you multiply or divide by powers of 10. A move from one prefix to another is either 10 times larger or 10 times smaller.

One meter is equal to 10 dm, 100 cm, and 1000 mm. For example, centimeters are 10 times larger than millimeters; therefore, 1 cm equals 10 mm. Because centimeters are larger than millimeters, it takes more millimeters to make up the same length.

For each "step" to the right along the metric line, you multiply by 10. For example, if you want to go from a base unit of liters (L) to centiliters (cL), use the following conversion:

$$2\,L = 20\,dL\,(2 \times 10 = 20) = 2\,cL\,(20 \times 10 = 200)$$

If you want to go from a base unit of grams (g) to milligrams (mg), use the following conversion:

$$4\,g = 40\,dg\,(4 \times 10 = 40) = 400\,cg\,(40 \times 10 = 400) = 4000\,mg\,(400 \times 10 = 4000)$$

Convert 4 L to Milliliters

Multiply 4 L by 1000.

$$4\,L \times 1000 = 4000\,mL$$

or

Move the decimal point three places to the right (you may need to fill in zeros to reach the new decimal point) to give you 4000 mL.

Box 28.1 Common Conversions Used in Health Care

1 oz = 30 mL
1 L = 1000 mL
1 g = 1000 mg
1 mg = 1000 mcg
1 kg = 2.2 lb or 1000 mL

Box 28.2 Common Abbreviations Used in Health are

kg = kilogram
g = gram
mg = milligram
mcg = microgram
mL[a] = milliliter
cc = cubic centimeter

[a]mL and cc are used interchangeably; "cc" is always written in lowercase, and the "L" in mL must be capitalized.

Table 28.1 The Metric Line

	KILO-	HECTA-	DECA-	METRIC BASE UNITS: METER (m) GRAM (g) LITER (L)	DECI-	CENTI-	MILLI-
Value	1000	100	10	1	1/10	1/100	1/1000

CONVERT 4000 MILLILITERS TO LITERS

Divide 4000 mL by 1000.

$$4000\,mL \div 1000 = 4\,L$$

or

Move the decimal point three places to the left to give you 4 L.

In answers that contain only a decimal (e.g., .5 mg), place a zero to the left of the decimal point. This will prevent any errors from occurring should the decimal point go unrecognized. The difference between administering a 5-mg dose and a 0.5-mg dose is significant. Answers containing a whole number, such as 5 mg, should be written as just 5 mg, not 5.0 mg. The difference between 5 mg and 50 mg would also be significant.

When you make a conversion within the metric system, you move the decimal point one place for each "step" that you move on the metric line. If you move to the right on the metric line, you move the decimal point to the right. If you move to the left on the metric line, you move the decimal point to the left.

An example of how to convert meters (m) to decimeters (dm), centimeters (cm), and millimeters (mm) follows:
Convert 5 m to dm.

$$5.0\,m \times 10 = 50\,dm$$

or
Move the decimal point one place to the right: 5.0 = 50.

$$Solution : 5\,m = 50\,dm$$

Convert 5 m to cm.

$$5.0\,m \times 100 = 500\,cm$$

or
Move the decimal point two places to the right: 5.0 = 500.

$$Solution : 5\,m = 500\,cm$$

Convert 5 m to mm.

$$5.0\,m \times 1000 = 5000\,mm$$

or

Move the decimal point three places to the right: $5.0 = 5000$

$$Solution: 5\,m = 5000\,mm$$

PRACTICE FOR METRIC UNITS

Convert the following measurements:
- 135 lb = _____ kg
- 340 cc = _____ mL
- 658 kg = _____ g
- 4 L = _____ mL
- 51 mL = _____ L
- 1000 g = _____ kg
- 2.1 m = _____ cm
- 32 g = _____ kg
- 1 mg = _____ mcg
- 1 mm = _____ cm
- 1 g = _____ mg
- 6400 mL = _____ L
- 4.97 g = _____ mg
- 6.7 cm = _____ mm
- 600 m = _____ km
- 64 kg = _____ lb

WEIGHT CALCULATIONS

In dialysis, patients are weighed most often in kilograms. Although a dialysis patient's weight is variable, an accurate weight is critical so that neither too much nor too little fluid is removed during treatment. If your patient is weighed in pounds, then conversion of pounds to kilograms would be needed.

$$1\ kilogram\ (kg) = 2.2\ pounds\ (lb)$$

$$1\ ounce\ (oz) = 30\ milliliters\ (mL)$$

The following are important definitions with regard to calculating weights and fluid removal in the dialysis patient.

Preweight: the patient's weight upon arrival to the dialysis clinic for treatment

Gain: the difference between the patient's weight after the last treatment and the weight before the current treatment begins

Estimated dry weight (EDW): the lowest weight a patient can tolerate without developing adverse symptoms or hypotension

Available weight (AW): the amount of fluid the patient has available to remove; it is the difference between the patient's pre-weight and EDW

Goal: the goal for fluid removal during treatment; usually this includes the AW plus any fluids that might be administered to the patient during treatment, such as any saline used for blood return, saline rinses, or medication

Lost: the amount of fluid lost during dialysis treatment; this is calculated by subtracting the patient's preweight from the weight after dialysis treatment (post-weight)

Example: Mrs. Jones arrives for her treatment on Friday, and her preweight is 52 kg. Her weight after her last treatment was 49 kg. To calculate her gain, use the following equation:

$$Preweight - Last\ weight = Gain$$

$$52\,kg - 49\,kg = 3\,kg\ gain$$

Mrs. Jones's EDW is 49.5 kg. To calculate her AW, use the following equation:

$$Preweight - EDW = AW$$

$$52\,kg - 49.5\,kg = 2.5\,kg\ AW$$

Mrs. Jones is receiving an antibiotic today that will be diluted with 150 mL of normal saline. To calculate her goal, use the following equation:

$$AW + \text{Additional intradialytic fluids} = \text{Goal}$$

$$2.5 \, kg + 150 \, mL = \text{Goal}$$

$$\text{Convert } 2.5 \, kg \text{ to mL} : 2.5 \times 1000 = 2500 \, mL$$

$$2500 \, mL + 150 \, mL = 2650 \, mL$$

CALCULATE THE PATIENT'S GAIN, AVAILABLE WEIGHT, AND GOAL

Mr. Smith arrived for his treatment today with a preweight of 74.5 kg. His ordered EDW is 72 kg. He left after his last treatment with a weight of 72.1 kg. He has brought with him a protein drink that he will consume during his treatment. The protein drink is 8 oz. Mr. Smith will be receiving vancomycin today, which will be reconstituted with 150 mL of normal saline. His rinseback when discontinuing treatment will be 350 mL.

1. Calculate gain.

$$\text{Preweight} - \text{Last weight} = \text{Gain}$$

$$74.5 \, kg - 72.1 \, kg = 2.4 \, kg \, gain$$

2. Calculate the AW.

$$\text{Preweight} - \text{EDW} = \text{AW}$$

$$74.5 \, kg - 72 \, kg = 2.5 \, kg \, AW$$

3. Calculate the goal.

$$AW + \text{Additional intradialytic fluids} = \text{Goal}$$

$$\text{Convert 8 oz to mL} : 8 \times 30 = 240 \, mL$$

$$\text{Convert } 2.5 \, kg \text{ to mL} : 2.5 \times 1000 = 2500 \, mL$$

$$2500 \, mL + 240 \, mL \, (\text{protein drink}) + 150 \, mL (\text{medication fluids}) + 350 \, mL \, (\text{rinseback}) = 3240 \, mL \, goal$$

PRACTICE FOR WEIGHT CALCULATIONS

Calculate the weights for the following patient situations:

Mrs. Renner arrives for her treatment on Monday with a preweight of 67.8 kg. Her last treatment was on Friday, and she left with a weight of 65.4 kg. Mrs. Renner's EDW is 65.0 kg. She is ordered one unit (250 mL) of packed red blood cells (PRBCs) to be given intradialytically. Her rinseback is 350 mL.

How much did Mrs. Renner gain between treatments?

What is her AW?

What is the goal for this treatment?

Mr. Whitmire arrives for his treatment with a preweight of 81.2 kg. His EDW is 77.0 kg. His rinseback will be 350 mL.

What is the goal for this treatment?

CALCULATING FLUID REMOVAL

Excess fluid is removed from patients during hemodialysis treatment by a process called ultrafiltration (UF). Most dialysis equipment used today provides volumetric control, which allows for very precise fluid removal. The dialysis machine is programmed to calculate the ultrafiltration rate (UFR) according to the patient's treatment goal and the number of hours he or she is scheduled to dialyze. The UFR can be calculated in mL/hr or L/hr. To calculate the UFR, you need to know the goal and length of treatment.

$$\text{Goal} \div \text{Treatment time} = \text{UFR}$$

Example:

Treatment time : 4 hours

Preweight : 87.7 kg

EDW : 84.2 kg

$$AW : 87.7 - 84.2 = 3.5\,kg$$

$$Rinseback : 300\,mL$$

$$Goal : 3.5 \times 1000 = 3500 + 300 = 3800\,mL$$

$$UFR : 3800\,mL \div 4\,hr = 950\,mL/hr\ or\ 0.95/hr$$

DETERMINING IF THE ULTRAFILTRATION GOAL IS LESS THAN OR EQUAL TO 13/mL/kg/hr

In Chapter 13, we talked about Centers for Medicare & Medicaid Services (CMS) guidelines that recommend fluid removal during hemodialysis to be no more than 13 mL/kg/hr. Let's review how to determine whether the UF goal meets the criteria.

1. Determine weight to remove = 1700 mL
   Dialyzer and line prime and rinse back = 300 mL
   Total fluid to be removed = 2000 mL
2. Divide total amount of fluid to be removed by treatment time
   2000 mL ÷ 4 hours = 500 mL/hr
3. Divide UFR in mL/hr by patient's target weight
   500 mL/hr ÷ 50 kg = 10 mL/kg/hr

This patient will remove fluid at a rate of 10 mL/kg/hr which meets the CMS criteria of ≤ 13/mL/kg/hr.

PRACTICE TO DETERMINE IF THE ULTRAFILTRATION IS LESS THAN OR EQUAL TO 13/mL/kg/hr

Calculate how much fluid will be removed and whether it will meet the CMS recommended guideline.

Mr. Wilson's EDW is 54.6 kg, and his treatment time is 3.5 hours. He reached his EDW after his last treatment. He arrived for his treatment today and weighed in at 56.6 kg. His prime and rinseback will be 300 mL, and he is getting 1 unit or 150 mL of PRBCs.

How much weight did Mr. Wilson gain between treatments?
How much total fluid is available for removal?
What is the amount of fluid to be removed per mL/kg/hr?
Will Mr. Wilson meet the goal of 13 mL/kg/hr or less?

RATIOS AND PROPORTIONS

Ratios and proportions can be used to calculate the dosages for some medications used in dialysis. A ratio may be used to describe the quantity of a medication in proportion to the quantity of the solution it is in. A proportion is two ratios that are equal. When using ratios and proportions to calculate dosages, you are actually solving for x. Heparin is one medication used in dialysis whose strength is measured by a ratio. Heparin is commonly found in dialysis units in the following strengths: 1:1000 or 1:5000. The 1:1000 strength means that there are 1000 units (U) of heparin per milliliter of solution. The 1:5000 strength means that there are 5000 U of heparin per milliliter of solution.
Example: The patient is ordered a loading dose of heparin of 8000 U. The heparin on hand is 1000 U/mL. How much heparin would you give?

$$Heparin\ on\ hand : 1000\,U/mL$$

$$Ordered\ dose : 8000\,U$$

$$1000 \times x = 8000 \times 1$$

$$1000x = 8000$$

$$8000 \div 1000 = 8\,mL$$

$$Answer : 8000\,U\ of\ 1 : 1000\ heparin = 8\,mL$$

Example: The patient is to receive 15,000 U of heparin. On hand is a vial containing 5000 U of heparin per milliliter. How many cubic centimeters (cc) would you administer?

$$5000 \times x = 15,000 \times 1$$

$$5000x = 15,000$$

$$15,000 \div 5000 = 3cc$$

Practice Problems for Heparin Dosing

Calculate the volume of heparin to administer for the following doses using a 1000-U/mL vial:
1. 6500 U = _____ mL
2. 10,000 U = _____ mL
3. 1500 U = _____ mL
4. 14,000 U = _____ mL
5. 3000 U = _____ mL

Calculate the volume of heparin to administer for the following doses using a 5000 U/mL vial:
1. 6500 U = _____ mL
2. 10,000 U = _____ mL
3. 1500 U = _____ mL
4. 14,000 U = _____ mL
5. 3000 U = _____ mL

SOLUTIONS

Practice for Metric Units

1. 135 lb = 61.36 kg (135 lb ÷ 2.2 = 61.36 kg)
2. 340 cc = 340 mL (cc and mL are used interchangeably)
3. 658 kg = 658,000 g (658 kg × 1000 = 658,000 g)
4. 4 L = 4000 mL (4 L × 1000 = 4000 mL)
5. 51 mL = 0.051 L (51 mL ÷ 1000 = 0.051 L)
6. 1000 g = 1 kg (1000 g ÷ 1000 = 1 kg)
7. 2.1 m = 210 cm (2.1 m × 100 = 210 cm)
8. 32 g = 0.032 kg (32 g ÷ 1000 = 0.032 kg)
9. 1 mg = 1000 mcg (1 mg × 1000 = 1000 mcg)
10. 1 mm = 0.1 cm (1 mm ÷ 10 = 0.1 cm)
11. 1 g = 1000 mg (1 g × 1000 = 1000 mg)
12. 6400 mL = 6.4 L (6400 mL ÷ 1000 = 6.4 L)
13. 4.97 g = 4970 mg (4.97 g × 1000 = 4970 mg)
14. 6.7 cm = 67 mm (6.7 cm × 10 = 67 mm)
15. 600 m = 0.6 km (600 m ÷ 1000 = 0.6 km)
16. 64 kg = 140.8 lb (64 kg × 2.2 = 140.8 lb)

Practice for Weight Calculations

How much did Mrs. Renner gain between treatments?

$$Preweight - Last\ weight = Gain$$

$$67.8 - 65.4 = 2.4\ kg\ gain$$

What is her AW?

$$Preweight - EDW = AW$$

$$67.8 - 65.0 = 2.8\ kg\ AW$$

What is the goal for this treatment?

$$AW + Additional\ intradialytic\ fluids = Goal$$

$$2.8\ kg + 250\ mL + 350\ mL = Goal$$

$$Convert\ 2.8\ kg\ to\ mL : 2.8 \times 1000 = 2800\ mL$$

$$2800\ mL + 250\ mL + 350\ mL = 3400\ mL\ goal$$

What is the goal for Mr. Whitmire's treatment?

$$Preweight - EDW = AW$$

$$81.2 - 77.0 = 4.2\ kg\ AW$$

$$AW + \text{Additional intradialytic fluids} = \text{Goal}$$

$$4.2\,\text{kg} + 350\,\text{mL} = \text{Goal}$$

$$\text{Convert 4.2 kg to mL}: 4.2 \times 1000 = 4200\,\text{mL}$$

$$4200\,\text{mL} + 350\,\text{mL} = 4550\,\text{mL}$$

PRACTICE TO DETERMINE IF ULTRAFILTRATION IS LESS THAN OR EQUAL TO 13/mL/kg/hr

How much weight did Mr. Wilson gain between treatments?

$$56.6\,\text{kg} - 54.6\,\text{kg} = 2.0\,\text{kg}$$

How much total fluid is available for removal?

$$2000\,\text{mL}\ (2\,\text{kg} = 2000\,\text{mL}) + 300\,\text{mL}\ (\text{prime}) + 150\,\text{mL}\ (\text{PRBC})$$

$$2000\,\text{mL} + 300\,\text{mL} + 150\,\text{mL} = 2450\,\text{mL}$$

What is the amount of fluid to be removed per mL/kg/hr?

$$2450\,\text{mL} \div \text{hours on dialysis}$$

$$2450 \div 3.5 = 700\,\text{mL/hr}$$

Will Mr. Wilson meet the goal of less than or equal to 13 mL/kg/hr?

$$700\,\text{mL/hr} \div \text{EDW}$$

$$700 \div 54.6 = 12.82\,\text{mL/kg/hr}$$

Will Mr. Wilson meet the goal of less than or equal to 13 mL/kg/hr?

$$\text{Yes, the goal is less than or equal to 13 mL/kg/hr.}$$

PRACTICE PROBLEMS FOR HEPARIN DOSING

Using a 1000-U/mL vial:
1. 6500 U = 6.5 mL (6500 U ÷ 1000 = 6.5 mL)
2. 10,000 U = 10 mL (10,000 U ÷ 1000 = 10 mL)
3. 1500 U = 1.5 mL (1500 U ÷ 1000 = 1.5 mL)
4. 14,000 U = 14 mL (14,000 U ÷ 1000 = 14 mL)
5. 3000 U = 3.0 mL (3000 U ÷ 1000 = 3.0 mL)
   Using a 5000-U/mL vial:
1. 6500 U = 1.3 mL (6500 U ÷ 5000 = 1.3 mL)
2. 10,000 U = 2.0 mL (10,000 U ÷ 5000 = 2.0 mL)
3. 1500 U = 0.3 mL (1500 U ÷ 5000 = 0.3 mL)
4. 14,000 U = 2.8 mL (14,000 U ÷ 5000 = 2.8 mL)
5. 3000 U = 0.6 mL (3000 U ÷ 5000 = 0.6 mL)

CHAPTER 29

TEST-TAKING GUIDELINES

Preparing to take any certification exam can produce a lot of anxiety. You may believe that the certification exam reflects all of the time and effort you have invested to be successful in your position. You may have already taken several steps to achieve success in your position and completed a specialty training program as preparation for your position, or you may have completed a review course in preparation for the certification exam. One method to achieve success is development of a plan for preparation, dedicated study time, and increasing your knowledge and skills in test taking. When that has been accomplished, the next step is development of a preparation plan to successfully pass the exam.

How Do I Develop a Plan?

First review your previous experiences in successful test taking. Think about the plan you developed to study for a particular test. What part of the study plan worked most successfully for you? Did you study best alone or in a group? Did you successfully set specific times to study? Were you able to balance time for work and family obligations? Did you have a comfortable study place at home or at another quiet location? Now that you have reviewed your previous study plans, develop a plan for successful completion of the certification exam. You should begin to study well before the exam is scheduled to be taken. Studying for a certification exam can take some individuals up to 6 months of study before they are comfortable with the material and confident that they can pass the exam. A good place to start is with the exam blueprint, which outlines all areas of the exam, including topics and how much weight is placed on each. You can make the most use of your studying time when you know which subject areas hold the most weight because these areas will have the highest number of questions. Take notes on areas which you are least familiar and spend extra time on those topics.

After reviewing the test blueprint, you can then develop a schedule, using a calendar to plan your work schedule, family obligations, study times, and the date when you will take the certification exam. Your calendar needs to include 2 to 3 hours of daily quality study time for at least 8 weeks before the day when you plan to take the exam. The most important thing is that you do not cram for the exam but instead stick with the schedule you created. Cramming causes confusion and makes it harder for you to focus on your study materials.

You may want to find a study partner or form a study group. Study groups work well if the group is small, approximately four to six members. It is best to establish a ground rule that each member will come prepared to study and share knowledge. Talking to someone who has already taken the exam might be helpful to receive some tips on how best to prepare and pass the exam.

What Is Quality Study Time?

Quality study time means uninterrupted daily quiet time spent studying for the certification exam. It involves finding a quiet and comfortable place at home or at another quiet location. Try to eliminate anything that may interrupt your study time; this includes turning off your cell phone and any other electronic devices so that you will not be disturbed. Let people around you know about your study needs and the importance of your study plan for successful completion of the certification exam. Review your study plan daily and make adjustments to it if necessary.

It is also helpful to practice taking tests that are similar to the certification exam. For example, if you will be taking the exam online, practice using the online testing system. Some organizations which offer certification exams offer online practice tests. Review books commonly include practice test questions.

What Is the Best Technique for Answering Multiple-Choice Questions?

Always carefully read the test directions. If the test is administered electronically, be sure you understand how to mark, change, and submit your answers. All multiple-choice questions have a scenario that contains essential information about the patient or situation followed by the stem or the question and several choices or answers. You may be asked to choose the one best answer or all answers that apply.

How Do I Select the Best Answer?

To select the best answer to a multiple-choice question, focus only on the information in the question. Avoid reading into the question or asking "What if?" The question provides all of the information necessary to choose the correct answer. Look for strategic words in the question, such as *immediate, initial, priority,* and *side effect*. These words give an indication of the answer (Box 29.1).

Always read the question twice and come up with the answer in your head. Then read all of the choices before you select an answer. Do not make the mistake of choosing an answer too quickly. Use the process of elimination and discard the answers you know are not correct. When you have eliminated choices, reread the question before selecting your final answer. Do not keep changing your answer; your first choice is usually correct unless you misread the question. Remember not to second guess yourself.

Box 29.1 Practice Question: Strategic Words

A patient arrives for her hemodialysis treatment complaining of flulike symptoms and says she has been vomiting. Which of the following laboratory values should be reported immediately to the physician?

1. Sodium, 148 mEq/L
2. Chloride, 102 mEq/L
3. Potassium, 3.2 mEq/L
4. Bicarbonate, 27 mEq/L

Correct choice: 3

Test-taking skill: The strategic word *immediately* indicates that one of the choices will contain an abnormal laboratory value that should be reported to the physician. Normal potassium ranges from 3.5 to 5.0 mEq/L. A value of 3.2 mEq/L is below the normal value and should be reported immediately.

How Do I Eliminate Wrong Choices?

Be aware of keywords that indicate a wrong choice. Absolute words, such as *never, always, only, all,* and *any,* are too broad and commonly indicate a wrong choice. If you cannot answer a question quickly or use logic to eliminate a wrong choice, move on to the next question and forget about the previous question. Most certification tests have a time limit. Do not use your valuable time trying to solve difficult questions or ones you cannot answer logically (Box 29.2).

What If the Test Includes True-or-False Items?

If the test includes true-or-false items, carefully read through each statement and pay attention to the qualifiers and keywords. Qualifiers, such as *usually, sometimes,* and *generally,* mean that the statement may be true or false depending on the information provided in the statement. It is common for these types of qualifiers to indicate a true answer. If any part of the statement is false, then the entire statement is false (Box 29.3).

What If I Have a Question That Requires Prioritizing?

When you read the scenario and stem of the question, look for strategic words that indicate the need to prioritize. Common strategic words that indicate a need to prioritize include *best, essential, first, immediate, initial, vital, most important,* and *most appropriate.* Remember that when a question asks about priority, all choices may be correct but you will need to determine which action should occur first (Box 29.4).

How Do I Reduce My Test-Taking Anxiety?

Review your test plan to determine whether you provided enough time to prepare for the exam. If you did not, make adjustments to your plan.

Box 29.2 Practice Question: Absolute Words

A patient is diagnosed with polycystic kidney disease. She requests information about the pathophysiology of her disease. Which of the following statements is correct about adult polycystic kidney disease?

1. The kidneys can become markedly enlarged.
2. Deterioration of kidney function is always rapid.
3. It is an immune-related disease.
4. Only invasive radiology tests can diagnose this disease.

Correct choice: 1

Test-taking skill: Adult polycystic kidney disease results in outpouching or distention of the wall, resulting in an enlarged kidney. Choices 2 and 4 contain absolute words and indicate wrong choices.

Box 29.3 Practice Question: True-or-False Items

Sodium polystyrene sulfonate (Kayexalate) is generally used for the treatment of hyperkalemia and is an effective treatment for severe hyperkalemia.

1. True
2. False

Correct choice: 2

Test-taking skill: The first part of the statement is true because Kayexalate is generally used for the treatment of hyperkalemia. However, it is *not* an effective method for treating severe hyperkalemia. Therefore, the second part of the statement is false, making the entire statement false.

Box 29.4 Practice Question: Prioritizing Items

A patient is experiencing an anaphylactic reaction to a new antibiotic. Which of the following actions should be performed immediately?

1. Maintaining a patent airway
2. Administering a corticosteroid
3. Administering epinephrine (adrenaline)
4. Instructing the patient on the importance of obtaining a Medic-Alert bracelet

Correct choice: 1

Test-taking skill: All of the choices should be performed, but the ABC (airway, breathing, circulation) of emergency situations indicates that maintaining a patent airway is the priority and requires immediate action.

A few days before the test, take some time to relax and recharge. If you must travel to a test center, you may want to take a test run to the center so that you will feel confident about the travel time needed and not feel anxious about reaching it late for the exam.

On the day before the exam, get a good night's sleep. Upon waking, follow your usual morning routine but do eat a nutritious meal before the test. It is difficult to concentrate if your stomach is rumbling. Finally, before the test begins, use the bathroom; it is difficult to concentrate if you are uncomfortable.

During the exam, read the test directions slowly and carefully. Stay relaxed and use positive self-talk; if you begin to get nervous, breathe deeply, try smiling (which is relaxing), and then refocus on the test. Write down any important formulas or definitions on a piece of paper given to you at the exam. Remember that you will most likely not be allowed to bring calculators, cell phones, or notes in the test area. Do not worry about how quickly other people finish the exam; concentrate on your own exam. Give yourself positive feedback and remember your plan for success.

NEPHROLOGY ORGANIZATIONS AND RESOURCES

For health care providers who are practicing within a dialysis unit or nephrology program, it becomes important to know where to turn for specific information for patients or for staff. Several organizations can be good resources for practitioners.

Knowing how to use these resources can be key to a successful practice. Most of us do not take full advantage of the educational and informational resources available to us from organizations and the manufacturers of the products we use every day. Product manufacturers have the best available information about their products. It is in the best interests of manufacturers to provide as much information as possible about their products, how to use the products, and other important information. Use these manufacturers as an important resource.

This appendix provides information about voluntary and professional organizations of interest to health professionals caring for patients with chronic kidney disease (CKD). These organizations are listed by category followed by an alphabetical listing that gives a description of each.

ORGANIZATIONS BY CATEGORY

CREDENTIALING ORGANIZATIONS

Board of Nephrology Examiners Nursing and Technology (BONENT): www.bonent.org
National Nephrology Certification Organization (NNCO): www.ptcny.com
Nephrology Nursing Certification Commission (NNCC): www.nncc-exam.org

EDUCATION RESOURCES

Baxter Healthcare: www.baxter.com
Centers for Medicare and Medicaid Services: https://www.cms.gov/Outreach-and-Education/Outreach-and-Education.html
Life Options: www.lifeoptions.org

PATIENT ORGANIZATIONS

American Association of Kidney Patients (AAKP): www.aakp.org
American Foundation for the Blind: https://www.afb.org
Dialysis Patient Citizens (DPC): https://www.dialysispatients.org
Hearing Loss Association of America: https://www.hearingloss.org
Home Dialysis Central: https://www.homedialysis.org/home-dialysis-basics
National Kidney Foundation (NKF): www.kidney.org
Renal Support Network: https://www.rsnhope.org

PROFESSIONAL ASSOCIATIONS

Association for the Advancement of Medical Instrumentation (AAMI): www.aami.org
American Nephrology Nurses Association (ANNA): www.annanurse.org
National Association of Nephrology Technicians/Technologists (NANT): www.dialysistech.net
National Renal Administrators Association (NRAA): www.nraa.org
Renal Physicians Association (RPA): https://www.renalmd.org/default.aspx

TRANSPLANTATION ORGANIZATIONS

American Society of Transplantation: https://www.myast.org
United Network for Organ Sharing (UNOS): www.unos.org
Organ Procurement and Transplantation Network: https://optn.transplant.hrsa.gov

OTHER ORGANIZATIONS

American Foundation of Urologic Disease: www.usrf.org/index.shtml
American Society of Artificial Internal Organs: https://asaio.com
American Society of Nephrology: https://www.asn-online.org
American Society of Pediatric Nephrology: https://www.aspneph.com
National Hospice and Palliative Care Organization: https://www.nhpco.org
Polycystic Kidney Research (PFR) Foundation: https://pkdcure.org

ORGANIZATIONS IN ALPHABETICAL ORDER

The following is an alphabetical listing of nephrology related organizations, with a brief explanation of their resources. Every effort has been made to provide each organization's mission statement or purpose.

American Association of Kidney Patients (AAKP) considers itself "the voice of all kidney patients" and was founded in 1969 by kidney patients for kidney patients. The purpose of this organization is to help patients and their families cope with the emotional, physical, and social impacts of kidney disease through education, advocacy, patient engagement, and cultivating patient communities. AAKP's goal is to educate and improve the health and well-being of CKD patients, those on hemodialysis and peritoneal dialysis, and transplant recipients, including children. Self-help and patient education are key elements of local chapter activities. AAKP publishes *Renalife* six times a year and provides access to information on issues affecting the care and treatment of kidney patients through its informational clearinghouse. Several electronic newsletters, kidney friendly recipes, and other kidney care–related articles are also published, and they can be accessed through the organization's website.

American Kidney Fund (AKF) is the leading nonprofit organization providing direct financial assistance to needy kidney patients. This organization publishes public and patient education brochures and other health-related education resources and many kidney health brochures are available to download directly from the website. The AKF provides financial assistance for low-income dialysis and transplant patients for health insurance premiums, transportation costs, medications, and other health-related expenses. The organization offers free medical screenings, fitness and nutrition presentations, and medical referrals at various venues. Topics on the website cover the spectrum of the AKF's programs and activities, as well as current nephrology issues.

American Nephrology Nurses Association (ANNA) is a nonprofit organization established in 1969. ANNA's stated purpose is to set forth and update high standards of patient care, educate its practitioners, stimulate research, disseminate new ideas through the nephrology nursing field, promote interdisciplinary communication and cooperation, and address issues encompassing the practice of nephrology nursing. The mission of ANNA is to improve members' lives through education, advocacy, networking, and science. ANNA has Specialty Practice Networks led by members with expertise in the areas of acute care, administration, advanced practice, chronic kidney disease, education, health policy, hemodialysis, home therapies, pediatrics, and transplant. Publications provided to members include the *Nephrology Nursing Journal* and a newsletter, *ANNA Update*. In addition to periodicals, ANNA publishes position papers and monographs devoted to nursing practice in nephrology, transplantation, and related therapies. For nurses interested in sitting for the Nephrology Nursing Certification Commission examination, ANNA has developed a *Nephrology Nursing Certification Review Guide* and a model Certification Review Course to assist nurses in their preparation.

Association for the Advancement of Medical Instrumentation (AAMI) is a nonprofit organization that provides continuing information needed by health care professionals to stay current with changes in health care technology. Its mission is the development, management, and safe use of medical technology to enhance patient care. AAMI was founded in 1967 and seeks to increase the understanding and beneficial use of medical instrumentation through effective standards, continuing education, certification programs, and publications. The organization publishes *Biomedical Instrumentation & Technology*, a bimonthly peer-reviewed journal with solutions, news, and advice on aspects of medical technology. *AAMI News Weekly* is a newsletter that presents information on government policies and regulations as well as national and international technology standards development. Other products offered include standards and quality management for water testing, dialysate, and water treatment equipment used in dialysis.

Board of Nephrology Examiners Nursing and Technology (BONENT) is a professional development and certification organization that promotes excellence in the quality of care of nephrology patients around the world. BONENT administers separate examinations in the individual nephrology specialties of hemodialysis technology, hemodialysis nursing, and peritoneal dialysis nursing. Registered nurses, licensed practical nurses, and dialysis technicians who are actively working in dialysis care and have a minimum of 1 year of experience are eligible to take the examination, for which BONENT provides a study outline that includes a comprehensive bibliography. Successful completion of the examination entitles the applicant to use Certified Hemodialysis Technician (CHT), Certified Hemodialysis Nurse (CHN), or Certified Peritoneal Dialysis Nurse (CPDN) as a credential after his or her name. BONENT is active in legislation involving the certification and credentialing of professionals working with kidney patients. BONENT's website provides information on regional seminars for dialysis technicians and nurses.

Home Dialysis Central is an online information site providing education and information on home dialysis modalities for patients and caregivers. A major goal of Home Dialysis Central is to increase the knowledge and interest in home modalities among patients and health care professionals and to increase the number of patients on a home modality. Patients can access information on home dialysis basics told through patient stories, videos, and articles. Health care providers can access educational materials on home dialysis and learn about and access the MATCH-D tool (see Chapter 19). An ultrafiltration rate calculator for provider or patient use can be found on this site to determine if the ultrafiltration rate is safe for the patient. Message boards and discussion forums can be accessed by patients and professionals to learn more about home dialysis.

Life Options is a nonprofit program of research, research-based education, and outreach founded in 1993 to help people live long and live well with kidney disease. A national panel of physicians, researchers, patients, nurses, social workers, dietitians, and ESRD Network directors reviews all Life Options materials and helps guide research. Life Options offers a resource library on their site. Kidney School can be found on the Life Options site, which provides interactive, web-based learning for dialysis patients and kidney professionals.

National Association of Nephrology Technicians/Technologists (NANT) is a nonprofit organization founded in 1983. NANT's goals are to provide educational opportunities for technical practitioners and other members of the integrated team, represent the technical professional in the regulatory and legislative arena, continue the development of technical professionals in leadership roles, and achieve recognition for the role and significant contribution of the technical practitioner to the total care of patients with CKD. The mission of NANT is to promote education and advance the professional role of the multidisciplinary team in delivering the highest quality of care to patients with CKD. NANT offers manuals and study guides on dialyzer reprocessing, water treatment, and dialysis technology, as well as selected reprints on technical aspects of dialysis. Members receive an electronic newsletter bimonthly, free webinars for content hours, and complimentary nephrology magazines.

National Hospice and Palliative Care Organization (NHPCO)'s mission is to lead and mobilize social change for improved care at the end of life. Hospice and palliative care information is located on their website along with policy and advocacy topics, advance care planning information, and an interactive map to locate local hospice providers.

National Kidney Foundation (NKF) is dedicated to increasing awareness of kidney disease, with a shared emphasis on prevention and treatment. NKF's goals are to support research and research training, continuing education of health care professionals, expanding patient services and community resources, educating the public, shaping health policy, and fundraising. Publications include the *American Journal of Kidney Diseases*, the official journal of the NKF, which includes peer-reviewed research papers as well as periodic position papers and proceedings from scientific symposia; *Advances in Chronic Kidney Disease*, a journal that provides in-depth, scholarly reviewed articles about the care and management of people with early kidney disease and kidney failure, as well as those at risk for kidney disease; *Journal of Renal Nutrition*, the official journal of the Council on Renal Nutrition; and *Journal of Nephrology Social Work*, the official journal of the Council of Nephrology Social Workers. Other publications include newsletters for the various councils, pamphlets for laypeople to educate the public about various kidney diseases, and other general kidney-related topics. The Patient Education Resource Center (PERC) contains continuing education courses for physicians, nurses, pharmacists, dietitians, and other health care providers. The NKF offers a KEEP Healthy program, which is a community-based initiative offering education about kidney disease as well as a KEEP Health check up which includes a risk survey, body mass index check, blood pressure check, and an albumine:creatinine ratio (ACR) test for albuminuria. A link to find a KEEP Healthy event can be found on the NKF's site.

The complete text of the NKF Kidney Disease Outcomes Quality Initiative (KDOQI) Clinical Practice Guidelines is available in a variety of formats. The key guidelines (Hemodialysis Adequacy, Peritoneal Dialysis Adequacy, Vascular Access, Treatment of Anemia of Chronic Kidney Failure, and Executive Summaries) and recommendations for the care of patients with CKD are available in summary form on the NKF's website. For guidelines, contact the NKF.

National Nephrology Certification Organization (NNCO) describes its mission as the development and administration of certification examinations in clinical and biomedical nephrology technology. Currently, there are three specialty examinations: (1) patient care technician, (2) biomedical (nephrology) technician, and (3) dialysis water specialist. Applicants who successfully complete the examinations can become a Certified Clinical Nephrology Technician (CCNT), a Certified Biomedical Nephrology Technician (CBNT), or the Certified Dialysis Water Specialist (CDWS). The NNCO offers practice online certification examinations for a fee. The NNCO offers a core curriculum for dialysis technicians that can be found on its website.

National Renal Administrators Association (NRAA) is a voluntary organization representing professional managers of dialysis facilities and centers throughout the United States. Through education, networking, information, and governmental representation, NRAA aims to maintain competence and enhance professionalism throughout the renal community, particularly the renal administrator. Publications include *NRAA Renal Watch* (a weekly email newsletter) and special NRAA reports to keep members informed of key legislative decisions and regulations affecting professionals, along with regional news from across the country.

Nephrology Nursing Certification Commission (NNCC) was established in 1987 to develop and implement certification exams for nephrology nursing. NNCC believes that certification serves as an added credential beyond nursing education and licensure and therefore designs the examination to test the specific knowledge of the nephrology nurse. NNCC's purpose is to improve and maintain the quality of professional nephrology nursing care through the development, administration, and supervision of a certification program in the field of nephrology nursing. Those who successfully complete the certification process by meeting the eligibility criteria and passing a multiple-choice written examination are entitled to display the designated certification of Certified Nephrology Nurse (CNN) or Certified Dialysis Nurse (CDN). The NNCC additionally offers the Certified Nephrology Nurse–Nurse Practitioner (CNN-NP) examination, the Certified Clinical Hemodialysis Technician (CCHT) examination, and the Certified Clinical Hemodialysis Technician–Advanced (CCHT-A).

United Network for Organ Sharing (UNOS)'s mission is to advance organ availability and transplantation by uniting and supporting its communities for the benefit of patients through education, technology, and policy development. UNOS manages the national transplant waiting list and matches donors to recipients through policy, education, and technology. Educational resources for professionals and an allocation calculator can be found on the website. Patient education and other resources for all organ transplants are provided. The Organ Procurement and Transplantation Network (OPTN) was established by the US Congress in 1984. The primary goals of the OPTN are to increase the effectiveness of organ sharing, ensure equity in the distribution, and increase the supply of donated organs available for transplantation. The UNOS administers the OPTN under contract.

By being aware of the resources available to practitioners in the dialysis unit setting, health care professionals will be better prepared to assist patients and their families to cope with living with CKD. Research has shown that patients with more extensive support systems live longer than those with little or no support. You play a key role in your patients' support system. Play this role wisely.

HIGH-POTASSIUM FOODS TO LIMIT OR AVOID[a]

INSTEAD OF THESE HIGHER POTASSIUM FOODS	CHOOSE THESE LOWER POTASSIUM FOODS
Beverages Grapefruit juice, orange juice, prune juice	Apple cider, cranberry juice cocktail, lemonade
Dairy Products Cheese, cow's milk, yogurt	Low-fat cottage cheese, nondairy whipped creamers, nondairy whipped topping, rice milk
Protein Dried beans, dark or packaged meats	Chicken (white meat), turkey (white meat), canned tuna, eggs
Vegetables Avocado, baked beans, Brussels sprouts (cooked), chard, collards, kale, potatoes, pumpkin, split peas, spinach, lentils, beans, sweet potatoes, tomatoes, winter squash, yams	Bell peppers, cabbage, carrots, cauliflower, celery, corn, cucumber, eggplant, green beans, kale, lettuce, onions, red bell pepper, summer squash
Fruits Fresh apricots, bananas, cantaloupe, dates, honeydew, nectarines, kiwi, plantains, prunes (whole and juice), oranges (and juice), raisins (dried fruit), spinach, star fruit	Apples, berries, cherries, cranberries, grapes, lemons, limes, mangos, papayas, pears, peaches, plums, pineapple, rhubarb, strawberries, tangerines, watermelon
Snacks Bran products and granola, chocolate	Jellybeans, lemon- or vanilla-flavored desserts, plain donuts
Other Foods Brown or wild rice	White rice, pita, tortillas, white bread

Modified from Potassium: tips for people with chronic kidney disease (CKD), National Kidney Disease Education Program, US Department of Health and Human Services, National Institute of Health, NIH Publication No. 11-7407, Revised September 2011.

[a]Avoid salt substitutes containing potassium chloride. Limit packaged foods that contain potassium chloride. Drain liquid from canned fruits and vegetables before eating. Season food with herbs and spices.

HIGH-SODIUM FOODS TO LIMIT OR AVOID[a]

INSTEAD OF THESE HIGHER SODIUM FOODS	CHOOSE THESE LOWER SODIUM FOODS
Beverages Carbonated beverages with sodium added, softened water, tomato juice (V8)	Coffee, fruit juices, water
Dairy Products Buttermilk, cottage cheese, processed cheese slices and spreads	Low-fat, low-sodium cheese; low-sodium cottage cheese
Protein Bacon; corned beef; hot dogs; lunch meats; sausage; canned chicken, fish, or meat	Fresh meat, poultry, seafood
Vegetables Canned beans, canned tomatoes, canned and pickled vegetables	Fresh or frozen vegetables
Snacks Pretzels, potato chips, crackers, nuts with salt	Unsalted air popped popcorn, unsalted crackers, unsalted nuts
Other Foods Bouillon, canned and instant soups or broths, frozen foods, olives, pickles, ramen noodles, relish, salt and salt seasonings, soy sauce, salad dressings, frozen dinners	Fresh seasonings and herbs, rice, noodles, cooked cereals without salt

Modified from Sodium: tips for people with chronic kidney disease (CKD), National Kidney Disease Education Program, US Department of Health and Human Services, National Institute of Health, NIH Publication No. 14-7407, Revised June 2014.

[a]Avoid foods that list salt or sodium in the first five ingredients. The following contain sodium: monosodium glutamate (MSG), sodium bicarbonate (baking soda), baking powder, disodium phosphate, sodium alginate, sodium citrate, sodium nitrate. Rinse canned vegetables and beans to remove excess sodium.

HIGH-PHOSPHORUS FOODS TO LIMIT OR AVOID[a]

INSTEAD OF THESE HIGHER PHOSPHORUS FOODS	CHOOSE THESE LOWER PHOSPHORUS FOODS
Beverages	
Milk	Rice milk (not enriched)
Colas and pepper-type sodas, flavored waters, bottled teas	Lemon lime soda, ginger ale, plain water, home-brewed iced tea
Dairy Products	
Yogurt	Regular and low-fat cream cheese
Hard cheese	
Ricotta or cottage cheese	
Fat-free cream cheese	
Protein	
Organ meats, walleye, sardines	Lean beef, pork, lamb, poultry, or other fish
Vegetables	
Dried peas (split, black eyed), beans (black, garbanzo, lima, kidney, navy, pinto) or lentils	Green peas (canned or frozen), green beans or wax beans, mixed vegetables
Snacks	
Pudding	Sherbet
Ice cream	Frozen fruit pops
Nuts and seeds	Popcorn
Chocolate	Hard candy, jellybeans
Other Foods	
Soups made with dried peas, beans, or lentils	Soups made with lower phosphorus ingredients such as broth or water based soups
Whole-grain breads, cereals, crackers, rice and pasta	Refined grains, including white bread, crackers, cereals, rice, and pasta
Peanut butter	Jam, jelly, or honey

Meat, poultry, and fish: A cooked portion should be 2 to 3 oz.
Dairy foods: Portions should be no more than ½ cup of milk or yogurt or one slice of cheese.
Beans and lentils: Portions should be about ½ cup of cooked beans or lentils.
Nuts: Keep portions to about ¼ cup.
Note: Packaged food may contain added phosphorus. Look for phosphorus on the food label or for words such as PHOS or phosphate.
Modified from Mayo Clinic: http://www.mayoclinic.org/food-and-nutrition/expert-answers/faq-20058408 and https://www.niddk.nih.gov/health-information/kidney-disease/chronic-kidney-disease-ckd/eating-nutrition#phosphorus.

[a]Eat smaller portions of foods high in protein at meals and for snacks.

DIALYSIS LABORATORY TESTS AT A GLANCE[a]

BLOOD TEST	NORMAL VALUES	TYPICAL VALUES FOR ESRD	SIGNS AND SYMPTOMS
Albumin	3.5–5.5 g/dL >4.0	BCG (preferred) Laboratory normal BCP	*Low:* malnutrition, weight loss, poor appetite, liver disease, medication side effects
Aspartate aminotransferase (AST) (formerly SGOT)	8–20 U/L	Same as normal	*High:* jaundice, nausea or vomiting, abdominal pain
Alanine aminotransferase (ALT) (formerly SGPT)	7–56 U/L	Same as normal	*High:* abdominal pain, nausea or vomiting, other medication side effects (e.g., muscle cramps)
Bicarbonate (CO_2)	21–30 mEq/L	>22 mEq/L	*High:* rapid breathing, shortness of breath
Bilirubin Direct Total	0.3 mg/dL 0.2–1.3 mg/dL	Same	*High:* jaundice, abdominal pain, fatigue, appetite changes
Blood cultures	Negative or no growth	Same	Depends on source: fever, malaise, rigors, hypotension, nausea, abdominal discomfort, cough, and so on
Blood urea nitrogen (BUN)	10–21 mg/dL Expect ratio of BUN:creatinine ~10:1	<90 mg/dL; depends on protein intake	*High:* fatigue, nausea, insomnia, dry or itching skin, urine-like body odor and breath
Calcium corrected for BCG albumin	8.5–10.5 mg/dL	Normal for laboratory Preferred upper level is <10 mg/dL	*Low:* muscle twitching or cramping, seizures, depression, hair loss, cataracts *High:* muscle weakness, fatigue, symptoms same as sodium, mental changes ranging from mild confusion to psychosis
Chloride (Cl)	95–108 mEq/L	Same	*High:* muscle weakness, fatigue, deep breathing *Low:* hyperexcitable nervous system, low blood pressure, shallow breathing, tetany

[a]**Stages of chronic kidney disease (CKD):**
Within this framework, the Kidney Disease Outcomes Quality Initiative classified CKD into five stages, as follows:
Stage 1: kidney damage with glomerular filtration rate (GFR) ≥90 mL/min/1.73 m^2
Stage 2: kidney damage with GFR 60–89 mL/min/1.73 m^2
Stage 3a: GFR 45–59 mL/min/1.73 m^2
Stage 3b: GFR 30–44 mL/min/1.73 m^2
Stage 4: GFR 15–29 mL/min/1.73 m^2
Stage 5: GFR <15 mL/min/1.73 m^2 or kidney failure treated by dialysis or transplantation

BLOOD TEST	NORMAL VALUES	TYPICAL VALUES FOR ESRD	SIGNS AND SYMPTOMS
Creatinine	0.5–1.4 mg/dL	12–20 mg/dL; varies with muscle mass	
Ferritin	*Male:* 12–300 ng/mL *Female:* 10–150 mg/mL	100–500 ng/mL CKD 1–4 and PD <500 ng/mL HD or evaluate	*If anemic:* pallor, fatigue, tachycardia, cold intolerance Level may be high because of infection or inflammation: abscess or wounds, fever
Glucose	*Fasting:* <126 mg/dL	Same as normal	*High:* excessive thirst *Low:* hunger, fatigue, vertigo, mood changes, sweating, anxiety, poor memory
Hemoglobin	*Male:* 13.2–16.2 g/dL *Female:* 12–15.2 g/dL	Minimize signs and symptoms, transfusions, and ESA risks	*Low:* fatigue, shortness of breath, chest pain, cold intolerance, weakness
Hemoglobin A$_{1c}$	<7%	Same as normal	May be inaccurate in ESRD due to decreased RBC life span
Hepatitis antibody (anti HBs)	Immune = ≥10 mIU/mL Susceptible = <10 mIU/mL	Same as normal	Patients are susceptible to infection by hepatitis B virus
Hepatitis B surface antigen (HbsAg) (formerly Australian antigen)	Negative	Same as normal	*Positive:* abdominal pain, anorexia, nausea or vomiting, jaundice, fatigue, or asymptomatic
Hepatitis C antibody (anti-HCV)	Negative	Same as normal	*Positive:* 80% of people have no signs or symptoms; symptoms may include jaundice, fatigue, dark urine; abdominal pain, loss of appetite, nausea
Magnesium (Mg)	1.5–2.5 mEq/L	Same as normal	*High or low:* muscle weakness, twitching, cramping, confusion
Mean corpuscular volume (MCV)	*Male:* 82–102 *Female:* 78–101	Same as normal	
Parathyroid hormone (PTH) level	Intact PTH, 10–65 pg/mL	*Adult:* 150–300 pg/mL (under review) *Pediatric:* 200–300 pg/mL	*High:* initially, asymptomatic; later, itching, bony changes on radiography, fractures
Phosphorus (PO$_4$)	3.0–5.0 mg/dL	*Goal:* 3.5–5.5 mg/dL	*High:* causes elevated PTH by lowering calcium *Abnormal:* bone fractures
Platelet count	140–450 × 103/μL	Same as normal	*Low:* increased risk of bleeding
Potassium (K)	3.5–5 mEq/L	Same, with some patients tolerating values ≤6.0 without problem	*High:* with ESRD, few symptoms below 7.0; extreme weakness preceding cardiac arrest
Reticulocyte count	0.5%–1.5%	Same but will be higher in states of increased RBC production	
Sodium (Na)	133–145 mEq/L	Same as normal	*High:* thirst and drinking more, fluid gain, elevated BP and shortness of breath *Low:* confusion, hallucination, coma, muscle spasms, muscle cramps, weakness, fatigue, loss of appetite, nausea, vomiting

Continued on following page

BLOOD TEST	NORMAL VALUES	TYPICAL VALUES FOR ESRD	SIGNS AND SYMPTOMS
Total protein	6–8 g/dL	Same as normal	*High:* chronic inflammation or infection, bone marrow disorders *Low:* liver disease, malnutrition or malabsorption disorders
Transferrin saturation (TSAT)	15%–50%	>20%	*Low:* anemia symptoms: fatigue, shortness of breath, cold intolerance
White blood count (WBC)	4.8–10.8 × 103/µL	Same as normal	*High:* signs of infection, fever

BCG, Bromocresol green; *BCP,* bromocresol purple; *BP,* blood pressure; *ESA,* erythropoietin-stimulating agent; *ESRD,* end-stage renal disease; *HD,* hemodialysis; *PD,* peritoneal dialysis; *RBC,* red blood cell.

References

American Diabetes Association: Clinical practice recommendations, 2019. Retrieved from http://care.diabetesjournals.org/content/42/Supplement_1.

Copstead LE, Banasik JL: *Pathophysiology,* ed. 6, St. Louis, 2019, Elsevier Saunders.

Centers for Disease Control and Prevention: Recommendations for preventing transmission of infections among chronic hemodialysis patients. *MMWR Recomm Rep* 50(RR-5):1–43, 2001.

FDA Drug Safety Communication: Modified dosing recommendations to improve the safe use of erythropoiesis-stimulating agents (ESAs) in chronic kidney disease, n.d. Retrieved from http://www.fda.gov/Drugs/DrugSafety/ucm259639.htm.

National Kidney Foundation. Retrieved from https://www.kidney.org/sites/default/files/01-10-7278_HBG_CKD_Stages_Flyer3.pdf.

National Kidney Foundation: KDOQI Clinical Practice Guidelines for chronic kidney disease: evaluation, classification, and stratification, guideline 2: evaluation and treatment. *Am J Kidney Dis* 39(2 suppl 1):S1–S266, 2002.

National Kidney Foundation: KDOQI Clinical Practice Guidelines and Clinical Practice Recommendations for anemia in chronic kidney disease. *Am J Kidney Dis* 47(5 suppl 3):S16–S85, 2006.

National Kidney Foundation: KDOQI Clinical Practice Guideline for Diabetes and CKD: 2012 update. *Am J Kidney Dis* 60(5):850–886, 2012.

Pagana KD, Pagana TJ, Pagana TN: *Mosby's diagnostic and laboratory test reference,* ed 12, St. Louis, 2015, Mosby.

Uribarri J, National Kidney Foundation: K/DOQI guidelines for bone metabolism and disease in chronic kidney disease patients: some therapeutic implications. *Semin Dial* 17(5):349–350, 2004.

GLOSSARY

ABO typing: A blood test used to determine red blood cell type.

action level: Term used by the Association for the Advancement of Medical Instrumentation that notes the concentration at which steps should be taken to prevent the levels of a substance, such as chlorine or chloramines, from increasing to the maximum allowable limits.

activated clotting time (ACT): A test to measure the clotting time of blood.

acute tubular necrosis (ATN): A kidney disorder involving damage to the tubular cells of the kidneys, resulting in acute kidney failure. In kidney transplant, it refers to reversible kidney damage resulting in delayed kidney function.

acute: An adjective used in two ways: to indicate that something is of a short duration or sudden onset and to indicate a high degree of severity.

adsorb: To cause particles or molecules in solution to stick to the surface of a solid material.

air embolus: An air bubble carried by the bloodstream to a vessel small enough to be blocked by the bubble.

AKI (acute kidney injury): Abrupt loss of kidney function, usually temporary.

albumin: A protein found in many body tissues. It disperses in water as a colloid and is an important fraction of blood plasma. The molecular weight is approximately 68,000 Da.

albuminuria: Presence of albumin in urine; this is usually a symptom of kidney disease.

allograft: A graft, such as a kidney, taken from another person (Greek *allo,* "other"). The donor may be a blood relative or unrelated.

amino acids: Building blocks of proteins. Amino indicates that one or more hydrogen ions of an acid have been replaced by the NH_2 radical. Amino acids also contain carbon, oxygen, and frequently sulfur.

amyloid: An abnormal protein material occurring as deposits in various body tissues in certain disorders. In patients with chronic kidney disease, it results from long-term accumulation of β_2-microglobulin.

analog: A structure whose function is similar to that of another organ or structure of a different kind and origin.

anaphylaxis: A particularly severe type of systemic reaction to a foreign protein or other substance. It results from previous sensitization to the particular substance and can be fatal.

aneroid: A pressure gauge (positive or negative) that contains no fluid.

aneurysm: A blood-filled sac formed by stretching and dilation of the wall of an artery.

angiogram: An x-ray film of a blood vessel obtained by injecting a liquid contrast material into the vessel.

anion: An ion carrying a negative ($-$) electric charge. Opposite electric charges attract one another; hence, the negatively charged particle is attracted to the positive pole (the anode).

anterior: In front or toward the front position.

antibody: A protein made by the body's immune system in response to a foreign substance.

anticoagulant: A medication or chemical to prevent clotting.

antigen: A molecule capable of binding specifically to an antibody, resulting in either an immune response or a specific tolerant state.

antiseptic: A chemical that stops the growth and reproduction of bacteria or germs; it does not necessarily destroy them.

anuria: Complete cessation of urine flow.

APN (advanced practice nurse): A registered nurse with advanced clinical and didactic education (e.g., nurse practitioners, nurse anesthetists, nurse midwives, or clinical nurse specialists).

APTT/PTT (activated partial thromboplastin time): Laboratory tests to determine the effects of heparin and the length of time necessary for the blood to clot.

arrhythmia: Any variation from the normal rhythmic heartbeat.

arterial: Related to an artery or arteries.

arteriovenous: Involving both arteries and veins.

artery: A blood vessel carrying blood under pressure from the heart to various parts of the body.

ascitic fluid (ascites): An accumulation of fluid in the abdominal cavity. Usually contains protein to a varying degree.

aseptic: Free of bacterial or infectious organisms; sterile.

aspirate: Remove something by suction or negative pressure.

assay: An analysis to determine the presence and amount of a substance.

Association for the Advancement of Medical Instrumentation (AAMI): An organization that sets the standards and recommended practices for dialysis machines, reuse of dialyzers, electrical safety, monitoring and culturing of machines and water systems, cleaning of machines, quality of water used for dialysis, and methodology for bacteriology and culturing samples.

atherosclerosis: A type of arteriosclerosis (hardening of the arteries) caused by degeneration and fatty changes in the walls of the arteries.

atony: Lack of normal tone or strength.

autoclave: A device for sterilizing materials using saturated steam under pressure.

autogenous: Produced within the organism itself.

azotemia: Retention of nitrogenous wastes (urea, creatinine) in blood and body fluid.

β_2M/β_2-microglobulin: A protein found on the surface of many cells.

bacteremia: Presence of bacteria in the bloodstream.

bacteria: Small, one-celled plantlike organisms that are widely prevalent everywhere. Many kinds are harmless or beneficial; certain kinds cause infections and may be dangerous.

bioavailability: The amount of an administered drug absorbed into the bloodstream that actually reaches the intended site of action in the body.

biocompatible: Not causing changes or reactions in living tissues. A biocompatible membrane would not damage blood cells, cause clotting, or release pyrogenic matter.

blood cells: Cellular elements of blood. Red blood cells are vital for the transport of oxygen from lungs to tissues; white blood cells act to combat infection and destroy bacteria.

bradycardia: Slow pulse rate or heart rate.

bruit: An abnormal sound or murmur heard by listening over a blood vessel with a stethoscope; expected sound heard over the vascular access of a dialysis patient produced by the blood flowing through it.

BUN (blood urea nitrogen): A chemical determination of the amount of nitrogen derived from urea present in blood. Actual urea is 2.2 times the BUN value. Normal BUN ranges from 9 to 15 mg/dL (3–6.5 mmol/L).

BUN:creatinine ratio: The normal ratio is 10:1.

cachexia: General ill health and malnutrition. Wasting.

cadaver donor: A person who has died and whose family has agreed to donate his or her organs for transplantation.

calcimimetic: A medication that mimics the effects of calcium. Recognized by the body as calcium, which helps to lower serum calcium levels.

calcium–phosphorus product: Calcium (in mg/dL) multiplied by phosphorus; the product should be less than 70.

calibrate: Adjust or accurately set a measuring device by comparison with a known standard.

cannula: A tube inserted into a body opening.

CAPD (continuous ambulatory peritoneal dialysis): A form of dialysis therapy that takes place throughout the day and uses the peritoneal membrane as a filter to remove toxicities.

carbohydrate: One of the three main categories of basic foodstuffs; composed of carbon, hydrogen, and oxygen and readily used by the body for energy. Starches and sugars are carbohydrates.

cardiomyopathy: Any weakness or dysfunction of the heart muscle. Usually there is dilation and enlargement of the heart.

caseation: Necrosis in which the tissue is changed into a dry mass resembling cheese. Typically seen with tuberculosis.

catabolism: Breakdown of body tissue at a rate faster than its restoration.

catheter: A hollow tube for withdrawing or introducing fluid into a cavity or passage of the body.

cation: An ion carrying a positive (+) charge that is attracted to the oppositely charged electric pole, the cathode.

caudad: Toward the tail or the tailbone.

CAVH (continuous arteriovenous hemofiltration): A treatment used in the management of acute kidney injury in hemodynamically unstable patients. This slow continuous form of ultrafiltration does not involve the use of a blood pump but uses the patient's mean arterial pressure to circulate blood through the extracorporeal circuit.

CAVHD (continuous arteriovenous hemodialysis): A treatment used in the management of acute kidney injury in critically ill patients. It does not involve the use of a blood pump but uses the patient's arterial blood pressure to circulate blood through the extracorporeal circuit.

CCHT (Certified Clinical Hemodialysis Technician): Credentialing for dialysis technicians who have passed a certification examination administered by the National Nursing Certification Commission.

CCNT: Certified Clinical Nephrology Technologist.

CCPD (continuous cycling peritoneal dialysis): A type of dialysis in which the patient is attached to a peritoneal dialysis automatic cycler for short exchanges throughout the night. During waking hours, the patient receives a long dialysis exchange without use of the machine.

CDC (Centers for Disease Control and Prevention): One of the major operating components of the Department of Health and Human Services. It functions to protect health through health promotion; prevention of disease, injury, and disability; and preparedness for new health threats.

cellulose: A complex carbohydrate polymer of the form $(C_6H_{10}O_5)N$. It is the fibrous support structure of plants. Treatment with heat and chemicals produces a semipermeable membrane.

centipoise: The amount of force necessary to move a layer of liquid in relation to another liquid. A unit of viscosity is equal to 1/100 poise.

cephalad: Toward the head.

CfCs (Conditions for Coverage): Guidelines health care organizations must meet to participate in Medicare and Medicaid programs.

chloramine: A chemical compound containing chlorine attached to nitrogen in the form of NCI groups.

CHT (Certified Hemodialysis Technician): Credentialing for dialysis technicians who have passed a certification examination administered by the Board of Nephrology Examiners Nursing and Technology.

CKD (chronic kidney disease): Gradual and progressive loss of kidney function over time, usually irreversible.

clearance: Mathematical expression of the rate at which a given substance is removed from a solution (e.g., the clearance of urea from blood by the natural or an artificial kidney). It is defined as the number of milliliters of solution that would be completely cleared of a given solute in 1 minute.

CLIA (Clinical Laboratory Improvement Act): United States federal regulatory standards that apply to clinical laboratory testing.

CMS (Centers for Medicare & Medicaid Services): A federal agency that administers the Medicare and Medicaid programs.

CNN (Certified Nephrology Nurse): Credentialing for dialysis registered nurses who have passed a certification examination administered by the National Nursing Certification Commission.

coagulation: Formation of a blood clot.

coagulopathy: A disease or condition affecting the blood's ability to coagulate.

colloid: A very finely divided substance, larger than a molecule, that spreads throughout a liquid as tiny particles. A colloid does not actually dissolve in the liquid or cross a semipermeable membrane. It does exert an osmotic effect proportionate to its concentration. Serum albumin is a colloid.

colony-forming units (CFU): A unit used to estimate the number of viable bacteria or fungal cells in a sample.

comorbid: A coexisting illness or disease process not directly related to the primary disorder. It may make the overall course more complicated or may adversely affect the outcome.

compliance: Capacity to yield or stretch. Also adherence to a plan of care, such as dietary and fluid restrictions.

compound: A distinctive substance formed by the chemical union of two or more elements in a definite proportion by weight.

concurrent: As applied to a dialyzer, the dialysis fluid and blood flow in the same direction.

conductivity: The ease with which an electric current is carried or conducted through something. The conductivity of the dialysis solution is proportional to its electrolyte content.

congestive heart failure (CHF): A condition in which the heart pumps less effectively because of excess body fluid.

conservative management: Treatment of end-stage kidney disease without dialysis.

contaminate: Make dirty, impure, or unsterile.

convection: Movement of solutes across a membrane caused by bulk flow of solution.

countercurrent: In a dialyzer, the directions of flow of the dialysis fluid and blood are 180 degrees opposite one another.

CQI (continuous quality improvement): A management philosophy focused on improving the quality of a product, program, or service.

creatinine clearance: A test that measures how efficiently the kidneys remove creatinine from blood.

creatinine: A nitrogenous waste product of normal muscle metabolism. It is produced at a fairly constant rate in the body.

Crit-Line monitor: An arterial in-line medical instrument that provides continuous measurement of absolute hematocrit, percent blood volume changes, and oxygen saturation in real time. It measures blood volume changes on the basis of the hematocrit because these two values have an inverse relationship. As fluid is removed from the intravascular space, blood density increases. This is displayed on the instrument's screen as a percent of blood volume change on a gridlike graph. With this device, it is possible to maximize ultrafiltration safely and prevent hypotension, cramping, and other intradialytic complications associated with volume depletion. A disposable blood chamber is attached to the arterial side of the dialyzer and photometric technology is used. This device also measures access recirculation.

cross-matching: Testing of blood and tissues to check the compatibility of a donor organ with a recipient. A positive cross-match indicates that the donor and recipient are incompatible.

CTS (carpal tunnel syndrome): A hand or arm condition that produces symptoms such as tingling, numbness, and weakness.

CVD (cardiovascular disease): A class of disease involving the heart or blood vessels.

CVVH (continuous venovenous hemofiltration): A slow process of removing fluid from a patient over a long period of time through a venous access.

CVVHD (continuous venovenous hemodialysis): A slow process of removing fluid and electrolytes from a patient over an extended period of time through a venous access.

cyclosporine A: An immunosuppressive medication, technically an undecapeptide. It is highly effective in controlling transplant rejection. However, it adversely affects kidney function.

cytomegalovirus (CMV): A group of species-specific herpetoviruses that infect humans and other animals. Infection is often asymptomatic but tends to exacerbate in immunosuppressed individuals, causing illness with cellular enlargement, cytoplasmic inclusion, and damage to various organs.

dalton (Da): One atomic mass unit. Named after John Dalton, a developer of the atomic concept.

debris: An accumulation of fragments of miscellaneous materials; rubbish or junk material.

degassing: Removing the gases (largely air) normally dissolved in tap water. Important in proportioning delivery systems.

deionize: Remove various solute ions from a solution. Usually it refers to a water treatment process that removes all electrolytes from the water.

delta: The Greek letter D (Δ) used in mathematics to indicate a difference or change between two points.

dementia: Progressive decline in cognitive function caused by brain damage or disease beyond what might be expected from normal aging.

dextran: A glucose polymer.

dextrose: A simple sugar readily used by body cells for metabolism.

dialysance: A term that indicates the capability of a dialyzer to clear a given solute. It represents the net rate of exchange of a substance between blood and bath per minute per unit of blood bath concentration gradient.

dialysate flow rate: The rate at which the dialysate flows through the dialyzer.

dialysate: A chemical bath used in dialysis to draw fluids and toxins out of the bloodstream and supply electrolytes and other chemicals to the bloodstream.

dialysis-quality water: Water that by LAL testing contains less than 1 EU/mL for mycobacteria and that meets the Association for the Advancement of Medical Instrumentation's chemical analysis standards for water used for dialysis.

diastole: Period of relaxation of the heart; its filling phase.

diastolic blood pressure: A blood pressure reading taken when the heart is relaxed.

diffusate: Dialysis fluid that has been used; it contains solutes not originally present. Often applied loosely to any dialysis fluid.

diffusion: Spreading out or scattering of different kinds of particles among each other.

dilate: Expand or make wider.

dilute: Thin out or weaken. A solution is diluted (made less concentrated) by the addition of more solvent.

disinfectant: Chemical that destroys bacterial organisms.

distal: In a direction away from the center of the body or from the point of attachment.

diuresis: Increased output of urine.

diuretic: Medications that increases the volume of urine that is passed.

diverticulum: A pocket or pouch off the side of a tube or hollow vessel.

dry weight: The weight of a dialysis patient when blood pressure is normal and all excess fluid has been removed.

dwell time: The length of time for which the dialysis solution stays in the peritoneal cavity during peritoneal dialysis.

dyspnea: Shortness of breath.

dyspraxia: Partial loss of the ability to perform coordinated movements.

ecchymosis: An extravasation or oozing of blood into the skin, as with a bruise.

edema: Collection of fluid in body tissues; swelling, often soft and compressible.

effluent: The outflow from something (usually liquid).

electrolyte: A substance that separates into ions after entering into solution.

embolus: A clot, or portion of a clot, carried by the blood flow from a distant vessel and forced into a small vessel, thereby blocking it.

encephalopathy: Any gross dysfunction of the brain, either temporary or permanent, that may result from anatomic damage, metabolic imbalance, or toxic agents.

endocarditis: Inflammation of the endocardium or interior lining of the heart. A serious condition that can be fatal.

endocrinologist: A physician who specializes in treating disorders of the endocrine glands, such as the pancreas.

endogenous: Originating within the body.

endotoxin: A toxic substance produced and held within bacterial cells until they die or are destroyed, whereupon it may be released.

endotoxin unit (EU): A measure of the activity of the endotoxin.

EPO (epoetin alfa): Medication used to treat anemia.

equilibrium: A state of balance between opposing forces.

erythrocyte: Red blood cell.

erythropoiesis: The process of production of red blood cells by the bone marrow.

erythropoietin: A hormone, normally produced by the kidneys, that causes the bone marrow to produce red blood cells (erythrocytes). A synthetic form of the hormone, recombinant human erythropoietin, is used to treat anemia.

ESRD (end-stage renal disease): The last stage of chronic kidney disease when maintenance dialysis or transplantation is required to survive.

ethylene oxide: A gas that may be used for sterilization of objects that might be damaged by heat. Articles must be dry and must be "aired" after sterilization with ethylene oxide.

euglycemia: Normal blood glucose value.

euvolemia: Normal intravascular volume.

exchange: The process of changing used dialysate for fresh solution in peritoneal dialysis.

exit site: Where a peritoneal dialysis catheter exits the skin.

exogenous: Originating outside the organism; due to external causes.

exsanguination: Extensive loss of blood by hemorrhage.

extracorporeal: Outside the body.

febrile: Feeling feverish; having an elevated temperature.

fecal: Relating to a bowel movement or excretion from the bowel.

feed water: Water that undergoes purification or processing and is then used for dialysate.

fibrin: Protein product, usually threadlike strands, formed during the clotting of blood.

fibrinolysin: A substance that lyses, or breaks up, fibrin.

fistula: Unnatural opening or passage. As related to dialysis, a surgical opening between an artery and vein to fill the vein with arterialized blood for blood access.

flowmeter: Device for indicating the rate of flow of a liquid past a given point.

flux: The rate of flow or change across or through a surface.

formalin: A disinfectant consisting of 40% formaldehyde gas in water.

gamma irradiation: Gamma rays are a form of high-frequency, high-energy radiation emitted from radioactive atomic nuclei. They are highly penetrating at a short distance and kill all bacteria, spores, and viruses that they strike.

gastroparesis: A disorder in which the stomach takes too long to empty its contents. It often occurs in people with type 1 or type 2 diabetes; also called delayed gastric emptying.

globulin: A class of proteins found in serum and tissue and of much larger molecular size than albumin. Certain serum globulins are involved in the immune response of the body and are called immunoglobulins (e.g., IgA, IgG, IgM).

glomerular filtration rate (GFR): The rate at which blood passes through the glomerulus in a given time.

glomerulonephritis: Inflammation of the glomeruli, which can cause kidney disease or failure.

glucose: Same as dextrose.

gradient: The rate of increase or decrease between two variables.

half-life: The time it takes for the amount of drug in the body to decrease by one half.

hematocrit: The cellular proportion of blood expressed as a percentage when blood is separated into its liquid and cellular elements by spinning in a centrifuge.

hematoma: Accumulation of blood that has escaped from a blood vessel into surrounding tissue.

hematuria: Presence of red blood cells or blood in the urine.

hemofiltration: Removal of water from the blood by ultrafiltration without dialysis. A volume of water with its solute load is removed by convective transfer. No osmolar gradient is generated between body fluid compartments because it might cause symptoms.

hemoglobin A$_{1c}$ (HbA$_{1c}$): A blood test that measures the average blood sugar level over the past 2 to 3 months. HbA$_1$c helps to diagnose, monitor, and treat diabetes.

hemoglobin: The red protein portion of red blood cells that has the capacity to bind oxygen temporarily while it is carried throughout the body.

hemolysis: Breakup of red blood cells so that hemoglobin is released into the surrounding fluid. Hemolysis may result from mechanical, chemical, or osmotic injury.

hemolytic uremic syndrome: An acute illness most common in children and usually brought on by toxic bacterial diarrhea. Involves breakup of red blood cells (hemolysis) with hemoglobin release, thrombocyte destruction, vascular endothelial injury, and acute kidney damage with azotemia and uremic symptoms and findings.

hemoperfusion: Removal of noxious substances by passing blood over a column of charcoal or special resin with a high binding capacity. No dialysis or ultrafiltration is involved.

hemothorax: Collection of blood in the space between the chest wall and the lung (the pleural cavity).

heparin: A chemical that slows the natural clotting of blood.

hepatitis: Inflammation of the liver; this is often caused by viral infection but can also be caused by toxic agents or medication.

HFAK: Hollow-fiber artificial kidney.

Hg: Chemical symbol for mercury (Latin, *hydrargyrum*).

high-efficiency dialysis: Nonconventional dialysis performed with a special dialyzer that uses a membrane with a very large surface area and therefore allows medium-molecular-weight solutes (up to 5000 Da) to diffuse across the membrane in significant amounts.

high-flux dialysis: Nonconventional dialysis performed with a special dialyzer that uses a highly permeable synthetic membrane that allows low- and high-molecular-weight solutes (up to 12,000 Da) to be convected across the membrane.

HLA (human leukocyte antigen): Molecule found on body cells that characterizes each person as unique. Determines whether a recipient will accept a donor organ.

hydrolysate: A substance produced from the breakdown of another substance by the addition of the elements of water.

hydrophilic: Water loving; a substance that blends or combines well with water.

hyper-: A prefix indicating higher than or greater than some standard.

hyperglycemia: Higher than normal blood sugar level.

hyperparathyroidism: A medical disorder in which the parathyroid gland produces too much parathyroid hormone (parathormone).

hypertension: Higher than normal blood pressure.

hypertrophy: Abnormal enlargement of a body part or organ.

hypo-: A prefix indicating lower or less than the normal.

hypobaric: Less than normal atmospheric pressure.

hypocalcemia: Less than normal serum calcium (normal, 9–11 mg/dL).

hypokalemia: Less than normal serum potassium (Latin, *kalium*) (normal, 3–5 mEq/L).

hyponatremia: Less than normal serum sodium (Latin, *natrium*) (normal, 135–145 mEq/L).

hypotension: Abnormally low blood pressure.

hypovolemia: Low volume within the vascular system.

iatrogenic: A condition resulting from therapy or medical treatment.

icterus: Jaundice.

idiogenic: Something separate or independent, originating with an organ or cells.

IDPN (intradialytic parenteral nutrition): A form of nutritional therapy that provides nutrients in the form of fats, protein, and carbohydrates administered through an infusion pump during the hemodialysis procedure.

immunosuppressant: A drug used to suppress the natural responses of the body's immune system; in transplant patients, it prevents organ rejection.

in vitro: A test done in a synthetic environment created for the particular test rather than in a living organism.

in vivo: A test done in a patient or living experimental animal.

infarction: An area of tissue destruction resulting from obstruction of local circulation, usually from embolism or thrombosis.

infuse: Introduce a fluid into something.

intima (tunica intima): The inner lining of blood vessels.

intravenous: Within a vein (abbreviated IV).

ion: An atom, or group of atoms, that has an electric charge.

IPD: Intermittent peritoneal dialysis.

ischemia: Temporary deficiency of blood supply.

isotonic: Having the same concentration or osmotic pressure (Greek *iso,* "same" or "equal").

jaundice: Deposition of bile pigments in the skin that produces a yellowish tinge; caused by liver disorder or disease.

K: Potassium (Latin, *kalium*).

KDOQI (Kidney Disease Outcomes Quality Initiative): Clinical practice evidence-based guidelines for all stages of chronic kidney disease.

kilogram: 1000 g; 1 kg equals 2.2 lb.

kinetic: Related to motion or movement.

kinetic modeling: Sometimes called urea kinetic modeling (UKM). A mathematical tool used to prescribe and monitor dialysis therapy and to assess protein intake.

Kt/V: A calculation result derived from urea kinetic modeling, identifying the adequacy of dialysis treatment.

k$_{UF}$: The ultrafiltration coefficient. It ranges from 0.5 to 80 mL/h/mm Hg, depending on the membrane.

labile: Unstable or easily changeable.

LAL test: Limulus amebocyte lysate; blood cells derived from the horseshoe crab used to detect and quantify bacterial endotoxins.

lateral: To one side or the other.

lesion: Any injury or wound or local area of degeneration.

leukocyte: A white blood cell.

lipid: A group of substances that includes fats and esters; a fatty or organic oily substance.

lot: In manufacturing terminology, a group of units manufactured at the same time, from the exact same material, or to the same specifications.

lumen: The open space within a tube or container.

lyse: To destroy or break up cells.

macerate: To soften or break up by immersion in water.

malrotate: To rotate or turn incorrectly or inappropriately.

manometer: An instrument or gauge to indicate pressure.

medial: Toward the middle or midline.

metabolic acidosis: Decreased pH and bicarbonate concentration in the body caused by the accumulation of acids.

metabolism: Chemical and physical processes by which living organisms produce and maintain their own substances and develop energy for their use.

metastatic: A disease or disorder that is transferred from one organ or tissue to another area not directly related to the primary site.

methemoglobin: Hemoglobin in which the iron is in ferric form rather than the ferrous form of normal hemoglobin. In this ferric form, hemoglobin cannot combine with oxygen to transport it in the normal way.

microalbuminuria: Screening tests for the presence of albumin or other proteins in the urine, such as the widely used "dipstick," generally do not detect protein in amounts less than 200 mg/dL. Sensitive analytic testing methodology measures much smaller or "micro" amounts.

modeling: Mathematical simulation using probability analysis to predict outcomes from changes in the known variables of a particular process. Usually done by a computer.

module: A self-contained unit that may be combined with others of the same type to form a larger unit.

molal: Abbreviation for millimoles per liter. A solution containing 1 mole of solute in 1 kg of solvent.

mole: One molecular weight of any given substance expressed in grams.

molecule: The smallest unit that a substance can be divided into without changing the chemical properties of the substance.

monitor: To supervise or check on something; a mechanical or electronic device that checks or supervises some operation.

mono-: A prefix indicating one (1).

mycotic: A disease or disorder caused by a fungus rather than by bacteria.

MΩ: Symbol for megaohm, an SI unit of electrical resistance equal to 10^6 ohms.

necrosis: Death of a tissue.

nephrectomy: Surgical removal of a kidney.

nephritis: A term that indicates inflammation of the kidneys.

nephrologist: A physician who specializes in kidney diseases and their treatment.

nephron: Basic functioning unit of a normal kidney.

nephropathy: Abnormal kidney function. It may result from trauma, inflammation, toxic agents, or metabolic disorder.

neuropathy: Damage to or disease of nerves.

NIPD (nocturnal intermittent peritoneal dialysis): A form of peritoneal dialysis in which the patient receives a nightly exchange of dialysis with the peritoneum left dry during the day.

normotensive: Having normal blood pressure.

obtund: Dull, stupid; poorly responsive.

obturator: A metal rod or stylus that fits inside the tube of a trocar. It carries a sharp point and can be withdrawn from the trocar after insertion.

occlude: Close off or shut off.

oliguria: Daily urine output of less than 400 mL, which is the minimum amount of normal urine that can carry the daily load of metabolic waste products.

omentum: Fold of peritoneum that hangs like an apron between the stomach and the anterior abdominal wall.

oncotic: Osmotic pressure resulting from the presence of nonionic solutes and suspended materials such as plasma proteins.

OSHA (Occupational Safety and Health Administration): A federal agency that edicts safety and health issues.

osmolality: Osmotic effect of a solute based on the molal concentration of the solution.

osmometer: An instrument for determining the osmolality of a solution. It operates by determining the precise depression of the freezing point of a solution, which is directly related to the concentration of particles of solute per unit amount of solvent.

osmosis: Passage of solvent through a semipermeable membrane that separates solutions of differing concentrations.

osteitis fibrosa cystica: Bone rarefaction with fibrous degeneration and cyst formation; a result of parathyroid overactivity.

osteoblast: A cell that lays down new bone structure.

osteoclast: A cell that resolves and removes bone structure.

osteodystrophy: A general term for defective bone formation that includes conditions such as osteomalacia and osteoporosis.

osteomalacia: Softening of bone caused by lack of calcium deposition.

osteoporosis: Bone rarefaction or thinning caused by inadequate new bone formation.

palpitation: Irregular jumping or pounding of the heart.

PAN (polyacrylonitrile): A dialyzer made of polyacrylonitrile (synthetic) membrane.

parameter: A quantity to which arbitrary values may be assigned; distinguished from a mathematical variable, which can assume only values determined by the form of the mathematical function. Parameters measured in dialysis work include blood pressure, flow rate, conductivity, and temperature.

parathyroid glands: Four small glands located on the posterior surface of the thyroid gland (*para,* "beside," "adjacent to"). The parathyroid hormone is concerned with the regulation of calcium in body fluid.

parathyroid hormone (PTH): A hormone produced by the parathyroid gland which helps to control serum levels of calcium. When the serum calcium is low, PTH is produced, causing calcium to be pulled from the bone into the blood.

patent: Open.

pathogenic: Causing a disease or abnormal process.

PCR (protein catabolic rate): Refers to a given patient's protein metabolism, expressed in grams of protein per kilogram.

peptide: A compound of two or more amino acids in which the carboxyl group of one is linked to the amino group of the other. A polypeptide is a chain of such peptides connected in a special sequence.

percutaneous: Through the skin.

pericarditis: Inflammation of the pericardium, the sac surrounding the heart.

peritoneal cavity: Space surrounding the abdominal organs (stomach, liver, bowels) located under the abdominal muscles.

peritoneal equilibration test (PET): A test to measure the membrane transport function of the peritoneal cavity. Used to assess the patient's suitability to different types of peritoneal dialysis.

peritoneum: The smooth, serous (and permeable) membrane that lines the abdominal cavity and covers the intestinal loops, liver, and other organs.

peritonitis: Inflammation of the peritoneum caused by an infection.

petechia: A small spot or freckle formed by blood leaking into the skin; usually occurs in crops (petechiae).

phlebitis: Inflammation involving the walls of a vein.

phlebotomy: Release of blood from a vein.

photocell: An electronic device sensitive to light; an electronic circuit that may be closed or opened by its response to light.

physiology: Life processes and functioning of living organisms.

PKD: Polycystic kidney disease.

plasma: The fluid portion of blood (without cellular elements) before clotting occurs.

plasmapheresis: *Pheresis* denotes "taking something away," derived from Greek. Special filter units, usually hollow fibers, permit removal of elements, such as antibodies and immunoglobulins, from serum.

platelet: A small circulating white blood cell, approximately 25% as large as a red blood cell, that is primarily concerned with instituting clot formation on contact with any abnormal surface of the circulatory system or a defect in the integrity of the system.

PMMA (polymethyl methacrylate): A dialyzer made of polymethyl methacrylate (synthetic) membrane.

pneumothorax: Presence of air in the chest cavity between the wall of the cavity and the lungs. Large volumes can constrict movement of the lungs and lead to respiratory failure.

polymer: A compound of the same elements in the same proportion as another but with different molecular weights (e.g., CNOH, $C_2N_2O_2H_2$, $C_3N_3O_3H_3$). Many plastics are polymers of simple compounds.

pore: A very small opening or hole.

posterior: Behind or toward the back of something.

PRA (panel reactive antibody): The percentage of cells from a panel of donors with which a potential recipient's blood serum reacts. A higher PRA indicates that more antibodies are being made.

premorbid: Before an illness.

product water: Water that is processed and ultrapure, which is used to mix the dialysate for dialysis treatments.

proportioning system: The system that mixes the electrolyte concentrate solution (or powder) with the purified water to produce the dialysis fluid.

protamine: A substance that neutralizes the anticoagulant action of heparin by combining with it.

protein: An essential constituent of all living cells that is formed from complex combinations of amino acids.

proteinaceous: Proteinlike, or a material derived from protein.

proteinuria: A condition in which the urine contains large amounts of protein.

proximal: Near a point or near the central area.

pruritus: Intense itching.

pseudoaneurysm (false aneurysm): Sac or outpouching on the wall of a vein.

Pseudomonas: A genus of bacteria found in soil, water, sewage, and air. These bacteria are often highly pathogenic and resistant to many antibiotics.

pulmonary edema: A serious medical condition in which fluids build up in the lungs.

pulsatile: Rhythmic throbbing; a rhythmic forward thrust.

pyrogen: Any substance or agent that causes fever.

QAPI (Quality Assurance and Performance Improvement): A dual approach to quality.

Q_b: Indication of blood flow rate.

Q_d: Indication of dialyzing fluid flow rate.

qualitative: Identifying a substance with regard to kind.

quantitative: Identifying a substance with regard to the amount present.

radial: Located on the side of the forearm near the radius, the forearm bone that ends at the wrist near the base of the thumb.

recombinant: Something manufactured by inserting the deoxyribonucleic acid (DNA) of a chosen or desired gene into the DNA of a bacterium, which reproduces itself to generate more of the desired gene.

renal: Pertaining to the kidneys (Latin *ren*, "kidney").

renin: A hormone produced in the kidney; it has important effects on the sodium and potassium balance and on blood pressure.

residual renal function: The remaining functional ability of the kidneys to remove wastes and excess fluids from the blood.

resin: A substance capable of chemically or physically binding another substance and rendering it inactive.

reticulocyte: An immature red blood cell.

retrograde: In a backward manner or opposite to the usual direction.

reverse filtration: During high-flux dialysis, a gradient from the dialysate to blood may occur, a reversal of the usual blood-to-dialysate gradient. This reversal of flow may carry bacterial or pyogenic material into blood.

rhabdomyolysis: Breakdown of muscle tissue along with the release of myoglobin into the circulation; it may result from trauma or toxic substances. Myoglobin is toxic to the kidneys and a cause of acute kidney injury.

RO (reverse osmosis): The process of removing almost all solute from a solution by applying high pressure on it against a membrane permeable only to the solvent; used to purify water.

sclerosis: An unusual hardening.

septicemia: Bacteremia with growth and multiplication of organisms in the blood. It is usually severe and may be life threatening.

serum: The fluid portion of blood remaining after a clot has formed.

shunt: A short circuit or bypass; in dialysis usage, the system of tubing that connects the flow of blood from the arterial cannula to the venous cannula when they are not needed for actual dialysis.

SI units: An extension of the metric system used by clinical laboratories. The amount of substance is reported as moles/L rather than g/L or mg/dL.

sodium modeling/variation: A technique of increasing sodium concentration in the dialysis bath for part of the treatment to minimize hypotension during fluid removal.

solute: A dissolved substance.

solvent: A liquid capable of dissolving a substance.

sorbent: An agent that acts through its adsorption effect.

sphygmomanometer: A device for measuring blood pressure by means of an inflatable cuff placed around an extremity.

SPM (semipermeable membrane): A selective membrane that allows some substances to pass through but not others.

Staphylococcus: A genus of bacteria, some species of which normally inhabit the skin or other body surfaces. Some species are pathogenic and may cause serious infection.

sterile: Completely free of any living microorganisms.

subcutaneous: Underneath the skin.

sump: Depression, or low point, for fluid collection.

syndrome: A complex or set of symptoms occurring together.

synthetic: Made by humans; artificial; not occurring naturally.

systemic: Affecting the entire body as a whole.

systole: Contraction of the heart; its emptying phase.

systolic blood pressure: A blood pressure reading measured when the heart is beating or blood is pushing against the arterial walls.

tachycardia: Excessively rapid heartbeat.

tamponade: Compression or pressure placement. Pericardial tamponade compresses the heart by the pressure of fluid in the pericardial sac.

The Joint Commission: An independent, not-for-profit organization that accredits and certifies nearly 21,000 health care organizations and programs in the United States.

thermistor: A small sensitive metal device that changes its electrical characteristics with temperature changes. These changes are sensed by electronic circuitry and displayed on an indicator or recorder.

thermocouple: A measuring device using a pair of coupled dissimilar metal conductors that bend when a temperature difference exists.

thrombosis: Clot formation.

thrombus: A clot formed in a blood vessel or blood passage.

tidal peritoneal dialysis: A form of peritoneal dialysis in which there is an incomplete drain of a portion of the infused dialysate fluid before refilling with the next cycle.

tight heparinization: Monitoring activated clotting time to maintain a clotting time of 90 to 120 seconds. This is used in the management of patients at risk for bleeding during hemodialysis treatment.

tissue typing: Matching of blood cells between transplant candidates and donors.

tortuous: Full of twists or turns; winding.

total dissolved solids (TDS): Refers to any minerals, salts, metals, cations or anions dissolved in water. Conductivity indicates the level of TDS in the water in terms of parts per million (ppm).

transducer: A device that transmits power from one system to another. For example, a pressure transducer converts the pressure (power) at its sensing surface to an electronic force that can be shown on an indicator or recorder.

transition of care (TOC): The coordination of and continuity of health care during a transition or movement from one health care setting to another or to home.

trauma: Injury or wound.

Trendelenburg position: A body position in which the head is placed at a 45-degree incline downward on a table with the legs elevated.

trocar: A tube with a sharp point for making puncture wounds.

turbulent: Characterized by agitated or irregular mixing action.

ulnar: Toward the ulna, the forearm bone on the inner side when the arm is held in the classic anatomic position.

ultrafiltration: Filtration by a pressure gradient between two sides of a porous (filtering) material.

urea reduction ratio (URR): A method to calculate the adequacy of dialysis. The formula yields a percentage of urea reduction = $100 \times (1 - Ct/Co)$.

urea: One of the chief nitrogenous waste products formed by metabolism or breakdown of proteins in the body.

uremia: The symptoms manifested when there is a buildup of excess water and waste products in the body as a result of kidney failure.

uric acid: The breakdown product of certain proteins known as nucleotides. Excessive amounts in the blood may cause acute inflammation of joints known as gout.

urticaria: An allergic skin reaction; hives.

vascular: Related to blood vessels.

veins: Blood vessels that return blood from various parts of the body to the heart. These vessels are usually under lower pressure and have thinner walls than arteries.

venospasm: Involuntary contraction or narrowing of a vein.

venous: Related to the veins.

vestibular: Related to the vestibule of the inner ear, which is concerned with maintaining balance.

virus: Submicroscopic, infectious living agents that are the causative factors of many illnesses. They are completely dependent on the cells of the host that they infect. They are not sensitive to antibacterial medications.

xenograft: A graft of tissue or an organ taken from a different animal species.

REFERENCES AND RECOMMENDED READINGS

Chapter 1

American Nephrology Nurses Association: *Nephrology nursing: scope and standards of practice,* ed. 8, Pitman, NJ, 2017, American Nephrology Nurses Association.

Board of Nephrology Examiners Nursing and Technology: *Candidate examination handbook [brochure],* Washington, DC, 2019, BONENT. Retrieved from https://bonent.org/wp-content/downloads/BONENT-Candidate-Handbook.pdf.

Centers for Medicare and Medicaid Services, Department of Health and Human Services: *ESRD: Conditions for Coverage: frequently asked questions about patient care technicians,* S&C-10-17-ESRD, 2010.

Gomez NJ: *Nephrology nursing scope and standards of practice,* Pitman, NJ, 2017, American Nephrology Nurses Association.

Parker J, Gallagher N: The certified dialysis nurse examination, *Dialysis Transplantation* 31(5):313–315, 2002.

Williams HF, Counts CS: Certification 101: the pathway to excellence, *Nephrology Nursing Journal* 40(3):197–208, 2013.

Chapter 2

Blagg CR: The early history of dialysis for chronic renal failure in the United States: a view from Seattle, *American Journal of Kidney Diseases* 49(3):482–496, 2007.

Cameron JS: *A history of the treatment of renal failure by dialysis,* Oxford, 2002, Oxford University Press.

DPC Education Center: *Dialysis patients' guide to the Medicare ESRD bundle,* 2005. Retrieved from https://www.dpcedcenter.org/news-events/news/dialysis-patients-guide-to-the-medicare-esrd-bundle/.

Eckardt KU, Berns JS, Rocco MV, Kasiske BL: Definition and classification of CKD: the debate should be about patient prognosis—a position statement from KDOQI and KDIGO, *American Journal of Kidney Diseases* 53(6):915–920, 2009.

Friedman EA: Willem Johan "Pim" Kolff: bionics for humans in any season, *Dialysis Transplantation* 38(5):180–182, 2009.

Hoffart N: The development of kidney transplant nursing, *Nephrology Nursing Journal* 36(2):127–134, 2009.

National Kidney Foundation: Current KDOQI projects, n.d. Retrieved from https://www.kidney.org/professionals/guidelines/current-KDOQI-projects.

Nobelprize.org: The Nobel prize in physiology or medicine 1990. Retrieved from http://nobelprize.org/nobel_prizes/medicine/laureates/1990/.

Quinn DJ: A brief history in nephrology pharmacotherapy, *Nephrology Nursing Journal* 36(2):223–227, 2009.

Szromba C: Anemia treatment through the years, *Nephrology Nursing Journal* 36(2):229–231, 2009.

Chapter 3

Hall JE, Guyton AC: *Guyton & Hall physiology review,* Philadelphia, 2011, Elsevier Saunders.

Laiken ND: *Fanestil, Best and Taylor's physiological basis of medical practice,* ed. 12, Baltimore, 1991, Williams & Wilkins.

Lewis SM, Dirksen SR, Heitkemper MM, Bucher L, Harding M: *Medical-surgical nursing: assessment and management of clinical problems,* St. Louis, 2015, Elsevier/Mosby.

Morris DG: *Calculate with confidence,* St. Louis, 2010, Elsevier.

Patton KT, Thibodeau GA: *Structure & function of the body,* St. Louis, 2008, Elsevier.

Chapter 4

Black JM, Hawks JH: *Medical-surgical nursing: clinical management for positive outcomes,* ed. 8, St. Louis, 2009, Saunders.

Brundage DJ: *Cancer and the kidney. Renal disorders,* St. Louis, 2013, Mosby.

Burrows L, Muller R: Chronic kidney disease and cardiovascular disease: pathophysiologic links, *Nephrology Nursing Journal* 34(1):55–63, 2007.

Centers for Disease Control and Prevention: *Chronic kidney disease initiative: protecting kidney health,* Atlanta, 2012, US Department of Health and Human Services.

Centers for Disease Control and Prevention: *National chronic kidney disease fact sheet: general information and national estimates on chronic kidney disease in the United States,* Atlanta, 2017, US Department of Health and Human Services.

Chang AR, Appel LJ: Blood pressure for cardiovascular disease prevention in patients with CKD, *Clinical Journal of American Society of Nephrology* 13(10):1572–1574, 2018.

Clarkson MR, Brenner BM, Magee C: *Pocket companion to Brenner & Rector's the kidney,* Philadelphia, 2010, Saunders.

Conway B, Phelan PJ, Stewart GD: *Davidson's principles and practice of medicine,* Philadelphia, 2018, Elsevier, pp 381–440.

Danesh F, Ho LT: Dialysis-related amyloidosis: history and clinical manifestations, *Seminars in Dialysis* 14(2):80–85, 2001.

Levey AS, de Jong PE, Coresh J, et al: The definition, classification and prognosis of chronic kidney disease: a KDIGO Controversies Conference report, *Kidney International* 80:17–28, 2010.

Levy MN, Koeppen BM, Stanton BA: *Berne and Levy principles of physiology,* ed. 4, Philadelphia, 2006, Elsevier.

Myers DJ, Myers SI, Stuart I: *Rutherford's vascular surgery and endovascular therapy,* Philadelphia, 2019, Elsevier, pp 555–566.

National Kidney Disease Education Program: *Making sense of CKD—a concise guide for managing chronic kidney disease in the primary care setting,* Bethesda, MD, 2014, National Institute of Diabetes and Digestive and Kidney Diseases.

National Institutes of Health: Making sense of CKD: a concise guide for managing chronic kidney disease in the primary care setting, 2014. Retrieved from https://www.niddk.nih.gov/-/media/Files/Health-Information/Communication-Programs/NKDEP/ckd-primary-care-guide-508.pdf.

National Kidney Foundation: Frequently asked questions about GFR estimates, n.d. Retrieved from http://www.kidney.org/professionals/kls/pdf/12-10-4004_KBB_FAQs_AboutGFR-1.pdf.

National Kidney Foundation: *One in seven American adults estimated to have chronic kidney disease*, 2017. Retrieved from https://www.kidney.org/news/one-seven-american-adults-estimated-to-have-chronic-kidney-disease.

Palevsky PM, Liu KD, Brophy PD, et al: KDOQI US commentary on the 2012 KDIGO clinical practice guidelines for acute kidney injury, *American Journal of Kidney Diseases* 61(5):649–672, 2013.

Rahman M, Fariha S, Smith MC: Acute kidney injury: a guide to diagnosis and management, *American Family Physician* 86(7):631–639, 2012.

Schatz SR: Diabetes and dialysis: nutrition care challenges, *Dialysis Transplantation* 39(4):144–147, 2010.

United States Renal Data System: *USRDS annual data report,* Bethesda, MD, 2015, National Institutes of Health, National Institute of Diabetes and Digestive and Kidney Diseases, Division of Kidney, Urologic, and Hematologic Diseases.

Wolf M: Update on fibroblast growth factor 23 in chronic kidney disease, *Kidney International* 82:737–747, 2012.

Chapter 5

American Heart Association: Cardiovascular disease and diabetes, 2018. Retrieved from https://www.heart.org/en/health-topics/diabetes/why-diabetes-matters/cardiovascular-disease–diabetes.

American Heart Association: *Understanding blood pressure readings*, 2010. Retrieved from http://www.heart.org.

Andersen MJ, Agarwal R: Kidney parenchymal hypertension. In Lerma EV, Sparks MA, Topf JM, eds: *Nephrology secrets*, Philadelphia, 2019, Elsevier.

Banasik J, Copstead-Kirkhorn LE: *Pathophysiology*, ed. 5, Philadelphia, 2014, Saunders.

Bliss D: Calciphylaxis: what nurses need to know, *Nephrology Nursing Journal* 29(5):433–444, 2002.

Bro S: How abnormal calcium, phosphate, and parathyroid hormone relate to cardiovascular disease, *Nephrology Nursing Journal* 30(3):275–278, 2003.

Centers for Disease Control and Prevention: Recommendations for preventing transmission of infections among chronic hemodialysis patients, *Morbidity and Mortality Weekly Report* 50(RR05):1–43, 2001.

Centers for Disease Control and Prevention: Decrease in reported tuberculosis cases—United States, 2009, *Morbidity and Mortality Weekly Report* 50(10):289–294, 2010.

Chang AR, Appel LJ: Target blood pressure for cardiovascular disease prevention in patients with CKD, *Canadian Journal of American Society of Nephrology* 13(10):1572–1574, 2018.

Conway B, Phelan PJ, Stewart GD: *Davidson's principles and practice of medicine*, Philadelphia, 2018, Elsevier, pp 381–440.

Cozzolino M: CKD-MBD KDIGO guidelines: how difficult is reaching the "target"? *Clinical Kidney Journal* 11(1):70–72, 2017.

Daugirdas JT, Blake PG, Ing TS: *Handbook of dialysis*, Philadelphia, 2007, Lippincott Williams & Wilkins.

Joint National Committee on Prevention, Detection, Evaluation, and Treatment of High Blood Pressure: *JNC 7 express: the seventh report of the Joint National Committee on Prevention, Detection, Evaluation, and Treatment of High Blood Pressure*, Bethesda, MD, 2003, US Department of Health and Human Services.

Kaushik A, Reddy SS, Umesh L, et al: Oral and salivary changes among renal patients undergoing hemodialysis: a cross-sectional study, *Indian Journal of Nephrology* 23(2):125–129, 2013.

Khan SS, Iraniha MR: Diagnosis of renal osteodystrophy among chronic kidney disease patients, *Dialysis Transplantation* 38(2):45–57, 2009.

Kidney Disease: Improving Global Outcomes (KDIGO) CKD-MBD Work Group: KDIGO clinical practice guideline for the diagnosis, evaluation, prevention and treatment of chronic kidney disease-mineral and bone disorder (CKD-MBD), *Kidney International* 76(suppl 113):S1–S130, 2009.

Kurella TM, Yaffe K: Dementia and cognitive impairment in ESRD: diagnostic and therapeutic strategies, *Kidney International* 79(1):14–22, 2011.

Linton A: *Introduction to medical-surgical nursing*, ed. 5, St. Louis, 2012, Saunders.

National Diabetes Information Clearinghouse: *National diabetes statistics*, Bethesda, MD, 2007, National Institutes of Health, US Department of Health and Human Services.

National Kidney Foundation KDOQI Clinical Practice Guideline and Clinical Practice Recommendations for Anemia in Chronic Kidney Disease: 2007 update of hemoglobin target, *American Journal of Kidney Diseases* 50(3):471–530, 2007.

Park JG, Ramar K: Sleep and chronic kidney disease. *Principles and practices of sleep medicine*, ed. 6, Philadelphia, 2017, Elsevier, 1323–1328.

Patton K, Thibodeau G: *Anatomy and physiology*, ed. 8, St. Louis, 2013, Mosby.

Romanowski K, Clark EG, Levin A, et al: Tuberculosis and chronic kidney disease: an emerging global syndemic, *Kidney International* 90(1):34–40, 2016.

Snively CS, Guitierres C: Chronic kidney disease: prevention and treatment of common complications, *American Family Physician* 70(10):1921–1928, 2004.

Sole ML, Klein DG, Moseley MJ: *Introduction to critical care nursing*, ed. 6, St. Louis, 2013, Elsevier.

Tangren J, Nadel M, Hladunewich MA: Pregnancy and end-stage renal disease, *Blood Purification* 45:194–200, 2018.

United States Renal Data System: *USRDS 2015 annual data report: atlas of chronic kidney disease and end-stage renal disease in the United States*, Bethesda, MD, 2010, National Institutes of Health, National Institute of Diabetes and Digestive and Kidney Diseases.

Wright J, Hutchison A: Cardiovascular disease in patients with chronic kidney disease, *Vascular Health and Risk Management* 5:713–722, 2009.

Chapter 6

AAMI Standards and Recommended Practices: *Dialysis edition, RD5–hemodialysis systems*, Arlington, VA, 2008, Association for the Advancement of Medical Instrumentation.

Desai N: Basics of base in hemodialysis solution: dialysate buffer production, delivery and decontamination, *Indian Journal of Nephrology* 25(4):189–193, 2015.

Fresenius Medical Care: Hemodialysis machine bibag system operator's instructions, 2008. Retrieved from https://fmcna.com/content/dam/fmcna/live/support/documents/operator%27s-manuals—hemodialysis-(hd)/2008t-operator%27s-manuals/490122_Rev_U.pdf.

Hoque MF, Fakir M: Adequacy of haemodialysis, *Journal of Armed Forces Medical College, Bangladesh* 7(2), 2011.

Ikizler TA, Serpil MD: Nutritional management of hemodialysis patients. In Nissenson AR, Fine RN, eds. *Handbook of dialysis therapy*, Philadelphia, 2017, Elsevier pp 501–510.

Lacson E, Lazarus JM: Dialyzer best practice: single use or reuse? *Seminars in Dialysis* 19(2):120–128, 2006.

Nissenson AR, Fine RN: *Handbook of dialysis therapy*, Philadelphia, 2017, Elsevier.

Skorecki K, Chertow GM, Marsden PA, et al: *Brenner and Rector's the kidney*, ed. 10, Philadelphia, 2016, Elsevier.

United States Renal Data System: *USRDS 2018 annual data report*, Bethesda, MD, 2018, National Institute of Diabetes and Digestive and Kidney Diseases, National Institutes of Health, US Department of Health and Human Services.

Chapter 7

Centers for Medicare & Medicaid Services, United States Department of Health and Human Services: Medicare and Medicaid programs; conditions for coverage for end-stage renal disease facilities. Final rule, *Federal Register* 73(73):20369–20484, 2008.

Centers for Medicare & Medicaid Services: *ESRD conditions for coverage: frequently asked questions (1-54)*, Baltimore, 2009, US Department of Health and Human Services.

Cosar AA, Cinar S: Effect of dialysate sodium profiling and gradient ultrafiltration on hypotension, *Dialysis Transplantation* 38(5):175–179, 2009.

Hall JE: *Guyton and Hall textbook of medical physiology*, ed.13, Philadelphia, 2016, Elsevier, pp 335–346.

Lacson E, Lazarus JM: Dialyzer best practice: single use or reuse? *Seminars in Dialysis* 19(2):120–128, 2006.

Yeun JY, Depner TA: *Chronic kidney disease, dialysis, and transplantation*, Philadelphia, 2017, Elsevier, pp 277–302.

Yung J: Optimal ultrafiltration profiling in hemodialysis, *Nephrology Nursing Journal* 35(3):287–289, 2008.

Chapter 8

Coulliette AD, Arduino MJ: Hemodialysis and water quality, *Seminars in Dialysis* 26(4):427–438, 2013.

Centers for Medicare & Medicaid Services (CMS): *ESRD survey training: ESRD core survey field manual*, version 1.2, 2014.

ESRD interpretive guidance version 1—cms.gov, 2014. Retrieved from https://www.cms.gov/Medicare/Provider-Enrollment-and-Certification/GuidanceforLawsAndRegulations/Downloads/esrdpgmguidance.pdf.

Forum of ESRD Networks: *Medical director toolkit*, 2012. Retrieved from https://esrdnetworks.org/resources/toolkits/mac-toolkits-1/medical-director-toolkit/medical-director-toolkit/view.

National primary drinking water regulations complete table, EPA 816-F-09-004, Washington, DC, 2009, United States Environmental Protection Agency.

Nissenson AR, Fine RN: *Handbook of dialysis therapy*, Philadelphia, 2017, Elsevier.

The National Forum of ESRD Networks: Welcome to the ESRD Network forum website, n.d. Retrieved from http://esrdnetworks.org.

Chapter 9

Centers for Medicare & Medicaid Services, United States Department of Health and Human Services: Medicare and Medicaid programs; conditions for coverage for end-stage renal disease facilities. Final rule, *Federal Register* 73(73):20369–20484, 2008.

Lacson E, Lazarus JM: Dialyzer best practice: single use or reuse? *Seminars in Dialysis* 19(2):120–128, 2006.

Nissenson AR, Fine RN: *Handbook of dialysis therapy*, Philadelphia, 2017, Elsevier.

United States Department of Labor, Occupational Safety and Health Administration: Formaldehyde: *OSHA fact sheet*, 2011. Retrieved from https://www.osha.gov/OshDoc/data_General_Facts/formaldehyde-factsheet.pdf.

Upadhyay A, Sosa MA, Jaber BL: Single-use versus reusable dialyzers: the known unknowns, *Clinical Journal of American Society of Nephrology* 2:1079–1086, 2007.

Chapter 10

Centers for Disease Control: Standard precautions for all patient care, n.d. Retrieved from https://www.cdc.gov/infectioncontrol/basics/standard-precautions.html.

Centers for Disease Control and Prevention: Recommendations for preventing transmission of infections among chronic hemodialysis patients, *Morbidity and Mortality Weekly Report* 50(RR05):1–43, 2001.

Centers for Disease Control and Prevention: Updated US public health service guidelines for the management of occupational exposures to HBV, HCV, and HIV and recommendations for postexposure prophylaxis, *Morbidity and Mortality Weekly Report* 50(RR11):1–42, 2001.

Centers for Disease Control and Prevention: Guidelines for the prevention of intravascular catheter-related infections, *Morbidity and Mortality Weekly Report* 51(RR10):1–26, 2002.

Centers for Disease Control and Prevention: Prevention of intravascular catheter-related infections, *Morbidity and Mortality Weekly Report* 51[RR-10], 2002.

Centers for Disease Control and Prevention: Infection control requirements for dialysis facilities and clarification regarding guidance on parenteral medication vials, *Morbidity and Mortality Weekly Report* 57(RR32):875–876, 2008.

Centers for Disease Control and Prevention: *Hepatitis B FAQs for the public*, 2009. Retrieved from http://www.cdc.gov/hepatitis/B/bFAQ.htm#statistics.

Centers for Disease Control and Prevention: CDC Dialysis Collaborative: Guide to hand hygiene opportunities in hemodialysis, version 11/30/2010. Retrieved from https://www.cdc.gov/dialysis/PDFs/collaborative/Hemodialysis-Hand-Hygiene-Observations.pdf.

Centers for Disease Control and Prevention: *TB elimination interferon-gamma release assays (IGRAs)—blood tests for TB infection*, 2011.

Centers for Disease Control and Prevention: Guidelines for vaccinating kidney dialysis patients and patients with chronic kidney disease. Recommendations of the Advisory Committee on Immunization Practices, 2012. Retrieved from http://www.cdc.gov/vaccines/pubs/downloads/dialysis-guide-2012.pdf.

Centers for Disease Control and Prevention: *Carbapenem-resistant Enterobacteriaceae (CRE) infection: clinician FAQs*, 2013. Retrieved from http://www.cdc.gov/hai/organisms/cre/cre-clinicianFAQ.html.

Centers for Disease Control and Prevention: *Clostridium difficile infection*, 2015. Retrieved from https://www.cdc.gov/hai/organisms/cdiff/cdiff_infect.html.

Centers for Disease Control and Prevention: *CRE toolkit: guidance for control of carbapenem-resistant Enterobacteriaceae (CRE)*, 2015. Retrieved from https://www.cdc.gov/hai/organisms/cre/cre-toolkit.

Centers for Disease Control and Prevention: *Viral hepatitis surveillance, United States*, 2015. Retrieved from https://www.cdc.gov/hepatitis/statistics/2015surveillance/Commentary.htm.

Centers for Disease Control and Prevention: *Occupational HIV transmission and prevention among health care workers*, 2016. Retrieved from https://www.cdc.gov/hiv/workplace/healthcareworkers.html.

Centers for Disease Control and Prevention: *Standard precautions for all patient care*, 2016. Retrieved from https://www.cdc.gov/infectioncontrol/basics/standard-precautions.html.

Centers for Disease Control and Prevention: *Hepatitis B questions and answers for health professionals*, 2017. Retrieved from https://www.cdc.gov/hepatitis/hbv/hbvfaq.htm#a1.

Centers for Disease Control and Prevention: *Reported tuberculosis in the United States*, 2017, Atlanta. US Department of Health and Human Services Retrieved from https://www.cdc.gov/tb/statistics/default.htm.

Centers for Disease Control and Prevention: HCV epidemiology in the United States, 2018.

Centers for Disease Control and Prevention: Information for healthcare personnel potentially exposed to hepatitis C virus (HCV) recommended testing and follow-up, 2018. Retrieved from https://www.cdc.gov/hepatitis/hcv/hcvfaq.htm.

Centers for Disease Control and Prevention, National Center for US Department of Health and Human Services, Public Health Service: *Recommended testing sequence for identifying current hepatitis C virus (HCV) infection*, 2013. Retrieved from https://npin.cdc.gov/publication/recommended-testing-sequence-identifying-current-hepatitis-c-virus-hcv-infection.

Centers for Medicare and Medicaid Services ESRD cores survey version 1.1, 2014. Retrieved from https://www.cms.gov/media/244396.

Centers for Medicare & Medicaid Services, United States Department of Health and Human Services: Medicare and Medicaid programs; conditions for coverage for end-stage renal disease facilities. Final rule, *Federal Register* 73(73):20369–20484, 2008.

ESRD interpretive guidance version 1—cms.gov. Retrieved from https://www.cms.gov/Medicare/Provider-Enrollment-and-Certification/GuidanceforLawsAndRegulations/Downloads/esrdpgmguidance.pdf.

Fenves AZ: Medical management of the dialysis patient: infectious complications, *Renal and Urology News*, 2016. Retrieved from https://www.renalandurologynews.com/home/decision-support-in-medicine/nephrology-hypertension/medical-management-of-the-dialysis-patient-infectious-complications.

Harris AM, Iqbal K, Schillie S, et al: Increases in acute hepatitis b virus infections—Kentucky, Tennessee, and West Virginia, 2006–2013, *Morb Mortal Wkly Rep* 65:47–50, 2016.

Hughes HY, Henderson DK: Postexposure prophylaxis after hepatitis C occupational exposure in the interferon-free era, *Current Opinion in Infectious Diseases* 29(4):373–380, 2016.

Immunization Action Coalition: Hepatitis B facts: testing and vaccination, n.d. Retrieved from https://www.immunize.org/catg.d/p2110.pdf.

Lewis JD, Enfield KB, Sifri CD: Hepatitis B in healthcare workers: transmission events and guidance for management, *World Journal of Hepatology* 7(3):488–497, 2015.

Moosavy SH, Davoodian P, Nazarnezhad MA, et al: Epidemiology, transmission, diagnosis, and outcome of hepatitis C virus infection, *Electronic Physician Journal* 9(10):5646–5656, 2017.

Chapter 11

Advanced Renal Technologies, n.d. Dialysis professionals. Retrieved from http://www.advancedrenaltechnologies.com/professionals/index.php.

United States Department of Health and Human Services, Food and Drug Administration: Heparin: change in reference standard, n.d. Retrieved from http://www.fda.gov/Safety/MedWatch/SafetyInformation/SafetyAlertsforHumanMedicalProducts/ucm184687.htm.

Chapter 12

Association for Professionals in Infection Control and Epidemiology: *Guide to the elimination of infections in hemodialysis*, Washington, DC, 2010, Association for Professionals in Infection Control and Epidemiology.

Ball LK: The buttonhole technique for arteriovenous fistula cannulation, *Nephrology Nursing Journal* 33(3):299–305, 2006.

Bhatt DL: *Cardiovascular intervention: a companion to Braunwald's heart disease*, Philadelphia, 2016, Elsevier.

Brouwer DJ: Cannulation camp: basic needle cannulation training for dialysis staff, *Dialysis Transplantation* 24(11):606–612, 1995.

Centers for Disease Control and Prevention: *Hemodialysis central venous catheter scrub-the-hub protocol. Institute for Healthcare Improvement. Scrub the hub: example posters*, 2011. Retrieved from http://www.ihi.org/resources/Pages/Tools/ScrubtheHubPosters.aspx.

Fistula First Breakthrough Initiative: *Assessment and monitoring of the newly placed AV fistula for maturation*, Midlothian, 2010, FFBI Coalition, Clinical Practice Workgroup.

Glickman MH: HeRO vascular access device, *Seminars Vascular Surgery* 24(2):108–112, 2011.

Jennings W, Ball L, Duval L: What you "know" about the "flow" is really important with reverse flow AVF's such as proximal radial artery fistulas, n.d. Retrieved from https://www.ncbi.nlm.nih.gov/pubmed/17486952.

McCann RL: Basilic vein transposition increases the rate of autogenous fistula creation. In Henry ML, ed. *Vascular access for hemodialysis*, vol. 7, Chicago, 2001, WL Gore & Associates and Precept Press.

National Kidney Foundation: Clinical practice guidelines for vascular access, *American Journal of Kidney Diseases* 48(suppl 1):S176–S247, 2006.

United States Renal Data System: *USRDS annual data report: epidemiology of kidney disease in the United States*, Bethesda, MD, 2016, National Institutes of Health, National Institute of Diabetes and Digestive and Kidney Diseases.

United States Renal Data System: *USRDS annual data report: epidemiology of kidney disease in the United States*, Bethesda, MD, 2018, National Institutes of Health, National Institute of Diabetes and Digestive and Kidney Diseases.

Chapter 13

Ball JW, Dains JE, Flynn JA, et al: Vital signs and pain assessment. In *Seidel's guide to physical examination*, St. Louis, 2019, Elsevier, pp 74–87.

Clarkson MR: *Pocket companion to Brenner and Rector's the kidney,* Philadelphia, 2010, Elsevier.

Department of Health and Human Services: Part 494: Conditions for coverage for end-stage renal disease facilities; interpretive guidance. 2008.

Feehally J, Floege J, Tonelli M, et al: *Comprehensive clinical nephrology,* 6 ed., Elsevier, 2019, Philadelphia.

Nissenson AR, Fine RN: *Handbook of dialysis therapy,* Philadelphia, 2008, Saunders.

Potter PA, Perry AG: *Fundamentals of nursing,* ed. 8, St. Louis, 2013, Mosby.

United States Centers for Medicare and Medicaid Services: *ESRD facilities conditions for coverage,* Baltimore, MD, 2008, Department of Health and Human Services.

Wilson SE: Dialysis disequilibrium syndrome, *Nephrology Nursing Journal* 28(3):348–349, 2001.

Chapter 14

Bickford A: Herbal therapies for kidney patients, *Renalife* 15(5), 2000.

De Mutsert R, Grootendorst DC, Axelsson J, et al: Excess mortality due to interaction between protein-energy wasting, inflammation and cardiovascular disease in chronic dialysis patients, *Nephrology Dialysis Transplantation* 23:2957–2964, 2008.

Feehally J, Floege J, Tonelli M, et al: *Comprehensive clinical nephrology,* 6 ed., Elsevier, 2019, Philadelphia.

Fouque D, Kalantar-Zadeh K, Kopple J, et al: A proposed nomenclature and diagnostic criteria for protein-energy wasting in acute and chronic kidney disease, *Kidney International* 73(4):391–398, 2008.

Gilbert SJ, Weiner DE: *National Kidney Foundation primer on kidney diseases,* Philadelphia, 2018, Elsevier, pp iv–iv.

León JB, Sullivan CM, Sehgal AR: The prevalence of phosphorus-containing food additives in top-selling foods in grocery stores, *Journal of Renal Nutrition* 23(4):265–270e2, 2013.

National Kidney Foundation: Clinical practice guidelines for nutrition in chronic renal failure, *American Journal of Kidney Diseases* 35(6 suppl 2):S1–S140, 2000.

National Kidney Foundation: K/DOQI clinical practice guidelines for bone metabolism and disease in chronic kidney disease, *American Journal of Kidney Diseases* 45(suppl 3):S1–S202, 2003.

National Kidney Foundation: Clinical practice guidelines for peritoneal dialysis adequacy, *American Journal of Kidney Diseases* 48(suppl 1): S99–S175, 2006.

National Kidney Foundation: KDOQI clinical practice guidelines for nutrition in children with CKD: 2008 update, *American Journal of Kidney Diseases* 53(3 suppl 2):S1–S108, 2008.

National Kidney Foundation: KDIGO 2012 clinical practice guidelines for the evaluation and management of chronic kidney disease, *Kidney International* 3(suppl 3), 2013.

National Kidney Foundation: KDIGO 2012 clinical practice guidelines for the evaluation and management of chronic kidney disease, *Kidney International supplements* 3, S5–S14, 2013.

National Kidney Foundation: KDOQI clinical practice guidelines for hemodialysis adequacy: 2015 update, *American Journal of Kidney Diseases* 67(3):534, 2016.

Renal Business Today: *The right diet may help prevent kidney disease, new study finds,* 2013. Retrieved from https://www.kidney.org/news/newsroom/nr/Right-Diet-May-Help-Prevent-KD.

Wells C: Optimizing nutrition in patients with chronic kidney disease, *Nephrology Nursing Journal* 30(6):637–646, 2003.

Wickman C, Kramer H: Obesity and kidney disease: potential mechanisms, *Seminars in Nephrology* 33(1):14–22, 2013.

Chapter 15

Askar AM: Hyperphosphatemia. The hidden killer in chronic kidney disease, *Saudi Medical Journal* 36(1):13–19, 2015.

Centers for Medicare and Medicaid Services: Dialysis lab tests at a glance (Version 1.4), 2014. Retrieved from http://www.cms.gov/Medicare/Provider-Enrollment-and-Certification/GuidanceforLawsAndRegulations/Dialysis.html.

Feehally J, Floege J, Tonelli M, et al: *Comprehensive clinical nephrology,* 6 ed., Philadelphia, 2019, Elsevier.

Gotch FA, Stennett AK, Ofsthun NJ: Method of calculating a phosphorus-protein ratio. Patent application. Publication date: 2012-07-19. Patent application number: 20120184036. 2012.

Macdougall IC, Eckardt K-U: Anemia in chronic kidney disease. In Feehally J, Tonelli M, et al, eds: *Comprehensive clinical nephrology,* 6 ed., Philadelphia, 2019, Elsevier, pp 958–966.

Mahan LM, Escott-Stump S, Raymond JL: *Krause's food & the nutrition care process,* ed. 13, St. Louis, 2012, Saunders.

National Kidney Foundation: K/DOQI clinical practice guidelines for anemia of chronic kidney disease: update 2000, *American Journal of Kidney Diseases* 37(suppl 1):S182–S238, 2001.

National Kidney Foundation: K/DOQI clinical practice guidelines for bone metabolism and disease in chronic kidney disease, *American Journal of Kidney Diseases* 42(suppl 3):S1–S202, 2003.

National Kidney Foundation: K/DOQI clinical practice guidelines for cardiovascular disease in chronic kidney disease, *American Journal of Kidney Diseases* 45(suppl 3):S1–S153, 2005.

National Kidney Foundation: *2006 Updates: clinical practice guidelines and recommendations.* National Kidney Foundation, New York, New York. Retrieved from https://www.kidney.org/sites/default/files/docs/12-50-0210_jag_dcp_guidelines-hd_oct06_sectiona_ofc.pdf.

National Kidney Foundation: *Cystatin C: what is the role in estimating GFR? Kidney learning systems,* 2009. Retrieved from www.kidney.org/professionals/tools/pdf/CystatinC.pdf.

National Kidney Foundation: *Parathyroid hormone and secondary hyperparathyroidism in chronic kidney disease stage 5D,* New York, 2012, National Kidney Foundation.

National Kidney Foundation: Clinical practice guidelines for hemodialysis adequacy, update 2015, *American Journal of Kidney Diseases* 67(3):L534, 2015.

Nissenson AR, Fine RN: *Handbook of dialysis therapy,* Philadelphia, 2017, Elsevier, pp 501–510.

Pagana KD, Pagana TJ: *Mosby's manual of diagnostic and laboratory tests,* St. Louis, 2013, Mosby.

Palit S, Kendrick J: Vascular calcification in chronic kidney disease: role of disordered mineral metabolism, *Current Pharmaceutical Design* 20(37):5829–5833, 2014.

Spectra Renal Management: *C-reactive protein: a test for assessing infection and inflammation,* Rockleigh, NJ, 2009, Spectra Renal Management.

Sridhar NR, Josyula S: Hypoalbuminemia in hemodialyzed end stage renal disease patients: risk factors and relationships—a 2 year single center study, *BMC Nephrology* 14(242), 2013.

Chapter 16

American Diabetes Association: Standards of medical care in diabetes—2019, *Diabetes Care* 42(suppl 1):S1, 2019.
National Diabetes Information Clearinghouse: *National diabetes statistics*, 2007. Retrieved from https://www.niddk.nih.gov/health-information/health-statistics/diabetes-statistics.
National Diabetes Information Clearinghouse 2017.
National Kidney Foundation: KDOQI clinical practice guideline for diabetes and CKD: 2012 update, *American Journal of Kidney Diseases* 60(5):850–886, 2012.
Ramirez SP, McCullough KP, Thumma JR, et al: Hemoglobin A(1c) levels and mortality in the diabetic hemodialysis population: findings from the Dialysis Outcomes and Practice Patterns Study (DOPPS), *Diabetes care* 35(12):2527–2532, 2012. https://doi.org/10.2337/dc12-0573.
United States Renal Data System: *USRDS 2017 annual data report*, Bethesda, MD, 2017, National Institute of Diabetes and Digestive and Kidney Diseases, National Institutes of Health, US Department of Health and Human Services.
United States Renal Data System: *USRDS 2010 annual data report: atlas of chronic kidney disease and end-stage renal disease in the United States*, Bethesda, MD, 2010, National Institutes of Health, National Institute of Diabetes and Digestive and Kidney Diseases.

Chapter 17

American Heart Association: *Understanding blood pressure readings*, 2013. Retrieved from http://www.heart.org/HEARTORG/Conditions/HighBloodPressure/AboutHighBloodPressure/Understanding-Blood-Pressure-Readings_UCM_301764_Article.jsp.
Amgen: Epogen: Highlights of prescribing information. Thousand Oaks, CA, 2012, Amgen, Inc. Retrieved from https://www.pi.amgen.com/~/media/amgen/repositorysites/pi-amgen-com/epogen/epogen_pi_hcp_english.pdf.
Amgen, Inc: *Epogen [package insert]*, 2014. Retrieved from http://druginserts.com/lib/rx/meds/epogen-1/.
Andrews L, Gibbs MA: Antihypertensive medications and renal disease, *Nephrology Nursing Journal* 29(4):379–382, 2002.
Brater DC: Dosing regimens in renal disease. In Jacobsen HR, Striker GE, Klahr S, eds: *The principles and practice of nephrology*, ed. 2, St. Louis, 1995, Mosby.
Cutler RE, Forland SC, Hammond PGS: Pharmacokinetics of drugs and the effect of renal failure. In Massry SG, Glasscock RJ, eds: *Textbook of nephrology*, vol. 2, ed. 3, Baltimore, 1995, Williams & Wilkins.
Goral S: Levocarnitine's role in the treatment of patients with end-stage renal disease: a review, *Dialysis Transplantation* 30(8):530–538, 2001.
KDIGO Anemia Work Group: KDIGO clinical practice guideline for anemia in chronic kidney disease, *Kidney International Supplements* 2:279–335, 2012.
Mirrakhimov AE, Barbaryan A, Gray A, Ayach T: the role of renal replacement therapy in the management of pharmacologic poisonings, *International Journal of Nephrology* 2016:3047329, 2016.
National Heart Lung and Blood Institute: Diseases and conditions index: high blood pressure, n.d. Retrieved from http://www.nhlbi.nih.gov/hbp.
National Kidney Foundation: Clinical practice guidelines and clinical practice recommendations for anemia in chronic kidney disease update, *American Journal of Kidney Diseases* 47(suppl 3):S1–S145, 2006.
National Kidney Foundation: KDOQI US commentary on the 2009 KDIGO Clinical Practice Guideline for the Diagnosis, Evaluation, and Treatment of CKD-Mineral and Bone Disorder (CKD-MBD), *American Journal of Kidney Diseases* 55(5):773–799, 2010.
Nielsen TM, Juhl MF, Feldt-Rasmussen B, Thomsen T: Adherence to medication in patients with chronic kidney disease: a systematic review of qualitative research, *Clinical Kidney Journal* 11(4):513–527, 2017.
Reilly RF: Attending rounds: a patient with intradialytic hypotension, *Clinical Journal of American Society of Nephrology* 9(4):798–803, 2014.
Rosner MH, Okusa MD: Drug-associated acute kidney injury in the intensive care unit. In DeBroe M, Porter G, Bennett W, Deray G, eds: Clinical nephrotoxins–renal injury from drugs and chemicals, ed. 3, New York, 2008, Springer.
Shahrbaf FG, Assadi F: Drug-induced renal disorders, *Journal of Renal Injury Prevention* 4(3):57–60, 2015.
Sharif-Askari FS, Syed Sulaiman SA, Saheb Sharif-Askari N, et al: Development of an adverse drug reaction risk assessment score among hospitalized patients with chronic kidney disease, *PloS One* 9(4), 2014. e95991.
Sinha AD, Agarwal R: Clinical pharmacology of antihypertensive therapy for the treatment of hypertension in CKD, *Clinical Journal of American Society of Nephrology* 14(5):757–764, 2018.
Skidmore-Roth L: *Mosby's drug guide for nurses*, ed. 5, St. Louis, 2004, Mosby.
Sommadossi JP, Bevan R, Ling T, et al: Clinical pharmacokinetics of ganciclovir in patients with normal and impaired renal function, *Reviews of Infectious Diseases* 10(suppl 3):S507–S514, 1998.
Uhlig K, Berns JS, Kestenbaum B, et al: KDOQI US commentary on the 2009 KDIGO Clinical Practice Guideline for the Diagnosis, Evaluation, and Treatment of CKD–Mineral and Bone Disorder (CKD-MBD), *American Journal of Kidney Diseases* 55(5):773–799, 2010.
US Food and Drug Administration: FDA modifies dosing recommendations for erythropoiesis-stimulating agents. US Food and Drug Administration, *FDA News Release*, June 24, 2011.
Zarama M, Abraham PA: Drug-induced renal disease. In Dipiro JT, ed. *Pharmacotherapy: a pathophysiologic approach*, ed. 3, Stamford, CT, 1997, Appleton & Lange.

Chapter 18

Ashley C, Morlidge C: *Introduction to renal therapeutics,* London, 2008, Pharmaceutical Press.
Brown JR, Rezae ME, Marshall EJ, Matheny ME: Hospital mortality in the United States following acute kidney injury, *Biomed Res Int* 2016:4278579, 2016.
Ghane SF, Assadi F: Drug-induced renal disorders, *Journal of Renal Injury Prevention* 4(3):57–60, 2015.
Golper TA, Schwab SJ, Sheridan AM: Continuous replacement therapy in acute kidney injury (acute renal failure), 2012. Retrieved from https://somepomed.org/articulos/contents/mobipreview.htm?20/8/20623/abstract/17.
Hoste EA, Clermont G, Kersten A, et al: RIFLE criteria for acute kidney injury are associated with hospital mortality in critically ill patients: a cohort analysis, *Critcal Care* 10(3):R73, 2006.

McPherson RA, Pincus MR: *Henry's clinical diagnosis and management by laboratory methods,* St. Louis, 2017, Elsevier.

Rahman M, Shad F, Michael MC: Acute kidney injury: a guide to diagnosis and management, *American Family Physician* 86(7):631–639, 2012.

Ramos P, Marshall MR, Golper TA: Acute hemodialysis prescription, 2013. Retrieved from https://www.uptodate.com/contents/acute-hemodialysis-prescription.

Schrier RW: *Diseases of the kidney and urinary tract,* vol. 11, ed. 8, Philadelphia, 2007, Lippincott Williams & Wilkins.

Sinha AD, Light RD, Agarwal R: Relative plasma volume monitoring during hemodialysis aids the assessment of dry weights, *Hypertension* 55:301–305, 2013.

Taal MW, Chertow GM, Marsden PA, et al: *Brenner & Rector's the kidney,* vol. 1, ed. 9, Philadelphia, 2012, Elsevier Saunders.

Urden LD, Stacy KM, Lough ME: *Critical care nursing diagnosis and management,* ed. 6, St. Louis, 2010, Mosby.

Chapter 19

Blake PG, Jain AK: Urgent start peritoneal dialysis: defining what it is and why it matters, *Clinical Journal of American Society of Nephrology* 13(8):1278–1279, 2018.

Clarkson MR, Brenner BM, Magee C: *Pocket companion to Brenner & Rector's the kidney,* Philadelphia, 2010, Saunders.

Crabtree JH: Selected best demonstrated practices in peritoneal dialysis access, *Kidney International* 70(suppl):S27–S37, 2006.

Curtis J: Daily short and nightly nocturnal home hemodialysis: state of the art, *Dialysis Transplantation* 33(2):64–71, 2004.

Hoy CD: Remote monitoring of daily nocturnal hemodialysis, *Hemodialysis International* 5:8–12, 2001.

Li PK, Szeto CC, deArteaga J, et al: ISPD peritonitis recommendations: 2016 update on prevention and treatment, *Peritoneal Dialysis International* 38(4), 313–313. doi: 10.3747/pdi.2018.00030

Li PK, Szeto CC, Piraino B, Bernardini J, et al: ISPD guidelines/recommendations: peritoneal dialysis-related infections recommendations: 2010 update, *Peritoneal Dialysis International* 30(4):393–423, 2010.

Medical Education Institute: Methods to assess treatment choices for home dialysis, 2007. Retrieved from http://www.homedialysis.org/documents/pros/MATCH-D-v4.pdf.

National Kidney Foundation: KDOQI update 2000, n.d. Retrieved from http://www.kidney.org/professionals/kdoqi/guidelines_updates/doqi_uptoc.html.

National Kidney Foundation: Clinical practice guidelines and clinical practice recommendations: Peritoneal dialysis adequacy, *American Journal of Kidney Diseases* 48(suppl):S91–S175, 2006.

Skorecki K, Chertow GM, Marsden PA, et al: *Brenner and Rector's the kidney,* ed. 10, Philadelphia, 2016, Elsevier.

Tian Y, Xie X, Xiang S, et al: Risk factors and outcomes of high peritonitis rate in continuous ambulatory peritoneal dialysis patients: a retrospective study, *Medicine* 95(49), 2016. e5569.

United States Renal Data System: *USRDS 2017 annual data report,* Bethesda, MD, 2017, National Institute of Diabetes and Digestive and Kidney Diseases, National Institutes of Health, US Department of Health and Human Services.

United States Renal Data System: *USRDS 2018 annual data report: atlas of chronic kidney disease and end-stage renal disease in the United States,* Bethesda, MD, 2018, National Institutes of Health, National Institute of Diabetes and Digestive and Kidney Diseases.

Urden LD: *Critical care nursing: diagnosis and management (with media),* ed. 6, St. Louis, 2010, Mosby.

Chapter 20

Amatya A, Florman S, Paramesh A, et al: HLA-matched kidney transplantation in the era of modern immunosuppressive therapy, *Dialysis Transplantation* 39(5):193–198, 2010.

Chilcot J, Wellsted D, Farrington K: Depression in end-stage renal disease: current advances and research, *Seminars in Dialysis* 23(1):74–82, 2010.

Drugs approved by the FDA: *Rapamune (sirolimus),* Boston, 2000, CenterWatch.

Floege J, Eitner F: Combined immunosuppression in high-risk patients with IgA nephropathy? *Journal of the American Society of Nephrology* 21(10):1604–1606, 2010.

Kasiske BL, Zeier MG, Chapman JR, et al: KDIGO clinical practice guideline for the care of kidney transplant recipients: a summary, *Kidney International* 77(4):299–311, 2010.

Mannon RB: Delayed graft function: the AKI of kidney transplantation, *Nephron* 140:94–98, 2018.

Nashan B, Abbud-Filho M, Citterio F: Prediction, prevention, and management of delayed graft function: where are we now? *Clinical Transplantation* 30:1198–1208, 2016.

National Kidney Foundation: *25 facts about organ donation and transplantation,* 2010. Retrieved from http://www.kidney.org/news/newsroom/fs_new/25factsorgdon&trans.cfm.

National Kidney Foundation: *Immunosuppressive drug coverage,* Washington, DC, 2011, NKF Government Relations Office.

National Kidney Foundation: *Immunosuppressive drug coverage,* 2013. Retrieved from https://www.kidney.org/content/immunosuppressive-drug-coverage.

National Kidney Foundation: *A to Z health guide,* 2017a. Retrieved from https://www.kidney.org/atoz.

National Kidney Foundation: *Kidney transplant,* 2017b. Retrieved from https://www.kidney.org/atoz/content/kidney-transplant.

Neyhart CD: Patient questions about transplantation: a resource guide, *Nephrology Nursing Journal* 36(3):279–285, 2009.

Organ Procurement and Transplantation Network: Transplants by donor type: kidney pancreas. US Department of Health and Human Services, 2018. Retrieved from http://optn.transplant.hrsa.gov.

Sprangers B, Nair V, Launay-Vacher V, et al: Risk factors associated with post–kidney transplant malignancies: an article from the Cancer-Kidney International Network, *Clinical Kidney Journal* 11(3):315–329, 2018.

US Department of Health and Human Services, Organ Procurement and Transplant Network: Educational guidance on patient referral to kidney transplantation, n.d. Retrieved from https://optn.transplant.hrsa.gov/resources/guidance/educational-guidance-on-patient-referral-to-kidney-transplantation.

US Department of Health and Human Services, Organ Procurement and Transplant Network: How organ allocation works, n.d. Retrieved from https://optn.transplant.hrsa.gov/learn/about-transplantation/how-organ-allocation-works.

United Network for Organ Sharing: Post transplant medications. *Transplant Living,* October 10, 2016.

United States Renal Data System: *USRDS 2014 annual data report,* Bethesda, MD, 2014, National Institute of Diabetes and Digestive and Kidney Diseases, National Institutes of Health, US Department of Health and Human Services.

United States Renal Data System: *USRDS 2017 annual data report,* Bethesda, MD, 2017, National Institute of Diabetes and Digestive and Kidney Diseases, National Institutes of Health, US Department of Health and Human Services.

United States Renal Data System: *USRDS 2018 annual data report,* Bethesda, MD, 2018, National Institute of Diabetes and Digestive and Kidney Diseases, National Institutes of Health, US Department of Health and Human Services.

Woodside KJ, Augustine JJ: Kidney transplant is no longer contraindicated for patients with well-controlled HIV, *MD News Clinical Notes,* 2012.

Chapter 21

Aldridge MD: How do families adjust to having a child with chronic kidney failure? A systematic review, *Nephrology Nursing Journal* 35(2):157–162, 2008.

Chand DH, Swartz S, Tuchman S, Valentini RP, Somers MJ: Dialysis in children and adolescents: the pediatric nephrology perspective, *American Journal of Kidney Diseases* 69(2):278–286, 2017.

KDOQI Clinical Practice Guidelines and Clinical Practice Recommendations for 2006 Updates: Hemodialysis adequacy, peritoneal dialysis adequacy and vascular access, *American Journal of Kidney Diseases* 48(suppl 1):S1–S322, 2006.

Kliger AS, Foley RN, Goldfarb DS, et al: KDOQI US commentary on the 2012 KDIGO clinical practice guideline for anemia in CKD, *American Journal of Kidney Diseases* 62(5):849–859, 2013.

National Kidney Foundation: 2006 Updates: clinical practice guidelines and recommendations. National Kidney Foundation, New York, NY. Retrieved from https://www.kidney.org/sites/default/files/docs/12-50-0210_jag_dcp_guidelines-hd_oct06_sectiona_ofc.pdf.

National Kidney Foundation: KDOQI clinical practice guidelines for nutrition in children with CKD: 2008 update, *American Journal of Kidney Diseases* 53(3 suppl 2):S1–S108, 2008.

National Kidney Foundation: KDOQI clinical practice guideline for nutrition in children with CKD: 2008 update, *American Journal of Kidney Diseases* 53(3):S11–S104, 2009.

Kliger AS, Foley RN, Goldfarb DS, et al: KDOQI US commentary on the 2012 KDIGO Clinical Practice Guideline for Anemia in CKD, *American Journal of Kidney Diseases* 62(5):849–859, 2013.

Pollart SM, Warniment C, Mori T: Latex allergy, *American Family Physician* 80(12):1413–1418, 2009.

Skorecki K, Chertow GM, Marsden PA, et al: *Brenner and rector's the kidney,* ed. 10, Philadelphia, 2016, Elsevier.

United States Renal Data System: *USRDS 2017 annual data report,* Bethesda, MD, 2017, National Institutes of Health, National Institute of Diabetes and Digestive and Kidney Diseases, Division of Kidney, Urologic, and Hematologic Diseases.

Warady BA, Neu AM, Schaefer F: Optimal care of the infant, child, and adolescent on dialysis: 2014 update, *American Journal of Kidney Diseases* 64(1):128–142, 2014.

Chapter 22

Sakacı T, Ahbap E, Koc Y, et al: Clinical outcomes and mortality in elderly peritoneal dialysis patients, *Clinics* 70(5):363–368, 2015.

Scherer J, Bitzer M: Geriatric issues in the elderly dialysis population, *American Society of Nephrology Kidney News:* 9, 2015.

Schmidt RJ: Advance care planning for patients approaching end-stage kidney disease, *Seminars in Nephrology* 37(2):173–180, 2017.

United States Renal Data System: *USRDS 2016 annual data report,* Bethesda, MD, 2016, National Institute of Diabetes and Digestive and Kidney Diseases, National Institutes of Health, US Department of Health and Human Services.

United States Renal Data System: *USRDS 2018 annual data report,* Bethesda, MD, 2018, National Institute of Diabetes and Digestive and Kidney Diseases, National Institutes of Health, US Department of Health and Human Services.

Wright S, Danziger J: *Peritoneal dialysis in elderly patients,* 2009. Retrieved from http://www.asn-online.org/education/distancelearning/curricula/geriatrics/Chapter22.pdf.

Chapter 23

Assimon MM, Nguyen T, Katsanos SL, Brunelli SM, Flythe JE: Identification of volume overload hospitalizations among hemodialysis patients using administrative claims: a validation study, *BMC Nephrology* 17(1), 2016.

Centers for Disease Control and Prevention: Don't fall behind on fall prevention, n.d. Retrieved from https://www.cdc.gov.

Centers for Medicare and Medicaid Services, Comprehensive ESRD care model fact sheet, 2014. Retrieved from https://www.cms.gov/newsroom/fact-sheets/comprehensive-esrd-care-model-fact-sheet.

Case Management Society of America: *Standards of practice for case management,* Little Rock, AK, 2016, Case Management Society of America.

Commission for Case Manager Certification: Definition and philosophy of case management, n.d. Retrieved from https://ccmcertification.org/about-ccmc/about-case-management/definition-and-philosophy-case-management.

Fraser SD, Roderick PJ, May CR, et al: The burden of comorbidity in people with chronic kidney disease stage 3: a cohort study, *BMC Nephrology* 16(1), 2015.

Galura G, Pai AB: Health literacy and medication management in chronic kidney disease, *Health Literacy Research and Practice* 1(3), 2017.

Mashayekhi F, Pilevarzadeh M, Rafati F: The assessment of caregiver burden in caregivers of hemodialysis patients, *Materia Socio Medica* 27(5):333, 2015.

Molnar AO, Hiremath S, Brown PA, Akbari A: Risk factors for unplanned and crash dialysis starts: a protocol for a systematic review and meta-analysis, *Systematic Reviews* 5(1), 2016.

Moran A: Factors influencing the introduction of a process of advance care planning in outpatient hemodialysis facilities, *Nephrology Nursing Journal* 45(1):43–60, 2018.

National Institutes of Health: Kidney disease statistics for the United States, 2016. Retrieved from https://www.niddk.nih.gov/health-information/health-statistics/kidney-disease.

Paliwal Y, Slattum PW, Ratliff SM: Chronic health conditions as a risk factor for falls among the community-dwelling US older adults: a zero-inflated regression modeling approach, *BioMed Research International* 1–9:2017.

Schmidt RJ: Advance care planning for patients approaching end-stage kidney disease, *Seminars in Nephrology* 37(2):173–180, 2017.

Schober GS, Wenger JB, Lee CC, Oberlander J, Flythe JE: Dialysis patient perspectives on CKD advocacy: a semistructured interview study, *American Journal of Kidney Diseases* 69(1):29–40, 2017.

Shirazian S, Grant CD, Aina O, Mattana J, Khorassani F, Ricardo AC: Depression in chronic kidney disease and end-stage renal disease: similarities and differences in diagnosis, epidemiology, and management, *Kidney International Reports* 2(1):94–107, 2017.

United States Renal Data System: *USRDS 2017 annual data report,* Bethesda, MD, 2017, National Institute of Diabetes and Digestive and Kidney Diseases, National Institutes of Health, US Department of Health and Human Services.

Wallace M, Shelkey M: Katz Index of independence in activities of daily living. *Assisted Living Consult*, March/April 2008.

Weiner DE, Seliger SL: Cognitive and physical function in chronic kidney disease, *Current Opinion in Nephrology and Hypertension* 23 (3):291–297, 2014.

Chapter 24

Chilcot J, Wellstead D, Farrington K: Depression in end-stage renal disease: current advances and research, *Seminars in Dialysis* 23(1):74–82, 2010.

Hedayati S, Yalamanchili V, Finkelstein F: A practical approach to the treatment of depression in patients with chronic kidney disease and end-stage renal disease, *Kidney International* 81(3):247–255, 2012.

National Council of State Boards of Nursing: *Professional boundaries,* Chicago, 2018, National Council of State Boards of Nursing.

National Institute on Aging: *End of life,* 2019. Retrieved from https://www.nia.nih.gov/health/end-of-life.

National Institute on Aging: *What are palliative care and hospice care?* n.d.. Retrieved from https://www.nia.nih.gov/health/what-are-palliative-care-and-hospice-care.

Robinson K: Does pre-ESRD education make a difference? The patients' perspective, *Dialysis Transplantation* 30(9):564–567, 2001.

Shirazian S, Grant CD, Aina O, Mattana J, Khorassani F, Ricardo AC: Depression in chronic kidney disease and end-stage renal disease: similarities and differences in diagnosis, epidemiology, and management, *Kidney International Reports* 2(1):94–107, 2016.

Shirazian S, Grant CD, Aina O, Mattana J, Khorassani F, Ricardo AC: Depression in chronic kidney disease and end-stage renal disease: similarities and differences in diagnosis, epidemiology, and management, *Kidney International Reports* 2(1):94–107, 2017.

Chapter 25

Agency for Healthcare Research and Quality: The patient education materials assessment tool (PEMAT) and user's guide, 2017. Retrieved from https://www.ahrq.gov/ncepcr/tools/self-mgmt/pemat.html.

Centers for Disease Control and Prevention: *Simply put: a guide for creating easy-to-understand materials,* ed. 3, 2009. Retrieved from http://www.cdc.gov/healthliteracy/pdf/Simply_Put.pdf.

Healthy People.gov: Health literacy, n.d. Retrieved from https://www.healthypeople.gov/2020/topics-objectives/topic/social-determinants-health/interventions-resources/health-literacy.

Miller WR, Rollnick S: *Motivational interviewing: helping people change,* The Guilford Press, 2013, New York.

Redman BK: *The practice of patient education: a case study approach,* St. Louis, 2007, Elsevier.

Resnicow K, McMaster F: Motivational interviewing: moving from why to how with autonomy support, *International Journal of Behavioral Nutrition and Physical Activity* 9:19, 2012.

US Department of Health and Human Services: *Health literacy,* n.d. Retrieved from https://www.healthypeople.gov/2020/topics-objectives/topic/social-determinants-health/interventions-resources/health-literacy.

Wingard R: Patient education and the nursing process: meeting the patient's needs, *Nephrology Nursing Journal* 32(2):211–215, 2005.

Chapter 26

Centers for Medicare and Medicaid Services: *ESRD network organizations,* 2013. Retrieved from http://www.cms.gov/Medicare/End-Stage-Renal-Disease/ESRDNetworkOrganizations.

Centers for Medicare and Medicaid Services: In-Center Hemodialysis CAHPS (ICH CAHPS), 2019. Retrieved from https://www.cms.gov/Research-Statistics-Data-and-Systems/Research/CAHPS/ICHCAHPS.

Centers for Medicare and Medicaid Services: *ESRD network organizations,* 2013. Retrieved from https://www.cms.gov/Medicare/End-Stage-Renal-Disease/ESRDNetworkOrganizations.

Kliger AS: Can we improve the quality of life for dialysis patients? *American Journal of Kidney Diseases* 54(6):993–995, 2009.

Pulliam J: Bundled payments for dialysis, *Renal and Urology News,* 2009. Retrieved from http://www.renalandurologynews.com/bundled-payments-for-dialysis/article/139957/.

United States Renal Data System: *USRDS 2018 annual data report,* Bethesda, MD, 2018, National Institute of Diabetes and Digestive and Kidney Diseases, National Institutes of Health, US Department of Health and Human Services.

US Centers for Medicare & Medicaid Services: 21244CAHPS for MIPS Survey, 2019.

Chapter 27

Billings DM, Halstead JA: *Teaching in nursing: a guide for faculty,* ed. 4, St. Louis, 2012, Elsevier.

Burns C, Beauchesne M, Ryan-Krause P, Sawin K: Mastering the preceptor role: challenges of clinical teaching, *Journal of Pediatric Health Care* 20(3):172–183, 2006.

Motacki K, Burke B: *Nursing delegation and management of patient care,* St. Louis, 2011, Mosby.

O'Connor AB: *Clinical instruction and evaluation: a teaching resource,* Sudbury, MA, 2001, Jones and Bartlett Publishers.

Chapter 28

Raines V: *Davis's basic math review for nurses with step-by-step solutions,* Philadelphia, 2010, FA Davis.

Stassi ME, Tiemann MA: *Math for nurses,* New York, 2009, Kaplan Publishing.

Chapter 29

Billings DM: Student extra: seven steps for test-taking success, *American Journal of Nursing* 107(4):72–172, 2007.

Lancaster LE: Systemic manifestations of renal failure. In *ANNA Core Curriculum for Nephrology Nursing,* ed. 4, Pittman, NJ, 2001 Anthony J. Jannetti.

Silvestri LA: Test-taking strategies. In *Saunders Comprehensive Review for the NCLEX-RN Examination,* ed. 4, Philadelphia, 2007, Saunders.

INDEX

Note: Page numbers followed by *f* indicate figures, *t* indicate tables, *b* indicate boxes, and *np* indicate footnotes.